Venous Thromboembolic Disease

CONTEMPORARY ENDOVASCULAR MANAGEMENT

Edited by Mark G. Davies and Alan B. Lumsden

The Contemporary Endovascular Management series is designed to be a focused, relevant, and timely review of the modern aspects of imaging and intervention in specific vascular beds. Each volume in the series addresses one vascular bed and equips readers with the current information necessary for vascular practice using a clear and easy-to-access format.

Please visit www.cardiotextpublishing.com for more information about this series.

Venous Thromboembolic Disease

CONTEMPORARY ENDOVASCULAR MANAGEMENT

Volume 2

editors

Mark G. Davies MD, PhD, MBA

Vice Chairman, Finance and Administration, Department of Cardiovascular Surgery; Program Director, Vascular Surgery Fellowship and Integrated Vascular Surgery Residency; Director of Research and Education, Methodist DeBakey Heart & Vascular Center, The Methodist Hospital, Houston, Texas; Senior Investigator, The Methodist Hospital Research Institute; Professor of Cardiovascular Surgery, Weill Cornell Medical College, New York, New York

Alan B. Lumsden MD

Chairman, Department of Cardiovascular Surgery; Medical Director, Methodist DeBakey Heart & Vascular Center, The Methodist Hospital, Houston, Texas; Professor of Cardiovascular Surgery, Weill Cornell Medical College, New York, New York

Daynene Vykoukal PhD   assistant editor

Scientific Editor, The Methodist Hospital Research Institute, Methodist DeBakey Heart & Vascular Center, The Methodist Hospital, Houston, Texas

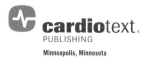
cardiotext.
PUBLISHING
Minneapolis, Minnesota

© 2011 Mark G. Davies and Alan B. Lumsden
Cardiotext Publishing, LLC
3405 W. 44th Street
Minneapolis, Minnesota 55410
USA

www.cardiotextpublishing.com

Any updates to this book may be found at:
www.cardiotextpublishing.com/titles/detail/9781935395225

Comments, inquiries, and requests for bulk sales can be directed to the publisher at:
info@cardiotextpublishing.com.

Unless otherwise stated, all figures and tables in this book are used courtesy of the authors.

Cover design by Brad Norr Design
Book design by Ann Delgehausen, Trio Bookworks

Library of Congress Control Number: 2011924295

ISBN: 978-1-935395-22-5

Printed in Canada
16   15   14   13   12   11   1   2   3   4   5   6   7   8   9   10

Contents

Contributors

Editors

Mark G. Davies MD, PhD, MBA   Vice Chairman, Finance and Administration, Department of Cardiovascular Surgery; Program Director, Vascular Surgery Fellowship and Integrated Vascular Surgery Residency; Director of Research and Education, Methodist DeBakey Heart & Vascular Center, The Methodist Hospital, Houston, Texas; Senior Investigator, The Methodist Hospital Research Institute; Professor of Cardiovascular Surgery, Weill Cornell Medical College, New York, New York

Alan B. Lumsden MD   Chairman, Department of Cardiovascular Surgery; Medical Director, Methodist DeBakey Heart & Vascular Center, The Methodist Hospital, Houston, Texas; Professor of Cardiovascular Surgery, Weill Cornell Medical College, New York, New York

Contributors

Frank R. Arko III MD   Associate Professor, Chief of Endovascular Surgery, Division of Vascular and Endovascular Surgery, Department of Surgery, University of Texas Southwestern Medical Center, Dallas, Texas

Gary Burns MBA, RHIA, CIRCC   Principal, Medical Asset Management, Inc., Atlanta, Georgia

Ruth L. Bush MD, MPH   Associate Professor of Surgery, Vascular Surgery, Scott & White Healthcare; Associate Dean for Education, Temple Campus, Texas A&M Health Science Center College of Medicine, Temple, Texas

Anthony J. Comerota MD, FACS, FACC   Director, Jobst Vascular Institute, Toledo, Ohio; Adjunct Professor of Surgery, University of Michigan, Ann Arbor, Michigan

Bo Eklöf MD, PhD   Emeritus Professor, Department of Surgery, University of Hawaii; Clinical Emeritus Professor, Lund University, Sweden

Hosam F. El Sayed MD, RVT   Department of Cardiovascular Surgery, Methodist DeBakey Heart & Vascular Center, The Methodist Hospital, Houston, Texas; Assistant Professor of Cardiovascular Surgery, Weill Cornell Medical College, New York, New York

Valerie B. Emery RN, ANP, BC   Department of Surgery, Section of Vascular Surgery, Center for Thoracic Outlet Syndrome, Washington University School of Medicine and Barnes-Jewish Hospital, St. Louis, Missouri

Joseph P. Hart MD, RVT, FACS   Assistant Professor of Surgery and Interventional Radiology; Chief of Endovascular Surgery, Division of Vascular Surgery, Department of Surgery, Medical University of South Carolina, Charleston, South Carolina

Peter K. Henke MD   Leland Ira Doan Professor of Surgery, Section of Vascular Surgery, University of Michigan, Ann Arbor, Michigan

Brandi Huf PharmD   Scott and White Anticoagulation Clinic, Scott and White Memorial Hospital and Clinics, Temple, Texas

Kaj H. Johansen MD, PhD, FACS   Swedish Heart & Vascular Institute, Swedish Medical Center, Seattle, Washington

Patricia Hightower Lambden MSN, CNS-BC, APN   McLennan Community College, Waco, Texas

Alan H. Matsumoto MD, FSIR, FACR, FAHA   Professor and Chair, Department of Radiology and Medical Imaging, University of Virginia Health System, Charlottesville, Virginia

Mark H. Meissner MD   Professor of Surgery, University of Washington School of Medicine, Seattle, Washington

L. Bernardo Menajovsky MD, MS   Associate Professor of Internal Medicine, Scott & White Healthcare, Temple, Texas

Erin H. Murphy MD   Division of Vascular and Endovascular Surgery, Department of Surgery, University of Texas Southwestern (UTSW) Medical Center, Dallas, Texas

Elina Quiroga MD   Division of Vascular Surgery, University of Washington, Seattle, Washington

Eduardo Ramacciotti MD, PhD   Section of Vascular Surgery, Department of Surgery, University of Michigan, Ann Arbor, Michigan

Michael J. Reardon MD   Department of Cardiovascular Surgery, Methodist DeBakey Heart & Vascular Center, The Methodist Hospital, Houston, Texas; Professor of Cardiothoracic Surgery, Weill Cornell Medical College, New York, New York

Wael E. A. Saad MBBCh, FSIR   Associate Professor of Radiology, Division of Vascular and Interventional Radiology, University of Virginia Health System, Charlottesville, Virginia

Saher Sabri MD   Assistant Professor of Radiology, Division of Vascular and Interventional Radiology, University of Virginia Health System, Charlottesville, Virginia

Claudio J. Schönholz MD   Heart & Vascular Center, Interventional Radiology, Medical University of South Carolina, Charleston, South Carolina

Robert W. Thompson MD   Professor of Surgery, Vascular Surgery, Radiology and Cell Biology and Physiology, Center for Thoracic Outlet Syndrome, Section of Vascular Surgery, Department of Surgery, Washington University School of Medicine and Barnes-Jewish Hospital, St. Louis, Missouri

CleAnn Toner PharmD   Scott and White Anticoagulation Clinic, Scott and White Memorial Hospital and Clinics, Temple, Texas

Thomas W. Wakefield MD   S. Martin Lindenauer Professor of Surgery, Section Head of Vascular Surgery, Department of Surgery, University of Michigan Health System, Cardiovascular Center, Ann Arbor, Michigan

Preface

Anthony J. Comerota and Thomas W. Wakefield

Venous thromboembolism (VTE) includes deep venous thrombosis (DVT) and pulmonary embolism (PE). VTE is a national health concern, with mortality exceeding that of acute myocardial infarction and acute stroke. VTE affects over 1,000,000 patients per year, with over 300,000 deaths per year in the United States. VTE fatalities have remained constant over the past 30 years, exceeding breast cancer and AIDS combined. The incidence of DVT has been increasing with the aging of the population. In those 85-89 years old, the incidence is reported to be as high as 310 people per 100,000 in the population. Additionally, treatment costs are in billions of dollars per year. The local consequence of DVT, termed postthrombotic syndrome (PTS), affects between 400,000 and 500,000 patients annually with pain, edema, pigmentation, and skin ulcerations. It has been reported that after having an iliofemoral DVT treated with anticoagulation alone, 95% of patients have chronic venous insufficiency, 40% have venous claudication and nearly all have reduced quality-of-life. Even asymptomatic DVT has been associated with PTS.

Although Virchow's triad of stasis, vessel wall injury, and hypercoagulability has defined the events that predispose individuals to DVT formation for the past 150 years, today the understanding of events that occur at the level of the vein wall, including the influence of the inflammatory response on thrombogenesis, is increasingly becoming recognized, although we still have much to learn.

The critical nature of venous thromboembolism to our nation and the world has been recognized, and a Surgeon General's conference held in Bethesda, Maryland, in May 2006 in conjunction with the National Institutes of Health led to a call to action against VTE in 2008. The fact that death due to pulmonary embolism remains the most common cause of in-hospital death today places this problem in stark perspective.

With the current emphasis that has been placed on VTE, the production of this excellent book which addresses all aspects of venous thromboembolic disease is very timely. In part 1, many different aspects of venous thromboembolic disease are covered, ranging from pathophysiology of DVT and PE to diagnosis and treatment of those conditions. Treatment involves not only pharmacologic agents, but also mechanical and pharmacomechanical approaches. Operative thrombectomy remains a good option for treating patients with iliofemoral DVT, and the well-designed Scandanavian trial illustrates the value of a strategy of thrombus removal in patients with iliofemoral DVT. However, VTE is not limited to the lower extremities. In part 2, upper extremity venous thrombosis related to thoracic outlet (thoracic inlet) syndrome is discussed. Part 3 involves issues of central venous disease with a major emphasis on dialysis access. The lifeline of patients with end-stage renal disease is a functional dialysis access. It is evident that the majority of successful accesses are dependent on good-quality venous outflow. Part 4 discusses practice management of venous disease.

Venous Thromboembolic Disease, volume 2 of Contemporary Endovascular Management, has contributions by leaders in the field, with evidence-based recommendations. We highly recommend this volume to those who are serious students of VTE and who want to update themselves on the current status of VTE pathophysiology, diagnosis, and treatment.

Acknowledgments

The editors would like to thank the following individuals for their kind contributions to the completion of this book: Yvette Whittier and Daynene Vykoukal, PhD, at The Methodist Hospital for organizational assistance, author relations, primary editing, and manuscript assembly; Steve Korn, Mike Crouchet, Caitlin Crouchet, and Carol Syverson at Cardiotext Publishing for their roles in series development, content management, and technical support; and Ann Delgehausen, Beth Wright, and Zan Ceeley at Trio Bookworks for their diligent execution of the publication and their contribution to the series designs and concepts. Without the time and effort of the contributors, no book can address its goals and we gratefully acknowledge the time and effort that each of the authors devoted to this project.

Mark G. Davies
Alan B. Lumsden

Introduction

Mark G. Davies

Acute venous disorders comprise the spectrum of deep venous thrombosis (DVT), superficial venous thrombophlebitis, and venous trauma.[1] This volume in the CEM series will provide a focused and timely review of the current state of the field in acute venous diseases.

Deep venous thrombosis has a variable estimated incidence of 56 to 160 cases per 100,000 population per year and appears to be linked with the convergence of multiple genetic and acquired risk factors. It is a significant problem in hospitalized patients. Acute venous thrombosis is followed by an inflammatory response in the thrombus and vein wall, leading to thrombus amplification, organization, and recanalization, which results in structural defects within the wall and in turn leads to luminal compromise and valvular dysfunction. Clinically, there is an exponential clearance of the thrombus by the body's inflammatory and fibrinolytic systems over the first 6 months, with most recanalization occurring over the first 6 weeks after thrombosis. Pulmonary embolism (PE) and the postthrombotic syndrome (PTS) are the most important acute and chronic complications of DVT. Due to the known risk profiles and ease of pharmacological intervention, thromboembolism prophylaxis is standard of care, but appropriate measures are utilized in as few as one-third of at-risk patients. DVT may present as fever or tachycardia, as leg swelling or pain, or as cardiopulmonary events secondary to acute pulmonary embolism. Duplex imaging and D-dimer testing remain integral to DVT imaging and diagnosis. Ventilation-perfusion (V/$\underline{Q}$) scans and computed tomography angiography (CTA) of the chest are the most common modalities employed to diagnose pulmonary embolism. Once diagnosed, anticoagulation constitutes the mainstay of management for a DVT, with the goal of preventing recurrent venous thromboembolism (VTE). However, anticoagulation is not a protection against

PTS because the valves and vessel wall are damaged as the thrombus is cleared by the body. Most recent guidelines recommend catheter-directed thrombolysis or combined pharmacomechanical thrombectomy for proximal DVT in the mobile and functional patient with no absolute contraindications. Effective lysis of these DVTs can reduce postthrombotic symptoms and improve quality of life after acute iliofemoral DVT. Inferior vena cava filters continue to have a role among patients with contraindications to, complications of, or failure of anticoagulation. The incidence of superficial venous thrombophlebitis is underreported and is considered to occur in approximately 125,000 patients per year in the United States. For lesions not encroaching on a deep system vein, conservative measures are adequate. For those lesions that encroach on a deep vein, recent investigations suggest that anticoagulation may be more effective than ligation in preventing DVT and PE. Venous injuries are similarly underreported, and current recommendations include repair of or bypass of injuries to the major proximal veins. If repair is not safe or possible, ligation should be performed.

Reference

1. Meissner MH, Wakefield TW, Ascher E, Caprini JA, Comerota AJ, Eklof B, et al. Acute venous disease: venous thrombosis and venous trauma. J Vasc Surg. 2007;46 (suppl) S: 25S-53S.

Venous Thromboembolic Disease

The occurrence of deep venous thrombosis (DVT) and pulmonary embolism continues be a significant problem in clinical practice. Guidelines for prevention of DVT have been updated by the American College of Chest Physicians (ACCP) and DVT prophylaxis remains a high-priority quality measure for hospitals and practitioners. Prevention of DVT and pulmonary embolism can save lives and decrease morbidity. As we refine our knowledge of the biology and progression of DVT, we will be able to develop better anticoagulants and alternative strategies to control DVT propagation. While the efforts to prevent DVT continue, the ability to clear existing DVTs has become more refined. While use of pharmacological lysis is a mainstay, introduction of mechanical declotting and ultrasound generating devices and combined pharmacomechanical techniques have accelerated treatment strategies and decreased lysis-related complications. In certain patients with limb-threatening DVT, open surgical embolectomy remains a viable and necessary option in the carefully selected patient. There has been a surge in the prophylactic placement of inferior vena cava filters, without any significant rise in the removal of retrievable filters, and the basic designs have not changed much since their introduction. Finally, a more aggressive stance has been taken when pulmonary embolism is detected and both lytic and mechanical devices are now available to facilitate a reduction in the cardiac and pulmonary sequelae of major pulmonary emboli. The evolution of the management of acute DVT and pulmonary embolism is well illustrated in this section.

Overview of Therapy for Venous Thromboembolic Disease

Eduardo Ramacciotti and Thomas W. Wakefield

Venous thomboembolism (VTE), a disease that includes deep venous thrombosis (DVT) and pulmonary embolism (PE), is serious and frequent. Nine hundred thousand cases of VTE are estimated to occur per year in the United States, with 300,000 deaths every year from PE.[1] Additionally, the development of long-term complications is common, despite appropriate acute phase treatment. Following the acute thrombotic process, damage to the vein wall and valves leads to a chronic condition called postthrombotic syndrome (characterized by pain and leg swelling, with eventual formation of distal ulcers). The incidence of postthrombotic syndrome is as high as 30% over 8 years.[2]

The ideal treatment should relieve the edema and pain, reduce or remove the thrombus, and prevent death by pulmonary embolism in the early stages of treatment. In the long term, treatment should prevent recurrence of DVT as well as avoid postthrombotic syndrome and chronic pulmonary hypertension secondary to PE. In the acute phase, treatment is targeted at:

- Arresting thrombus growth, thereby preventing recurrent thrombotic disease in the chronic phase
- Preventing embolization, thereby preventing PE and secondary hypertension in the chronic phase
- Dissolving or removing the clot, thereby preventing venous dysfunction and chronic venous insufficiency
- Limiting progressive swelling of the leg, thereby preventing an increase in compartmental pressure

Venous Thromboembolic Disease. Contemporary Endovascular Management series. © 2011 Mark G. Davies MD and Alan B. Lumsden MD, eds. Cardiotext Publishing, ISBN 978-1-935395-22-5.

Once the diagnosis is confirmed, immediate systemic anticoagulation should be started, unless contraindicated. A therapeutic dose is required, due to a 4- to 6-fold risk of recurrence with insufficient anticoagulation in the first 24 hours.[3] Adequate anticoagulation has been shown to prevent the development of fatal PE both during the initial treatment and after treatment is complete.[4] However, the recurrence rates are still high. It is expected that one-third of properly treated patients will present recurrent DVT after an 8-year follow-up period.[5]

Historically, intravenous unfractionated heparin (UFH) was the initial standard therapy. Due to large individual variation in heparin effect response, frequent adjustment of the dose is required and the treatment is maintained for an average of 5 days. Patients usually have to be hospitalized to undergo the frequent monitoring and dose adjustments necessary to maintain therapeutic plasma concentrations of UFH. Monitoring of activated partial thromboplastin time (aPTT) is crucial during the initial phase of treatment. Patients who fail to achieve therapeutic levels of heparin within 24 hours of starting treatment have a 15 times higher risk of recurrence than patients who achieve heparin concentrations within the target therapeutic range, aPPT 1.5 to 2.5 x control.[6] In this period, treatment with oral vitamin K antagonist (VKA) is instituted (usually warfarin, 5 mg/day) and an international normalized ratio (INR) therapeutic (usually above 2) is required before stopping heparin infusion. The usual minimum time for heparin initial therapy is 5 days.

Recently, the treatment of VTE has been markedly simplified by the introduction of low-molecular-weight heparins (LMWHs). LMWHs are derived from standard heparin after exposure to different chemical processes. However, in comparison with UFH, the small molecular weight of LMWH means that it has a more predictable anticoagulant effect, can be given subcutaneously, causes less platelet activation and bleeding, and is associated with a lower rate of heparin-induced thrombocytopenia.[7] In addition, LMWH may be administered subcutaneously in a weight-based manner (q.d. or b.i.d.), and in many instances, may be administered in the outpatient setting. These compounds do not require monitoring except in certain circumstances such as renal failure and morbid obesity, and during pregnancy.[8] However, its use in the outpatient settings usually requires a team approach and a coordinated effort of multiple healthcare providers. There is also limited evidence that LMWH may decrease the incidence of postthrombotic syndrome.

There are different LMWHs available for the treatment of VTE. Since they are biologic preparations, they are not interchangeable. Moreover, the regimen and doses for the compounds differ, as listed in Table 1.1.

Prevention of Recurrent Venous Thromboembolism

Warfarin (and other VKAs) remains the only available oral anticoagulant proven to reduce the risk of recurrent VTE. Several studies have established that for the vast majority of patients, anticoagulation results in an annual risk of recurrence of less than 2%.[9,10] Because warfarin has a narrow therapeutic index, monitoring the INR is necessary. A target INR value of 2 to 3 is appropriate for patients with VTE.

Warfarin should be started only after heparinization is therapeutic to prevent war-

Table 1.1. **FDA-Approved Anticoagulant Agents for Treatment of VTE**

Agent	Route of Administration	Dose	Need for Monitoring
UFH	IV	80 U/kg initial bolus, followed by 18 U/kg/h maintenance	Adjusted to achieve aPTT 1.5 –2.5 x control
UFH	SQ	333 IU/kg SQ initially, followed by 250 IU/kg SQ	No. However, reserved as second-line therapy
LMWH			
Enoxaparin	SQ	1.0 mg/kg b.i.d. or 1.5 mg/g q.d.	No
Dalteparin	SQ	100 mg/kg b.i.d. or 200 mg/kg q.d.	No
Tinzaparin	SQ	175 IU/kg q.d.	No
PENTASACCHARIDE			
Fondaparinux	SQ	7.5 mg q.d. (5–10 mg q.d. based on weight)	No

UFH = unfractionated heparin IV, LMWH= low-molecular-weight heparin. IV= intravenous, SQ= subcutaneous, aPTT= activated partial thromboplastin time. Taking all of the evidence together, LMWH is now preferred over standard UFH for the initial treatment of VTE with a level of evidence 1A.
Source: van Dongen CJ, van den Belt AG, Prins MH, Lensing AW. Fixed dose subcutaneous low molecular weight heparins vs. adjusted dose unfractionated heparin for venous thromboembolism. Cochrane Db Syst Rev. 2004(4):CD001100.

farin-induced skin necrosis, usually on the first day of therapy. This condition occurs due to transient hypercoagulability, which occurs for the first few days after warfarin is administered. Warfarin causes inhibition of protein C and protein S before most coagulation factors are inhibited by warfarin, leading to a transient prothrombotic state.

After a first episode of VTE, the recommended duration of anticoagulation is 3 to 6 months.[11] For patients with VTE that occurred in association with a well-defined, "time-limited" risk factor (eg, major surgery, pregnancy, trauma), the future risk of recurrent thrombosis appears to be lower than 5%,

with shorter administration (3 months) of VKA.[12] Calf-level thrombi may be treated for shorter periods, ranging from 6 to 12 weeks of warfarin. Patients with a second episode of VTE require prolonged warfarin therapy, unless contraindicated, due to high rates of recurrence.

The warfarin therapy length in other clinical situations is controversial. Inherited or acquired hypercoagulable states, such as the presence of homozygous factor V Leiden (FVL) and prothrombin G20210A mutations (FII), protein C/S or antithrombin III deficiency, antiphospholipid syndrome, and active cancer, significantly increase the risk of VTE recurrence, and prolonged oral anticoagulation is warranted. However, first episodes of VTE in patients with heterozygous mutations of FVL/ FII do not carry the same high risk as those in their homozygous counterparts, shortening the required length of oral anticoagulation.

Another particularly controversial treatment situation involves patients experiencing unprovoked VTE. These subjects are at substantial risk for recurrent disease after warfarin discontinuation. During 3 years following warfarin discontinuation, approximately 20% of such patients will suffer recurrent VTE, particularly on the same vascular site as the index event.[13] The actual length of therapy and dose of warfarin best suited for this particular group are not known. The PREVENT multicenter trial suggested that, for idiopathic DVT, low-dose warfarin (INR 1.5–2.0) is superior to placebo over a 4-year follow-up period with a 64% risk reduction for recurrent DVT after the completion of an initial 6 months of standard warfarin therapy.[14] However, a second study has suggested that full-dose warfarin (INR 2–3) is superior to low-dose warfarin in these same patients, without a difference in bleeding.[15] Taken together, this data suggest that long-term therapy is required for unprovoked VTE patients, with INR targeting 2 to 3.

When estimating the risk of recurrent disease for an individual patient, certain factors have been linked to a higher likelihood of future events: an unprovoked initial clot, and if the index event is PE, rather than DVT.[16] Recently, one additional criterion has been used to determine the length of anticoagulation. This validated criterion involves D-dimer testing obtained 1 month after warfarin is completed. If the D-dimer level is elevated above normal, warfarin should be continued, as this result suggests that the patient is still prothrombotic and

at an increased risk for VTE recurrence.[17] Moreover, another recent study has demonstrated a statistically significant advantage to resuming Coumadin if the D-dimer assay is positive compared to remaining off Coumadin during an average 1.4-year follow-up period (odds ratio [OR] 4.26, $P = 0.02$).[18] One other factor that impacts the recurrence rates is the quality of anticoagulation. One trial has demonstrated that patients exposed to an INR <1.5 during the first 3 months of treatment presented higher risk for recurrent VTE.[19]

Decisions about the duration of anticoagulant therapy are further complicated by the need to individualize the hazards associated with anticoagulation by weighing the risks vs. the benefits of anticoagulation. After estimating both the risk of thrombosis without warfarin as well as the risk of bleeding with treatment, the clinician should consider factors such as adherence history, risk of falling, and underlying diseases before making a recommendation about when or if to discontinue anticoagulation.[20] In addition, if the anticoagulation is not discontinued, decreasing risk of bleeding dose adjustments and using anticoagulation clinics are emphasized.

Thus, the decisions for discontinuation of oral anticoagulation should include thrombosis risk assessment, evaluation of residual thrombus burden, and coagulation system activation (as suggested by D-dimer measurements). These criteria are given a level of evidence of 1A.[17-19]

Complications of Anticoagulant Therapy

The most common complication of anticoagulation is bleeding. Increasing the anticoagulant effect of a pharmacological agent increases the risk of bleeding. By decreasing the anticoagulant effect of the compound, the risk of bleeding decreases, but the risk of recurrence or even treatment failure increases. For UFH, the risk of bleeding during the initial 5 days is around 10%. With the addition of warfarin at an INR between 2 and 3, the annual bleeding risk is 6%.

Another complication associated with heparin use is heparin-induced thrombocytopenia (HIT). This immune-mediated disorder occurs in 0.6% to 30.0% of patients exposed to heparin. Heparin-dependent antibodies mediated by platelet factor 4 (PF4) bind to platelets, activating them. This activation leads initially to platelet aggregation and release of thrombogenic microparticles, which can produce thrombosis, both arterial and venous. Thrombocytopenia due to consumption occurs, increasing the risk of bleeding. Both UFH and LMWH have been associated with HIT, although the incidence is lower with LMWH. Clinically, the patient presents a drop on platelet count greater than 50% of baseline, or below 100,000/μL during heparin therapy. Eventually, thrombosis occurs.[21] The test of choice for diagnosis is an enzyme-linked immunosorbent assay (ELISA) that detects the antiheparin antibody in the patient's plasma. Cessation of heparin is mandatory. LMWH should not be used as substitute, due to a strong immunogenic cross-reactivity. In addition, warfarin alone is also contraindicated. The initial drop in protein C/S associated with beginning VKA treatment in conjunction with HIT may produce severe paradoxal thrombosis. Direct thrombin inhibitors hirudin (lepirudin/Refludan) and argatroban are the treatments approved by the FDA, although other agents such as fondaparinux have been found to treat this syndrome as well.[22] Fondaparinux, a synthetic penthassacharide, does not produce this immune-

mediated reaction, and it seems to be safe as a substitute anticoagulant for HIT patients.[22] The use of these alternative agents is given a 2C and 1C level of evidence.

Prolonged Anticoagulation in Cancer Patients

The safety of LMWH compared with that of warfarin has led to a consideration of the long-term use of LMWH as a replacement for oral vitamin K antagonists. Rates of recanalization have been reported to be higher in certain venous segments using LMWH vs. traditional oral agents.

Cancer patients are reported to have longer periods out of the therapeutic INR range compared to patients free of cancer. Additionally, the use of LMWH has been found to result in improved outcomes in cancer patients compared with standard heparin or LMWH/warfarin therapy when used for 6 months, without differences in major bleeding.[23] The use of LMWH in selected cancer patients for prolonged anticoagulation is given a 1A level of evidence.

LMWH has also been found to provide better DVT prophylaxis compared with placebo for extended 4-week prophylaxis in patients undergoing abdominal/pelvic cancer surgery, decreasing by half the incidence of postoperative VTE, with similar bleeding rates.[24]

Standard Therapy for VTE Algorithm

The algorithm in Figure 1.1 summarizes the standard pharmacological therapy for DVT.

Venous Thromboembolic Disease

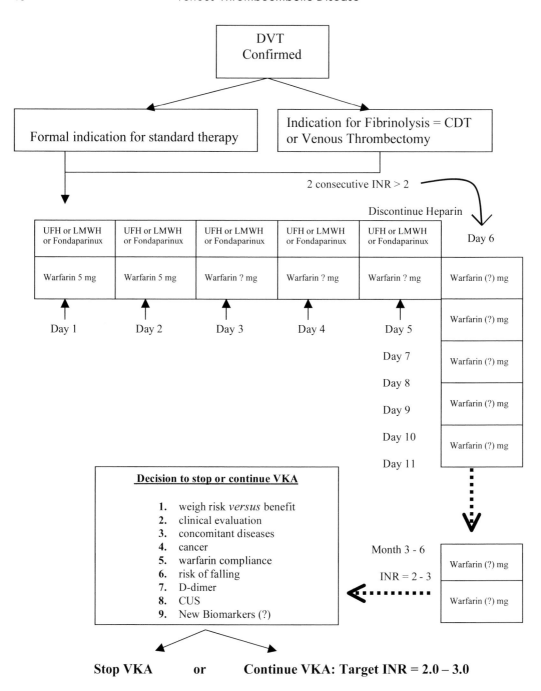

FIGURE 1.1. Algorithm for the standard pharmacological therapy for DVT.

Nonpharmacological Treatments

Pain and swelling after an above-the-knee DVT can be decreased by approximately 50% by the use of strong compression stockings. Additionally, walking with good compression does not increase the risk of PE, while significantly decreasing the incidence and severity of pain and swelling after DVT. It is recommended that once patients are therapeutic on anticoagulants, they ambulate while wearing compression stockings. The use of strong compression and early ambulation after initiation of DVT treatment can significantly reduce the long-term morbidity of pain and swelling resulting from the DVT and carries a 1A level of evidence.[25]

Invasive Therapies for Acute DVT and PE

Proximal DVT, particularly of the iliofemoral system, is a severe form of venous occlusion that in the long term leads to severe postthrombotic morbidity in a large number of patients. Ninety percent of iliofemoral DVT patients who are treated with anticoagulation therapy alone will have ambulatory venous hypertension, resulting in severe chronic venous insufficiency. Up to 40% will have symptoms of venous claudication, and within 5 years, up to 15% may develop venous ulceration. In addition, the severity of the acute venous thrombotic event is predictive of the degree of postthrombotic morbidity, with consequent impact on quality of life. This is especially true in patients with iliofemoral DVT. Recent studies are providing solid evidence that a strategy of thrombus removal is the preferred management for

patients with iliofemoral DVT and offers the best long-term outcome.

Rationale for Thrombolytic Therapy

In gathering the reported data of the pathophysiology of postthrombotic syndrome, as well as the reported series of venous thrombectomy and randomized trials of venous thrombectomy vs. anticoagulation for acute iliofemoral DVT, a persistent observation surfaces. Patients in whom thrombosed venous segments are restored to patency have the lowest ambulatory venous pressure and the fewest postthrombotic symptoms.[26] Those patients with persistent venous obstruction have the most severe postthrombotic symptoms, and this is associated with the highest venous pressures. Therefore, it is apparent that the long-term benefits of treatment are directly related to maintenance of a patent deep venous system.

There are 4 major pathophysiology concepts that support aggressive fibrinolytic or thrombus removal for treatment of proximal DVT of the lower extremities:

1. Residual thrombus (thrombus burden) increases the odds of rethrombosis
2. Thrombus burden is related to increased thrombus activity
3. Persistent thrombus activity favors rethrombosis
4. Rethrombosis increases postthrombotic morbidity

Various authors have led strong advocacy of early thrombus removal worldwide. Thrombus removal strategies promote early restoration of patency and improved venous return. Recently, new evidence-based data have encouraged a more aggressive approach to remove proximal thrombus, rather than a conservative treatment based upon anticoagulation alone.

The 2004 Seventh ACCP consensus conference section stated that "there is no evidence that supports the use of thrombolytic agents for the initial treatment of DVT in the large majority of patients."[27] Recommendations were against the routine use of catheter-directed thrombolysis (CDT) (grade 1C). In addition, it was emphasized that thrombolytic therapy should be confined to patients requiring limb salvage (grade 2C).

More recently, the 2008 Eighth ACCP consensus conference changed its statements. The recommendations regarding CDT for acute DVTs are: "In selected patients with extensive acute proximal DVT (eg, ileofemoral DVT, symptoms for <14 days, good functional status, life expectancy of ≥1 year) who have a low risk of bleeding, we suggest that catheter-directed thrombolysis may be used to reduce acute symptoms and postthrombotic morbidity if appropriate expertise and resources are available (grade 2B). After successful CDT, we suggest correction of underlying venous lesions using balloon angioplasty and stents (grade 2C)."[28] Additionally, pharmacomechanical thrombolysis (eg, with inclusion of thrombus fragmentation or aspiration) in preference to CDT alone to shorten treatment time if appropriate expertise and resources are available, is given a grade 2C recommendation.

Treatment Options

Several methods for removal of thrombus are available, including catheter-directed thrombolysis, percutaneous pharmacomechanical thrombolysis, and operative venous thrombectomy.

Catheter-Directed Thrombolysis

The initial attempts to dissolve DVT were based on systemic infusion of plasminogen activators. Higher rates of bleeding complications associated with poor reduction in postthrombotic morbidity were frustrating. However, some of these patients achieved good results, preserving their valvular function, with reduced postthrombotic morbidity.

The concept of directly delivering smaller amounts of thrombolytic agents into the thrombus results in higher rates of clot dissolution, shorter treatment times, and reduced bleeding complications. Many reports have documented good outcomes of catheter-directed thrombolysis for acute DVT. Generally, success rates in the 75% to 90% range can be anticipated. Bleeding complications have been reported in up to 11% of cases; however, in the majority of the reports published within the past 6 years, bleeding complications are 5% or less, with very few intracranial bleeds. Symptomatic PE during thrombolytic infusion is uncommon and fatal PE is a rarity.

Pharmacomechanical Thrombolysis

Good results have been reported with CDT. However, reports indicate an average treatment time for CDT of 71 hours. This duration of acute care is logistically difficult for many practitioners and medical centers.

Percutaneous mechanical techniques alone or in combination with thrombolysis have been developed to more rapidly clear the venous system. These techniques include catheters with 2 occluding balloons, drug infusion holes between the balloons, and mechanical drug dispersion capabilities. This pharmacomechanical combination enables focused treatment of thrombus within a targeted vessel. Other modalities include catheters with microsonic (ultrasound emission) capabilities to facilitate fibrin dissolution, and catheters that utilize the Venturi effect.

The effectiveness of mechanical thrombectomy alone or in combination with pharmacologic thrombolysis was recently compared. Mechanical thrombectomy alone was successful for removing a thrombus that developed intraprocedurally (which is generally gelatinous and not cross-linked with fibrin). However, in patients with thrombosis already installed, only 26% of the thrombus was removed by mechanical thrombectomy. The addition of a plasminogen activator solution to the mechanical technique removed 82% of the thrombus.[29]

Operative Venous Thrombectomy

Contemporary venous thrombectomy for iliofemoral venous thrombosis has been shown to be effective in both short- and long-term follow-ups. The long-term benefits of venous thrombectomy relate to its ability to achieve proximal patency and maintain distal valve competency. Both outcomes are influenced by the initial technical success and the avoidance of recurrent thrombosis. Therefore, attention to operative detail in terms of complete thrombus removal, correcting underlying venous stenoses, and maintaining therapeutic anticoagulation postoperatively is crucial. Pooled data from a number of contemporary reports on iliofemoral venous thrombectomy demonstrate that early and long-term patency of the iliofemoral venous segment is 70% to 80% compared with 30% of patients treated with anticoagulation alone.[1]

The indication for venous thrombectomy in proximal DVT patients was reviewed in the latest (2008) ACCP consensus: patients with proximal DVT (eg, symptoms for <7 days, good functional status, and life expectancy of >1 year) can be treated with operative venous thrombectomy to reduce acute symptoms and postthrombotic morbidity, if appropriate expertise and resources are available (grade 2B). If such patients do not have a high risk of bleeding, CDT is usually preferable to operative venous thrombectomy, with a grade 2C recommendation.[28]

Future Medical Treatments for DVT/PE

The evolution of anticoagulant drugs for VTE from the 1930s to the present day is a series of agents with increasing specificity. Traditional therapy has been standard intravenous unfractionated heparin, which is a good drug for preventing fatal PE. However, heparin has a number of potential problems, including bleeding, the development of osteoporosis and alopecia with high doses over long periods of time, the development of HIT (heparin-induced thrombocytopenia), and importantly, the need for IV administration and frequent monitoring. Additionally, contaminated heparins were a problem earlier in 2008. Low-molecular-weight heparins (LMWHs) are an alternative to standard unfractionated heparin, which has become the gold standard for the prophylaxis and treatment of VTE. LMWHs work more on inhibiting factor Xa than on inhibiting factor IIa (thrombin). Advantages of LMWHs include an improved pharmacokinetic profile, a half-life that is not dose-dependent, less physiologic antiplatelet activity, more constant anti-factor Xa activity, less protein C antigen decrease, less complement activation, less inhibition of physiologic platelet aggregation, and importantly the ability for subcutaneous administration with no monitoring necessary (except in renal failure, pregnancy, or morbid obesity).[30] LMWH is a little better than standard unfractionated heparin regarding recurrent venous thromboembolic events, major hemorrhage, and even mortality compared to standard heparin. Even proximal above-knee thrombi are associated with improvements with LMWH therapy. In fact, the latest 2008 ACCP guidelines give LMWH a 1A recommendation for the initial treatment of VTE.[28]

Newer drugs include fondaparinux, among others. This indirect thrombin inhibitor is a synthetic pentasaccharide that is identical to the antithrombin III binding sequence of heparin. Fondaparinux is useful for the prophylaxis and treatment of VTE, and it has been FDA-approved for the prophylaxis of DVT, which may lead to PE in patients undergoing abdominal surgery, hip fracture surgery, extended prophylaxis for hip fracture surgery, hip replacement surgery, and knee replacement surgery. Additionally, it is indicated for the treatment of acute DVT when administered in conjunction with warfarin sodium and for the treatment of PE when administered in conjunction with warfarin sodium and initial therapy is given in the hospital. A cousin of fondaparinux, Idraparinux, has a 10-day half-life. However, it did not meet the noninferiority target against PE in a recent study and was also associated with significant intracranial bleeding. Thus, its development was halted. The drug has been biotinylated so that its effects can be reversed by avidin. This drug is called SSR126517 and is undergoing evaluation.

Other new drugs target specifically either factor Xa or IIa and are oral agents. These include rivaroxaban, apixaban, and dabigatran.[31] A comparison of these 3 drugs reveals that they all are orally administered, they have varying bioavailability, and their half-lives are not the same. Rivaroxaban is an oral direct factor Xa inhibitor that inhibits free and fibrin-bound factor Xa activity and thrombotic activity. It has potent anticoagulant effects, and it does not directly inhibit thrombin but instead inhibits thrombin generation via inhibition of factor Xa activity. It has a rapid onset of action (within 2–4 hours), high bioavailability (greater than 80%), and does not affect agonist-induced platelet aggregation and therefore has no direct effects on primary hemostasis. It does not require a cofactor such as antithrombin, it may be safely administrated with concomitant agents, and there are no dosage requirement adjustments needed for gender, age, or extreme body weight. It has been evaluated in treatment studies and prophylaxis studies, where it has been found to be quite effective in reducing the risk for VTE, between approximately 30% and 80%. Apixaban, another factor Xa inhibitor, has also successfully undergone both treatment and prophylaxis protocols. Finally, dabigatran etexilate is a new oral direct thrombin inhibitor. This drug has predictable anticoagulant effects, no need for monitoring, and binds directly to thrombin with high affinity and specificity. This drug was approved for prophylaxis in total hip replacement and total knee replacement in Western Europe and Canada, but approval will require additional trials in the United States as testing against LMWH 30 mg b.i.d. failed to meet the noninferiority target. This drug shows a low rate of bleeding comparable to LMWH, demonstrates elevated liver enzymes in only a small portion of patients (comparable with LMWH treatment), and offers oral dosing without coagulation monitoring.

HIT requires special components for its treatment. Agents available for patients with HIT include direct thrombin inhibitors lepirudin (Refludan), argatroban, and fondaparinux.[32] Refludan is a 65-amino-acid protein that is the most potent thrombin inhibitor, can be difficult to monitor, and undergoes renal excretion. Bivalirudin (Angiomax) is an alternative, a shorter-acting agent requiring a drip. Argatroban is a synthetic thrombin inhibitor with little or no effect on factor Xa and that is metabolized by the liver. There is a fairly predictable aPPT nomogram starting with infusion of 2 to 4 µg/kg/h, with a maximum of 10 µg/kg/h. With Argatroban and Coumadin administration, the INR must be greater than 4 before stopping therapy due to a false elevation of INR with Argatroban. Moreover, fondaparinux has also been used successfully in HIT, but it has not been approved by the FDA for this indication.

Other antithrombotic agents are being evaluated, including plasminogen activation inhibitors (PAI-1), P-selectin inhibitors, and PSGL-1 inhibitors (the ligand for P-selectin). The use of P-selectin and PSGL-1 inhibitors is an area of intense ongoing research in our laboratory. Such an anti-inflammatory approach uses an antithrombotic agent that does not cause direct anticoagulant activities and thus raises the possibility of a therapeutic compound without bleeding potential. Preclinical studies are promising. Aptamers that can bind P-selectin, thereby reducing inflammation and thrombus progression, are under development. Without directly targeting the coagulation cascade, and therefore dramatically reducing the risk of bleeding, these new compounds are focused on safety: with an aptamer, a corresponding strand of genetic material can be made to immediately reverse the effects of the drug.

References

1. Wakefield TW, Caprini J, Comerota AJ. Thromboembolic diseases. Curr Prob Surg. 2008;45(12):844-99.

2. Prandoni P, Lensing AW, Prins MR. Long-term outcomes after deep venous thrombosis of the lower extremities. Vasc Med. 1998;3(1):57-60.

3. Hull RD, Raskob GE, Brant RF, Pineo GF, Valentine KA. The importance of initial heparin treatment on long-term clinical outcomes of antithrombotic therapy. The emerging theme of delayed recurrence. Arch Intern Med. 1997;157(20):2317-21.

4. Douketis JD, Kearon C, Bates S, Duku EK, Ginsberg JS. Risk of fatal pulmonary embolism in patients with treated venous thromboembolism. JAMA. 1998;279(6):458-62.

5. Prandoni P, Lensing AW, Cogo A, Cuppini S, Villalta S, Carta M, et al. The long-term clinical course of acute deep venous thrombosis. Ann Intern Med. 1996;125(1):1-7.

6. Hull RD, Raskob GE, Hirsh J, Jay RM, Leclerc JR, Geerts WH, et al. Continuous intravenous heparin compared with intermittent subcutaneous heparin in the initial treatment of proximal-vein thrombosis. N Engl J Med. 1986;315(18):1109-14.

7. Weitz JI. Low-molecular-weight heparins. N Engl J Med. 1997;337(10):688-98.

8. Ageno W, Turpie AG. Low-molecular-weight heparin in the treatment of pulmonary embolism. Semin Vasc Surg. 2000;13(3):189-93.

9. Agnelli G, Prandoni P, Santamaria MG, Bagatella P, Iorio A, Bazzan M, et al. Three months versus one year of oral anticoagulant therapy for idiopathic deep venous thrombosis. Warfarin Optimal Duration Italian Trial Investigators. N Engl J Med. 2001;345(3):165-9.

10. Kearon C, Gent M, Hirsh J, Weitz J, Kovacs MJ, Anderson DR, et al. A comparison of three months of anticoagulation with extended anticoagulation for a first episode of idiopathic venous thromboembolism. N Engl J Med. 1999;340(12):901-7.

11. Hyers TM, Agnelli G, Hull RD, Morris TA, Samama M, Tapson V, et al. Antithrombotic therapy for venous thromboembolic disease. Chest. 2001;119(1 suppl):176S-193S.

12. Schulman S, Rhedin AS, Lindmarker P, Carlsson A, Larfars G, Nicol P, et al. A comparison of six weeks with six months of oral anticoagulant therapy after a first episode of venous thromboembolism. Duration of Anticoagulation Trial Study Group. N Engl J Med. 1995;332(25):1661-5.

13. Eichinger S, Weltermann A, Minar E, Stain M, Schonauer V, Schneider B, et al. Symptomatic pulmonary embolism and the risk of recurrent venous thromboembolism. Arch Intern Med. 2004;164(1):92-6.

14. Ridker PM, Goldhaber SZ, Danielson E, Rosenberg Y, Eby CS, Deitcher SR, et al. Long-term, low-intensity warfarin therapy for the prevention of recurrent venous thromboembolism. N Engl J Med. 2003;348(15):1425-34.

15. Kearon C, Ginsberg JS, Kovacs MJ, Anderson DR, Wells P, Julian JA, et al. Comparison of low-intensity warfarin therapy with conventional-intensity warfarin therapy for long-term prevention of recurrent venous thromboembolism. N Engl J Med. 2003;349(7):631-9.

16. Agnelli G, Prandoni P, Becattini C, Silingardi M, Taliani MR, Miccio M, et al. Extended oral anticoagulant therapy after a first episode of pulmonary embolism. Ann Intern Med. 2003;139(1):19-25.

17. Prandoni P, Lensing AW, Prins MH, Bernardi E, Marchiori A, Bagatella P, et al. Residual venous thrombosis as a predictive factor of recurrent venous thrombo-embolism. Ann Intern Med. 2002;137(12):955-60.

18. Palareti G, Cosmi B, Legnani C, Tosetto A, Brusi C, Iorio A, et al. D-dimer testing to determine the duration of anticoagulation therapy. N Engl J Med. 2006;355(17):1780-9.

19. Palareti G, Legnani C, Cosmi B, Guazzaloca G, Cini M, Mattarozzi S. Poor anticoagulation quality in the first 3 months after unprovoked venous thromboembolism is a risk factor for long-term recurrence. J Thromb Haemost. 2005;3(5):955-61.

20. Garcia DA, Spyropoulos AC. Update in the treatment of venous thromboembolism. Sem Resp Crit Care M. 2008;29(1):40-6.

21. Alving BM. How I treat heparin-induced thrombocytopenia and thrombosis. Blood. 2003;101(1):31-7.

22. Kovacs MJ. Successful treatment of heparin induced thrombocytopenia (HIT) with fondaparinux. Thromb Haemost. 2005;93(5):999-1000.

23. Lee AY, Levine MN, Baker RI, Bowden C, Kakkar AK, Prins M, et al. Low-molecular-weight heparin versus a coumarin for the prevention of recurrent venous thromboembolism in patients with cancer. N Engl J Med. 2003;349(2):146-53.

24. Bergqvist D, Agnelli G, Cohen AT, Eldor A, Nilsson PE, Le Moigne-Amrani A, et al. Duration of prophylaxis against venous thromboembolism with enoxaparin after surgery for cancer. N Engl J Med. 2002;346(13):975-80.

25. Prandoni P, Lensing AW, Prins MH, Frulla M, Marchiori A, Bernardi E, et al. Below-knee elastic compression stockings to prevent the post-thrombotic syndrome: a randomized, controlled trial. Ann Intern Med. 2004;141(4):249-56.

26. Eklof B, Kistner RL. Is there a role for thrombectomy in iliofemoral venous thrombosis? Semin Vasc Surg. 1996;9(1):34-45.

27. Büller HR, Agnelli G, Hull RD, Hyers TM, Prins MH, Raskob GE. Antithrombotic therapy for venous thromboembolic disease: the Seventh ACCP Conference on Antithrombotic and Thrombolytic Therapy. Chest. 2004;126(3 suppl):401S-28S.

28. Kearon C, Kahn SR, Agnelli G, Goldhaber S, Raskob GE, Comerota AJ. Antithrombotic therapy for venous thromboembolic disease: American College of Chest Physicians Evidence-Based Clinical Practice Guidelines (8th ed.). Chest. 2008;133(6 suppl):454S-545S.

29. Vedantham S, Vesely TM, Parti N, Darcy M, Hovsepian DM, Picus D. Lower extremity venous thrombolysis with adjunctive mechanical thrombectomy. J Vasc Interv Radiol. 2002;13(10):1001-8.

30. Ramacciotti E, Araujo GR, Lastoria S, Maffei FH, Karaoglan de Moura L, Michaelis W, et al. An open-label, comparative study of the efficacy and safety of once-daily dose of enoxaparin versus unfractionated heparin in the treatment of proximal lower limb deep-vein thrombosis. Thromb Res. 2004;114(3):149-53.

31. Gross PL, Weitz JI. New anticoagulants for treatment of venous thromboembolism. Arterioscl Throm Vas. 2008;28(3):380-6.

32. Baldwin ZK, Spitzer AL, Ng VL, Harken AH. Contemporary standards for the diagnosis and treatment of heparin-induced thrombocytopenia (HIT). Surgery. 2008;143(3):305-12.

Deep Venous Thrombosis and Pulmonary Embolism Pathophysiology

Peter K. Henke

Acute Venous Thrombosis

Venous thromboembolism (VTE) is a significant healthcare problem in the United States, with an estimated 900,000 cases of deep venous thrombosis (DVT) and pulmonary embolism (PE) reported yearly, with approximately 300,000 deaths.[1] For the past 150 years, the pathogenesis of VTE centered on Virkow's triad of stasis, changes in the vessel wall, and thrombogenic changes in the blood. Stasis is probably not a direct cause, while infection and systemic inflammation may be more causal than previously thought.[2,3] Beyond prevention, which is the best-case scenario, understanding the basic

Venous Thromboembolic Disease. Contemporary Endovascular Management series. © 2011 Mark G. Davies MD and Alan B. Lumsden MD, eds. Cardiotext Publishing, ISBN 978-1-935395-22-5.

pathophysiology of thrombosis is important for furthering medical and surgical therapies.

Venous Thrombosis Pathways

Hemostasis is often initiated by damage to the vessel wall and disruption of the endothelium, although it may be initiated in the absence of vessel wall damage, particularly in venous thrombosis (VT),[4] and new paradigms are emerging.[5] Vessel wall damage simultaneously results in release of tissue factor (TF), a cell membrane protein, from injured cells and the circulation, with subsequent activation of the extrinsic pathway of the coagulation cascade (Figure 2.1). These 2 events are critical to the activation and acceleration of thrombosis. Tissues also vary with regard to their susceptibility to thrombosis, and the local mechanisms may be somewhat different.[6]

The adhesion of platelets to exposed subendothelial collagen is one mechanism

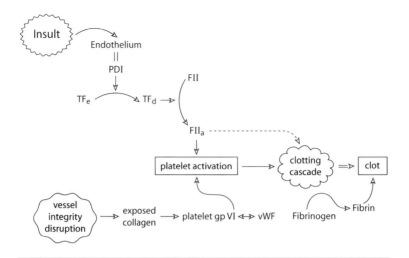

FIGURE 2.1   Pathways of thrombosis. Two primary pathways that initiate thrombosis are shown with the primary factors of platelets, tissue factor, and thrombin. These converge on the coagulation pathway, and fibrin is formed, with thrombus produced. PDI = protein disulfide isomerase; TF = tissue factor; gp = glycoprotein; vWF = von Willebrand factor. Based on Furie and Furie, New Engl J Med. 2008;359:938(5).

for an effective hemostatic "platelet plug" to form, resulting in platelet activation. This interaction is mediated by von Willebrand factor (vWF), whose platelet receptor is glycoprotein (Gp) Ib, and Gp VI and IX are also involved. Direct TF de-encryption can occur by endothelial protein disulfide isomerase, leading to platelet activation. Activation of platelets also leads to the release of the prothrombotic contents of platelet granules, containing receptors for coagulation factors Va and VIIIa, as well as fibrinogen, vWF, and ADP. Fibrinogen forms bridges between platelets by binding to the GpIIb/IIIa receptor, resulting in further platelet aggregation. Platelet activation also leads to the elaboration of arachidonic acid metabolites such as thromboxane A_2, further promoting platelet aggregation.

The extrinsic clotting pathway begins with TF complexing with factor VII, causing activation (VIIa). The TF-VIIa complex then activates factors IX and X to IXa and Xa

in the presence of calcium. Feedback amplification occurs as VIIa, IXa, and Xa are all capable of activating VII to VIIa, especially when bound to TF.[7] Factor Xa is also capable of activating factor V to Va. Factors Xa, Va, and II (prothrombin) form on the platelet phospholipid surface in the presence of Ca^{2+} to initiate the prothrombinase complex, which catalyzes the formation of thrombin from prothrombin. Thrombin feedback amplifies the system not only by activating factor V to Va, but also factors VIII (normally circulating bound to vWF) to VIIIa and XI to XIa. After activation, factor VIIIa dissociates from vWF and assembles with factors IXa and X on the platelet surface in the presence of Ca^{2+} to form a complex called the Xase complex, which catalyzes the activation of factor X to Xa. It is important to recognize that these events occur at the vessel wall–platelet interface.

Thrombin (factor II) is central to coagulation by its action of cleavage and release of fibrinopeptide A (FPA) from the α-chain of fibrinogen and fibrinopeptide B (FPB) from the β-chain of fibrinogen. This causes fibrin monomer polymerization and cross-linking, stabilizing the thrombus and the initial platelet plug. Thrombin also activates factor XIII to XIIIa, which catalyzes this cross-linking of fibrin as well as that of other plasma proteins, such as fibronectin and α_2-antitrypsin. In addition, factor XIIIa activates platelets as well as factors V and VIII, further amplifying thrombin production.

The physiologic importance of the intrinsic pathway is not completely clear and is probably not as physiologically important in the venous system as the extrinsic system. Intrinsic pathway activation occurs with activation of factor XI to XIa, which subsequently converts factor IX to IXa, promoting formation of the Xase complex and ultimately thrombin. Another mechanism by which this occurs in vitro is through the contact activation system, in which factor XII (Hageman factor) is activated to XIIa when complexed to prekallikrein and high-molecular-weight kininogen (HMWK) on a negatively charged surface; factor XIIa then activates factor XI to XIa.

Inflammation and Thrombosis

In the early 1970s, the relationship between thrombosis and inflammation was first suggested.[8] Inflammation increases TF, membrane phospholipids, platelet reactivity, and fibrinogen, while decreasing thrombomodulin (TM) and inhibiting fibrinolysis.[9] Coincidently, cell adhesion molecules (CAM) are up-regulated on inflamed endothelium and allow leukocyte transmigration. The selectins (P- and E-selectin) are integrally involved in venous thrombosis.[10] P-selectin is up-regulated in the vein wall as early as 6 hours after thrombus induction, while E-selectin has been found up-regulated at later time points.[11]

Microparticles (MPs) are involved in the initiation and amplification of thrombosis. MPs are small (< 1μm) phospholipid vesicles shed from platelets, leukocytes, and endothelial cells in a calcium-dependent fashion.[12-14] MPs lack DNA and RNA but are protein rich, and subpopulations of MPs rich in TF and phosphatidylserine have been identified.[15] Fusion of MPs with activated platelets is another mechanism that results in decryption of TF and the initiation of thrombosis.[16] Several circulating markers of inflammation once thought to be soluble are actually carried by MPs.[17]

In veins, CAMs and MPs interface in promoting thrombosis and inflammation. Both venous stasis and hypoxia result in the up-regulation of P-selectin, which localizes prothrombotic MPs to the area of stasis and promotes DVT formation.[18-20] The P-selectin receptor, P-selectin glycoprotein ligand 1(PSGL-1), is expressed on leukocytes and platelets, as well as on their derived MPs. Indeed, MPs coexpressing TF and leukocyte markers have been shown to accumulate in growing thrombi in a P-selectin:PSGL-1–dependent fashion.[10] Further, P-selectin: PSGL-1 interactions stimulate the production of thrombogenic MPs from leukocytes, along with platelets and endothelial cells.[21]

The importance of P-selectin:PSGL-1 to thrombosis also depends on the nature of the stimulus and the role of TF, which is normally abundant in the outer portion of the vessel wall. With significant vascular injury and the exposure of vein wall TF, this TF is likely more important in the thrombogenic process than the TF that is brought to the point of thrombogenesis by activated MPs, in contrast to arterial thrombosis.[22] Furthermore, monocyte-derived MPs deliver TF to areas of injury and inflammation by binding to P-selectin mobilized to the surface of activated platelets and endothelial cells, resulting in the generation of fibrin.

Natural Anticoagulants

Physiologic anticoagulants balance thrombin formation and localize thrombotic activity to sites of vascular injury by several mechanisms. Antithrombin (AT) is a central anticoagulant protein that binds to thrombin, and interferes with coagulation by 3 major mechanisms. First, inhibition of thrombin prevents the removal of FPA and FPB from fibrinogen, limiting fibrin formation. Second, thrombin becomes unavailable for factor V and VIII activation, slowing the coagulation cascade. Third, thrombin-mediated platelet activation and aggregation are inhibited. In the presence of heparin, inhibition of thrombin by AT is accelerated, resulting in systemic anticoagulation. Antithrombin has been shown to directly inhibit factors VIIa, IXa, Xa, XIa, and XIIa.

A second natural anticoagulant mechanism is activated protein C (APC), which is produced on the surface of intact endothelium when thrombin binds to its receptor, thrombomodulin (TM), and endothelial protein C receptor (EPCR). The thrombin-TM complex inhibits the actions of thrombin and also activates protein C to APC. APC, in the presence of its cofactor protein S, inactivates factors Va and VIIIa, therefore reducing Xase and prothrombinase activity.

The third innate anticoagulant is tissue factor pathway inhibitor (TFPI). This protein binds the TF-VIIa complex, thus inhibiting the activation of factor X to Xa and formation of the prothrombinase complex. Finally, heparin cofactor II is another inhibitor of thrombin whose action is in the extravascular compartment. The activity of heparin cofactor II is augmented by glycosaminoglycans, including both heparan and dermatan sulfate, but its deficiency is not associated with increased VTE risk.[23]

Fibrinolysis

In addition to preventing thrombus generation, controlled thrombolysis serves to limit thrombus extension as well as to metabolize the thrombus to allow scar tissue to form. The central fibrinolytic enzyme is plasmin, a serine protease generated by the proteolytic cleavage of the proenzyme plasminogen. Its main substrates include fibrin, fibrinogen, and other coagulation factors. The degradation of fibrin polymers by plasmin ultimately results in the creation of fragment E and 2 molecules of fragment D, which are released as a covalently linked dimer (D-dimer).[24]

Activation of plasminogen occurs by several mechanisms. In the presence of thrombin, vascular endothelial cells produce and release tissue plasminogen activator (tPA) as well as α_2-antiplasmin, a natural inhibitor of excess fibrin-bound plasmin. In contrast to free-circulating tPA, fibrin-bound tPA is an efficient activator of plasminogen.

A second endogenous activator of plasminogen is the urokinase-type plasminogen activator (uPA), also produced by endothelial cells, but with less affinity for fibrin. The activation of uPA in vivo is not completely understood. However, it is hypothesized that plasmin in small amounts (produced through tPA) activates uPA, leading to further plasminogen activation and amplification of fibrinolysis.[25] This protease is most important for experimental DVT resolution, as compared with tPA.[26]

The third mechanism of plasminogen activation involves factors of the contact activation system; activated forms of factors XII, kallikrein, and XI can each independently convert plasminogen to plasmin.

These activated factors may also catalyze the release of bradykinin from HMWK, which further augments tPA secretion. Finally, APC has been found to proteolytically inactivate plasminogen activator inhibitor type 1 (PAI-1), an inhibitor of plasmin activators, released by endothelial cells in the presence of thrombin.[27]

In plasma, plasminogen activator inhibitor (PAI-1) is the primary inhibitor of plasminogen activators and is stored in the alpha-granules of quiescent platelets.[25] It is secreted in an active form from liver and endothelial cells, and stabilized by binding to vitronectin (and inhibits thrombin in this form).[28] Plasminogen activator inhibitor-1 levels are elevated by hyperlipidemia, and PAI-1 elevation appears to synergize with factor V Leiden genetic abnormalities, possibly contributing to pathological thrombosis.

Endothelium and Hemostasis

Most of the thrombosis-thrombolysis processes occur in juxtaposition to the endothelium; hence, the endothelium is one of the pivotal regulators of homeostasis (Figure 2.2). Under normal conditions, endothelial cells maintain a vasodilatory and local fibrinolytic state in which coagulation, platelet adhesion, and activation are suppressed. A nonthrombogenic endothelial surface is maintained through a number of mechanisms, including: (1) endothelial production of TM and subsequent activation of protein C; (2) endothelial expression of heparan sulfate and dermatan sulfate, which accelerate AT and heparin cofactor II activity; (3) constitutive expression of TFPI; and (4) local production of tPA and uPA. In addition, the production of nitric oxide (NO) and prostacyclin by the endothelium inhibits the adhesion and activation of leukocytes and produces vasodilation.[29]

During states of endothelial disturbances, a prothrombotic and proinflammatory state of vasoconstriction is supported by the endothelial surface. Release of platelet-activating factor and endothelin-1 promotes vasoconstriction, while production of vWF,

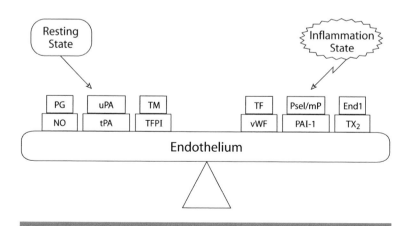

FIGURE 2.2 Counterbalancing pro- and antithrombotic endothelial functions. At rest, the balance is tipped toward an anticoagulant milieu. With inflammation or with local damage, the balance tips to a procoagulant state by several mechanisms.

TF, PAI-1, and factor V augment thrombosis.[30] Indeed, vWF is expressed to a greater extent on the endothelium of veins as compared with arteries, and tPA is less commonly expressed in venous endothelium. Loss of endothelium likely also contributes to the vein wall fibrosis, as well as the predisposition to recurrent venous thrombosis. Experimental DVT was associated with decreased expression of homeostatic endothelial genes such as NO and TM, as compared with controls, and correlated with loss of vWF positive cell luminal staining.[31] Other investigators have found that prolonged venous stasis is associated with decreased plasminogen activators, probably related to loss of endothelium.[32]

Experimental Pulmonary Embolism

Pulmonary embolism is the fatal complication of DVT, primarily related to acute right heart failure and less so to hypoxemia.[33] While the basic processes of thrombolysis in all vascular beds are similar, several experimental studies have suggested that pulmonary artery (PA) injury is different from in the inferior vena cava (IVC). In an experimental study in rats using an in vivo–generated thromboembolism, the early PA response is associated with elevated monocyte chemotactic protein-1 (MCP-1), early monocyte influx, and later intimal hyperplasia.[34] Little elevation in PA selectins is observed, in contrast to the IVC response.[35] Interestingly, the mechanical obstruction in the PA induces significant injury, and the resulting intimal hyperplasia is independent of the thrombus effect.[36] Moreover, LMWH, but neither tPA nor a gIIb/IIIa antagonist, was associated with attenuated intimal hyperplasia.[37] Consistent with what is observed in the IVC, uPA

is the primary fibrinolytic mechanism in the PA, including the arterioles.[38] Although animal models can mimic the acute to chronic PE pathophysiology, DVT characteristics that predispose to PE as compared to no PE have not yet been forthcoming, but would be of significant clinical interest.

Differential Risk of DVT vs. PE

Approximately 50% of patients with a DVT may suffer a PE, although many of the PEs are asymptomatic and of small magnitude.[33] Conversely, pulmonary symptoms often point the physician to a suspected PE. Defining those at risk for PE after DVT is diagnosed, given similar levels of risk, and anticoagulation, is important, and data are lacking. Adequate anticoagulation certainly reduces the risk, but some patients present with primary PE without a DVT source defined and may have symptoms related to failure of local DVT resolution.

From a large epidemiological study, several factors including age and corticosteroid use are independently associated with PE, but not DVT.[2] From a large patient registry, predictors of fatal PE in patients with incident DVT included older age (>75 years), cancer, and immobility related to neurological disease.[39] Recent studies also suggest that very high D-dimer levels may be predictive of PE over isolated DVT, with a threshold of >4000 ng/mL.[40] Similarly, those patients whose initial clinical event was a PE rather than simply a DVT are at higher risk of recurrent PE.[41] In hospitalized patients, the postoperative state may also confer an increased risk of PE, but studies specifically defining the DVT prior to PE are few.[42] It is likely that the differences are related to the balance of thrombolysis, thrombus–vein wall adherence, and thrombus composition related to undefined genetic factors.

Factors That Increase VTE Risk

Most clinical VTEs have a proximate cause, including environmental risks and genetic predispositions, which may account for most of the VTEs that manifest clinically. The most common risk factors for VTE are prior DVT, malignancy, immobility, intravenous catheters, increased age, major surgery, trauma, infections such as pneumonia and urinary tract, and certain chemotherapies.[2,41,43] Some medications such as oral contraceptives and hormonal replacement therapies also increase the risk of VTE. A particularly aggressive acquired hypercoagulable state is antiphospholipid antibody syndrome.

Although beyond the scope of this chapter, it is important to emphasize that under specific circumstances, evaluating for an inherited thrombophilic state is warranted.[44] Clinical scenarios include early age of VTE (<40 years), recurrent unprovoked VTE, thrombosis at unusual sites, and a strong family history of VTE. The intersection of environmental stressor (eg, postsurgery) with an inherited thrombophilia is common; a form of the 2-hit hypothesis.

The most common inherited thrombophilias are divided among the deficiencies of the natural anticoagulants, the genetic factor abnormalities, and a miscellaneous category (Table 2.1). The suggested screening tests to evaluate for the most common thrombophilias are as follows: antithrombin, protein C/S; factor V Leiden; prothrombin 20210A; homocysteine; factor VIII; and antiphospholipid antibody panel.

Biomarkers for VTE

While atherosclerotic disease has numerous biomarkers for clinical symptom risk, such as C-reactive protein (CRP), cholesterol subtypes, Lipoprotein a, and more, markers for VT occurrence have been less forthcoming. Part of this has been a lack of understanding of VT pathophysiology and the nature of VTE occurrence as compared with arterial events. Venous thrombosis biomarkers would be most useful to determine primary risk, risk for recurrence, and perhaps defining therapy duration of VTE.

Venous thrombosis biomarkers are several and are variably studied clinically[45] (Table 2.2). Some of these, such as factor VIII, may be etiologic for VTE, whereas others such as D-dimer and thrombin-antithrombin complex (TAT) may reflect the thrombotic process.[46] D-dimer is cur-

TABLE 2.1   **Inherited Thrombophilias**

Natural Anticoagulant Deficiencies	Factor Genetic Abnormalities	Miscellaneous
Antithrombin	Factor V Leiden	Hyperhomocysteimia
Protein C	PT G20210A	Factor VIII
Protein S		Factor IX
		Antiphospholipid syndrome

TABLE 2.2   **Selected Biomarkers for Acute VTE**

Biomarker	Etiologic Association	VTE dx Sens/Spec (%)	Clinically Available?
D-dimer[47]	No	100/78	Yes
P-selectin[53]	Yes	71/81	No
Microparticles[53]	Yes	59/62	No
Factor VIII[45]	Yes	UNK	Yes
Thrombin antithrombin[45]	No	100/18 (>1.6 ng/mL)	Yes (not all)
Brain natriuretic peptide*[55]	No	> 80%/40% for major complications	Yes
Troponin*[55]	No	OR=5.2, 95% CI = 3.3–8.4 for cardiac death	Yes

*These are specific for PE patients.

rently used to define the likelihood of VTE probability in the clinical setting.[47] Studies are well established, confirming its use to effectively rule out, but not rule in, a VTE. Defining VTE recurrence risk has been improved with D-dimer measurement and now is included in the AACP guidelines.[48] For example, longer duration of VTE oral anticoagulation therapy is suggested by significantly elevated D-dimer levels after 3 months of oral coagulant therapy.[49] Thrombin-antithrombin complex, although not widely available, is also useful for acute VTE probability[46] and prediction of VTE recurrence.[50] Other measures, such as assessment of fragment 1 + 2, may further improve these predictions.[51]

Soluble P-selectin is an etiological factor in VTE,[52] and studies suggest its utility as additive for VTE prediction.[53] Elevated P-selectin levels correlate highly in patients with malignancy.[41] Inhibition of P-selectin can confer protection against VTE as suggested by nonhuman primate studies.[54] Specific anti-P-selectin agents are being developed for human trials and may offer prophylaxis benefit with anticoagulation risks. Although E-selectin plays a role in DVT, it has not been examined as a biomarker in humans.

Both probrain natriuretic peptide (BNP) and troponin are useful biomarkers reflecting the physiological stress of a PE. For example, a low BNP is associated with good clinical outcome, whereas BNP 1000 ng/mL is associated with a 12-fold increased risk of cardiac complications in combination with an abnormal ECHO.[55] Similarly, those patients with significantly elevated troponin-I have a 5.9-fold increased risk of in-hospital mortality. These biomarkers may be helpful in selecting those who would benefit from aggressive thrombus removal and close clinical support.[56]

On the horizon is potentially more specific VTE biomarker risk assessment by proteonomic evaluation.[57,58] Limiting this will be ease of use and rapidity of test results. However, refinements in technology may make this very useful in the future for assessment of VTE risk, particularly if specific enough to allow risk prediction in asymptomatic patients.

Commonalities of Arterial and Venous Thrombosis

Several epidemiologic and basic science studies have suggested a common interface between venous and arterial vascular pathology. In a prospective study of nearly 300 patients with DVT and a control group of 150 subjects, evaluation of carotid plaque progression was done. Patients with a spontaneous DVT had a 2.3-fold increased incidence of atherosclerosis progression, as compared with control subjects, which was independent of other atherosclerotic risk factors.[59] Similarly, those patients with a spontaneous VTE had a 1.6-fold increased incidence of symptomatic atherosclerosis,[60] suggesting overlap in vascular inflammation and risk. Interestingly, the proven effectiveness for antiplatelet therapy in preventing arterial thrombotic events does not translate to prevention of VTE,[48,61] despite the fact that platelets play a role.

The concept that VTE and atherosclerosis may share common risk factors has also been assessed by a recent meta-analysis.

The risk of VTE was increased 2.0-fold for obesity, 1.5-fold for hypertension, 1.4 for diabetes, 1.2 for smoking, and 1.2 for hypercholesterolemia.[62] Interestingly, mean HDL levels were lower in patients with VTE as compared with controls, although this finding is not universal.[63] Reports are forthcoming that HMG-CoA reductase inhibitors (statins) may be associated with decreased DVT incidence. Registry cohort patient data suggest a 22% risk reduction of symptomatic VTE in patients on a statin, as compared to matched patients not on a statin.[64] More impressive are results of a randomized clinical trial of patients with normal cholesterol but elevated hsCRP who were assigned to rosuvastatin or placebo. A 45% highly significant reduction of incident VTE was observed.[65] In addition to the endothelial protective effects of statins, these agents may increase TM expression and enhance APC activity, tipping the balance of endothelium toward a more anti-inflammatory and anticoagulant state. Future research will better define the vascular biology of venous thrombosis, which may reveal further similarities in arterial and venous risk factors and possibly response to therapy.

References

1. Heit JA, Cohen AT, Anderson FJ. Estimated annual number of incident and recurrent, non-fatal venous thromboembolism (VTE) events in the US. Blood. 2005;106(11): 910.

2. Gangireddy C, Rectenwald JR, Upchurch GR, Wakefield TW, Khuri S, Henderson WG, et al. Risk factors and clinical impact of postoperative symptomatic venous thromboembolism. J Vasc Surg. 2007;45(2):335-41.

3. Meissner MH, Wakefield TW, Ascher E, Caprini JA, Comerota AJ, Eklof B, et al. Acute

venous disease: venous thrombosis and venous trauma. J Vasc Surg. 2007;46 suppl S:25S-53S.

4. Mackman N, Tilley RE, Key NS. Role of the extrinsic pathway of blood coagulation in hemostasis and thrombosis. Arterioscl Throm Vas. 2007;27(8):1687-93.

5. Furie B, Furie BC. Mechanisms of thrombus formation. N Engl J Med. 2008;359(9):938-49.

6. Mackman N. Tissue-specific hemostasis in mice. Arterioscl Throm Vas. 2005;25(11): 2273-81.

7. Dahlback B. Blood coagulation. Lancet. 2000;355(9215):1627-32.

8. Stewart GJ. Neutrophils and deep venous thrombosis. Haemostasis. 1993;23 suppl 1:1 27-40.

9. Esmon CT. Inflammation and thrombosis. J Thromb Haemost. 2003;1(7):1343-8.

10. Celi A, Pellegrini G, Lorenzet R, De Blasi A, Ready N, Furie BC, et al. P-selectin induces the expression of tissue factor on monocytes. P Natl Acad Sci USA. 1994;91(19):8767-71.

11. Myers D Jr, Farris D, Hawley A, Wrobleski S, Chapman A, Stoolman L, et al. Selectins influence thrombosis in a mouse model of experimental deep venous thrombosis. J Surg Res. 2002;108(2):212-21.

12. Gilbert GE, Sims PJ, Wiedmer T, Furie B, Furie BC, Shattil SJ. Platelet-derived microparticles express high affinity receptors for factor VIII. J Biol Chem. 1991;266(26):17261-68.

13. Mesri M, Altieri DC. Endothelial cell activation by leukocyte microparticles. J Immunol. 1998;161(8):4382-7.

14. Sabatier F, Roux V, Anfosso F, Camoin L, Sampol J, Dignat-George F. Interaction of endothelial microparticles with monocytic cells in vitro induces tissue factor-dependent procoagulant activity. Blood. 2002;99(11):3962-70.

15. Falati S, Liu Q, Gross P, Merrill-Skoloff G, Chou J, Vandendries E, et al. Accumulation of tissue factor into developing thrombi in vivo is dependent upon microparticle P-selectin glycoprotein ligand 1 and platelet P-selectin. J Exp Med. 2003;197(11):1585-98.

16. Osterud B. The role of platelets in decrypting monocyte tissue factor. Semin Hematol. 2001;38(4 suppl 12):2-5.

17. Ahn ER, Lander G, Jy W, Bidot CJ, Jimenez JJ, Horstman LL, Ahn YS. Differences of soluble CD40L in sera and plasma: implications on CD40L assay as a marker of thrombotic risk. Thromb Res. 2004;114(2):143-8.

18. Myers DD, Hawley AE, Farris DM, Wrobleski SK, Thanaporn P, Schaub RG, et al. P-selectin and leukocyte microparticles are associated with venous thrombogenesis. J Vasc Surg. 2003;38(5):1075-89.

19. Myers DD, Wakefield TW. Inflammation-dependent thrombosis. Front Biosci. 2005;10:2750-7.

20. Polgar J, Matuskova J, Wagner DD. The P-selectin, tissue factor, coagulation triad. J Thromb Haemost. 2005;3(8):1590-6.

21. Andre P, Hartwell D, Hrachovinova I, Saffaripour S, Wagner DD. Pro-coagulant state resulting from high levels of soluble P-selectin in blood. P Natl Acad Sci USA. 2000;97(25):13835-40.

22. Day SM, Reeve JL, Pedersen B, Farris DM, Myers DD, Im M, et al. Macrovascular thrombosis is driven by tissue factor derived primarily from the blood vessel wall. Blood. 2005;105(1):192-8.

23. Corral J, Aznar J, Gonzalez-Conejero R, Villa P, Minano A, Vaya A, et al. Homozygous deficiency of heparin cofactor II: relevance of P17 glutamate residue in serpins, relationship with conformational diseases, and role in thrombosis. Circulation. 2004;110(10):1303-7.

24. Hassouna HI. Laboratory evaluation of hemostatic disorders. Hematol Oncol Clin N. 1993;7(6):1161-249.

25. Sidelmann JJ, Gram J, Jespersen J, Kluft C. Fibrin clot formation and lysis: basic

mechanisms. Semin Thromb Hemost. 2000;26(6):605-18.

26. Singh I, Burnand KG, Collins M, Luttun A, Collen D, Boelhouwer B, et al. Failure of thrombus to resolve in urokinase-type plasminogen activator gene-knockout mice: rescue by normal bone marrow-derived cells. Circulation. 2003;107(6):869-75.

27. Esmon CT. The regulation of natural anticoagulant pathways. Science. 1987;235(4794):1348-52.

28. Stoop AA, Lupu F, Pannekoek H. Colocalization of thrombin, PAI-1, and vitronectin in the atherosclerotic vessel wall: a potential regulatory mechanism of thrombin activity by PAI-1/vitronectin complexes. Arteriosc Throm Vas. 2000;20(4):1143-49.

29. Becker MD, O'Rourke LM, Blackman WS, Planck SR, Rosenbaum JT. Reduced leukocyte migration, but normal rolling and arrest, in interleukin-8 receptor homologue knockout mice. Invest Ophth Vis Sci. 2000;41(7):1812-7.

30. Aird WC. Phenotypic heterogeneity of the endothelium: I. Structure, function, and mechanisms. Circ Res. 2007;100(2):158-73.

31. Moaveni DK, Lynch EM, Luke C, Sood V, Upchurch GR, Wakefield TW, et al. Vein wall re-endothelialization after deep vein thrombosis is improved with low-molecular-weight heparin. J Vasc Surg. 2008;47(3):616-24.

32. Stenberg B, Bylock A, Risberg B. Effect of venous stasis on vessel wall fibrinolysis. Thromb Haemost. 1984;51(2):240-2.

33. Tapson VF. Acute pulmonary embolism. N Engl J Med. 2008;358(10):1037-52.

34. Eagleton MJ, Henke PK, Luke CE, Hawley AE, Bedi A, Knipp BS, et al. Southern Association for Vascular Surgery William J. von Leibig Award. Inflammation and intimal hyperplasia associated with experimental pulmonary embolism. J Vasc Surg. 2002;36(3):581-8.

35. Henke PK, DeBrunye LA, Strieter RM, Bromberg JS, Prince M, Kadell AM, et al. Viral IL-10 gene transfer decreases inflammation and cell adhesion molecule expression in a rat model of venous thrombosis. J Immunol. 2000;164(4):2131-41.

36. Zagorski J, Debelak J, Gellar M, Watts JA, Kline JA. Chemokines accumulate in the lungs of rats with severe pulmonary embolism induced by polystyrene microspheres. J Immunol. 2003;171(10):5529-36.

37. Rectenwald JE, Deatrick KB, Sukheepod P, Lynch EM, Moore AJ, Moaveni DM, et al. Experimental pulmonary embolism: effects of the thrombus and attenuation of pulmonary artery injury by low-molecular-weight heparin. J Vasc Surg. 2006;43(4):800-8.

38. Bdeir K, Murciano JC, Tomaszewski J, Koniaris L, Martinez J, Cines DB, et al. Urokinase mediates fibrinolysis in the pulmonary microvasculature. Blood. 2000;96(5):1820-6.

39. Laporte S, Mismetti P, Decousus H, Uresandi F, Otero R, Lobo JL, et al. Clinical predictors for fatal pulmonary embolism in 15,520 patients with venous thromboembolism: findings from the Registro Informatizado de la Enfermedad TromboEmbolica venosa (RIETE) registry. Circulation. 2008;117(13):1711-6.

40. Tick LW, Nijkeuter M, Kramer MH, Hovens MM, Buller HR, Leebeek FW, et al. High D-dimer levels increase the likelihood of pulmonary embolism. J Intern Med. 2008;264(2):195-200.

41. Zhu T, Martinez I, Emmerich J. Venous thromboembolism: risk factors for recurrence. Arteriosc Throm Vas. 2009;29(3):298-310.

42. Henke PK, Ferguson E, Varma M, Deatrick KB, Wakefield GT, Woodrum DT. Proximate versus nonproximate risk factor associated primary deep venous thrombosis: clinical spectrum and outcomes. J Vasc Surg. 2007; 45(5):998-1003; discussion 1003-4; quiz 1005-7.

43. Heit JA. The epidemiology of venous thromboembolism in the community. Arterioscl Throm Vas. 2008;28(3):370-2.

44. Middeldorp S, Levi M. Thrombophilia: an update. Semin Thromb Hemost. 2007;33(6):563-72.

45. Pabinger I, Ay C. Biomarkers and venous thromboembolism. Arterioscl Throm Vas. 2009;29(3):332-6.

46. Bozic M, Blinc A, Stegnar M. D-dimer, other markers of haemostasis activation and soluble adhesion molecules in patients with different clinical probabilities of deep vein thrombosis. Thromb Res. 2003;108:107-14.

47. Wells PS, Anderson DR, Rodger M, Forgie M, Kearon C, Dreyer J, et al. Evaluation of D-dimer in the diagnosis of suspected deep-vein thrombosis. N Engl J Med. 2003;349(13):1227-35.

48. Geerts W. Antithrombotic and thrombolytic therapy. Chest. 2008;133 (8th ed: ACCP Guidelines):381s-451s.

49. Palareti G, Cosmi B, Legnani C, Tosetto A, Brusi C, Iorio A, et al. D-dimer testing to determine the duration of anticoagulation therapy. N Engl J Med. 2006;355(17):1780-9.

50. Hron G, Kollars M, Binder BR, Eichinger S, Kyrle PA. Identification of patients at low risk for recurrent venous thromboembolism by measuring thrombin generation. JAMA. 2006;296(4):397-402.

51. Poli D, Antonucci E, Ciuti G, Abbate R, Prisco D. Combination of D-dimer, F1+2 and residual vein obstruction as predictors of VTE recurrence in patients with first VTE episode after OAT withdrawal. J Thromb Haemost. 2008;6(4):708-10.

52. Hrachovinova I, Cambien B, Hafezi-Moghadam A, Kappelmayer J, Camphausen RT, Widom A, et al. Interaction of P-selectin and PSGL-1 generates microparticles that correct hemostasis in a mouse model of hemophilia A. Nat Med. 2003;9(8):1020-5.

53. Rectenwald JE, Myers DD Jr, Hawley AE, Longo C, Henke PK, Guire KE, et al. D-dimer, P-selectin, and microparticles: novel markers to predict deep venous thrombosis. A pilot study. Thromb Haemost. 2005;94(6):1312-7.

54. Myers DD Jr, Wrobleski SK, Longo C, Bedard PW, Kaila N, Shaw GD, et al. Resolution of venous thrombosis using a novel oral small-molecule inhibitor of P-selectin (PSI-697) without anticoagulation. Thromb Haemost. 2007;97(3):400-7.

55. Binder L, Pieske B, Olschewski M, Geibel A, Klostermann B, Reiner C, et al. N-terminal pro-brain natriuretic peptide or troponin testing followed by echocardiography for risk stratification of acute pulmonary embolism. Circulation. 2005;112(11):1573-9.

56. Piazza G, Goldhaber SZ. Acute pulmonary embolism: part II: treatment and prophylaxis. Circulation. 2006;114(3):e42-7.

57. Hong CC, Kume T, Peterson RT. Role of crosstalk between phosphatidylinositol 3-kinase and extracellular signal-regulated kinase/mitogen-activated protein kinase pathways in artery-vein specification. Circ Res. 2008;103(6):573-9.

58. Ganesh SK, Sharma Y, Dayhoff J, Fales HM, Van Eyk J, Kickler TS, Billings EM, Nabel EG. Detection of venous thromboembolism by proteomic serum biomarkers. PLoS One. 2007;2(6):e544.

59. Prandoni P, Bilora F, Marchiori A, Bernardi E, Petrobelli F, Lensing AW, et al. An association between atherosclerosis and venous thrombosis. N Engl J Med. 2003;348(15):1435-41.

60. Prandoni P, Ghirarduzzi A, Prins MH, Pengo V, Davidson BL, Sorensen H, et al. Venous thromboembolism and the risk of subsequent symptomatic atherosclerosis. J Thromb Haemost. 2006;4(9):1891-6.

61. Glynn RJ, Ridker PM, Goldhaber SZ, Buring JE. Effect of low-dose aspirin on the occurrence of venous thromboembolism:

a randomized trial. Ann Intern Med. 2007;147(8):525-33.

62. Ageno W, Becattini C, Brighton T, Selby R, Kamphuisen PW. Cardiovascular risk factors and venous thromboembolism: a meta-analysis. Circulation. 2008;117(1):93-102.

63. Chamberlain AM, Folsom AR, Heckbert SR, Rosamond WD, Cushman M. High-density lipoprotein cholesterol and venous thromboembolism in the Longitudinal Investigation of Thromboembolism Etiology (LITE). Blood. 2008;112(7):2675-80.

64. Ray JG, Mamdani M, Tsuyuki RT, Anderson DR, Yeo EL, Laupacis A. Use of statins and the subsequent development of deep vein thrombosis. Arch Intern Med. 2001;161(June 11):1405-10.

65. Glynn RJ, Danielson E, Fonseca FA, Genest J, Gotto AM Jr, Kastelein JJ, et al. A randomized trial of rosuvastatin in the prevention of venous thromboembolism. N Engl J Med. 2009;360(18):1851-61.

Deep Venous Thrombosis

Prevention and Treatment

Mark G. Davies

Introduction

Venous thromboembolic diseases comprise the spectrum from deep venous thrombosis (DVT) to pulmonary embolism (PE), and occur with an incidence of approximately 1 per 1000 annually in adult populations.[1] Rates are slightly higher in men than in women. About two-thirds of episodes manifest as DVT, and one-third as PE with or without DVT. The major outcomes of venous thrombosis are death, recurrence, postthrombotic syndrome, and major bleeding due to anticoagulation. Thrombosis is also associated with impaired quality of life, particularly when postthrombotic syndrome develops.[2] Death occurs within 1 month of an episode in about 6% of those with DVT and

10% of those with PE.[3] The mortality rate for PE has been estimated to be as high as 30% in studies that included autopsy-based PE diagnosis.[4] Mortality rates are lower among patients with idiopathic venous thrombosis and highest among those whose thrombosis occurs in the setting of cancer. Venous thrombosis increases in incidence with age, with a low rate of about 1 per 10,000 annually before the fourth decade of life, rising rapidly after age 45 years and approaching 5 to 6 per 1000 annually by age 80.[5,6] The morbidity impact of thrombosis on the elderly appears to be greater, with a steeper rise in incidence of PE as compared to DVT with aging.[5]

Lower Limb

There are more than a quarter of a million hospital admissions each year in the United States for acute lower extremity deep venous thrombosis and pulmonary embolism.[7-9] In hospital patients without prophylaxis, it is

Venous Thromboembolic Disease. Contemporary Endovascular Management series. © 2011 Mark G. Davies MD and Alan B. Lumsden MD, eds. Cardiotext Publishing, ISBN 978-1-935395-22-5.

estimated that the incidence of isolated calf DVT and proximal DVT is 25% and 7%, respectively.[9,10] When thrombosis is proximal to the calf, there is a 50% likelihood of pulmonary embolism. There are geographical differences in reports on DVT, with up to twice the reported incidence of calf DVT being reported in Europe compared to North America.[10]

Upper Limb

Upper extremity venous thrombosis represents 0.5% to 1.5% of all venous thromboses. The primary form of the disease also is known as "effort thrombosis" or Paget-Schroetter disease. The secondary form of the disease is most commonly a result of central venous catheterization for central venous or cardiac access. Iatrogenic causes of secondary venous thrombosis account for up to 30% of symptomatic subclavian venous thromboses.[11] In addition, studies have shown that clinically silent thrombosis may occur in 20% to 30% of patients after central venous catheter insertion.[12,13]

Risk Factors

Multiple studies have consistently identified risk factors for the development of DVT, which are outlined in the following list:

- Age >40 years
- Male sex
- Obesity
- Presence of malignancy
- Presence of varicose veins
- Prior deep venous thrombosis or pulmonary embolism
- Type of procedure
  - Orthopedic
  - Neurosurgical

- Urologic
- Gynecological
- Any procedure >2 hours long
- Use of oral contraceptives
- Pregnancy
- Presence of hypercoagulable disorder

Commonly identified risk factors include age >40 years, prolonged immobility, prior venous thrombotic disease, malignancy, major surgery, obesity, varicose veins, congestive heart failure, myocardial infarction, orthopedic trauma, and estrogen use. An increasing concern during the workup for a DVT is identification of a hypercoagulable disorder (Table 3.1). Primary disorders involve a specific defect of a hemostatic protein, while secondary disorders result in an indirect effect on the hemostatic pathways.[14-17] All patients with thrombosis at an early age (<45 years), with a positive family history of thrombotic disease, thrombosis at an unusual site (mesenteric vein, cerebral vein), or recurrent thromboses without predisposing factors should be screened for hypercoagulability. In considering who needs prophylaxis, patients may be categorized into levels of risk: low, moderate, high, and highest (Table 3.2). In these categories, the incidence of calf vein DVT is 2%, 10% to 20%, 20% to 40% and 40% to 80%, whereas for proximal DVT, the incidence is 0.4%, 2% to 4%, and 4% to 8% and 10% to 20%, respectively.

Pathogenesis

One or more of 3 conditions cause thrombi to form in the systemic veins: reduced blood flow in the systemic veins, injury to the vein wall, and the presence of hypercoagulability. These factors remain important in the

TABLE 3.1   **Hypercoagulable States**

Primary

Antithrombin III deficiency	Heparan cofactor II deficiency
	Protein C deficiency
	Protein S deficiency
	Factor V Leiden
	Fibrinolysis deficiencies (dysplasminogenemia, decreased plasminogen activator or increased plasminogen activator inhibitors, dysfibrinogenemia)
Factor VII deficiency	

Secondary   Defects of coagulation and fibrinolysis
        Malignancy
        Pregnancy
        Use of oral contraceptives
        Nephrotic syndrome
        Lupus anticoagulant
Defects of platelets
        Myeloproliferative disorders
        Paroxysmal nocturnal hematuria
        Diabetes mellitus
        Hyperlipidemia
        Cushing's syndrome
        Heparin-induced thrombocytopenia
Defects of blood vessels and rheology
        Immobilization
        Postoperative care
        Vasculitis
        Chronic obliterative arterial disease
        Homocystinemia
        Hyperviscosity
        Thrombocytopenic thrombotic purpura

pathogenesis of pulmonary embolism and are known as Virchow's triad.[18,19]

Lower Limb

Venous stasis is the most important feature predisposing to venous thrombosis. The venous sinuses of the veins are especially vulnerable to stasis and thrombosis. Propagation of the thrombus may then follow upstream, or the process may spread retrograde.

Thrombi found in veins when blood flow is reduced are composed predominantly of fibrin and entrapped blood cells with relatively few platelets and are often termed "red thrombi." The friable ends of these thrombi are the source of the material that eventually becomes pulmonary emboli. Formation of venous thrombi is typically asymptomatic and may involve the superficial or deep venous systems. Deep venous thrombi can propagate into the superficial system.

TABLE 3.2 **Risk Stratification**

Low Risk	Uncomplicated minor surgery
	Age ≤40 years
	No risk factors
Moderate Risk	Age 40–60 years and no additional risk factors
	Age ≤40 years, major surgery, and no additional risk factors
	Minor surgery with additional risk factors
High Risk	Age >60 years and major surgery, with no additional risk factors
	Age 40–60 years and major surgery with additional risk factors, patients with myocardial infarction, and medical patients with risk factors
Highest Risk	Age >40 years and major surgery, plus prior thromboembolism, malignancy, or hypercoagulable state
	Major lower extremity orthopedic surgery
	Hip fracture
	Stroke
	Multiple trauma
	Spinal cord injury

Upper Limb

Primary axillosubclavian venous thrombosis is related to chronic venous compression and stenosis in the axillary-subclavian vein at the level of the costoclavicular space. It is seen most commonly in young individuals following vigorous exercise or activity involving hyperabduction of the affected extremity.[20,21] In the most common form of the disease, the vein is compressed between a hypertrophied scalene tendon and the first rib. Secondary axillosubclavian venous thrombosis is generally associated with instrumentation of the central venous circulation, direct venous trauma, or the presence of a hypercoagulable disorder. Secondary axillosubclavian venous thrombosis is an important clinical issue that requires attention. Iatrogenic causes of secondary venous thrombosis account for up to 30% of symptomatic subclavian venous thromboses.[11] In addition, studies have shown that clinically silent thrombosis may occur in 20% to 30% of patients after central venous catheter insertion.[12,13] Although it has not been clearly delineated, there are several inciting possibilities for secondary axillosubclavian vein thrombosis; they include endothelial trauma during insertion of the catheter, trauma from the indwelling catheter, venous stasis and fibrin deposition upon the catheter surface, and the effects of infusates on the surrounding vessel. Venous stenosis occurs in 30% to 40% of patients with central venous catheters.[22,23]

Natural History

In isolated calf thrombosis, proximal propagation occurs in up to 23% of untreated patients and 10% of patients treated with intravenous heparin. Propagation to a new segment has been documented in 30% of initially involved limbs and rethrombosis of partially occluded or recanalized segments in 31% of extremities. After completion of a course of anticoagulation, the theoretical rate of recurrence is 0.9% per month.[24] Following venous thrombosis, the venous lumen is most often reestablished. Recanalization occurs in an exponential manner over 6 months.[25] Up to 40% of occluded segments recanalized within 7 days, while 100% recanalization occurs within 90 days.[26] It appears that venous valvular incompetence occurs after deep venous thrombosis. This is supported by natural history studies that have demonstrated a correlation between segment thrombosis and subsequent valvular incompetence.[27] The development of reflux is highest within the first 6 to 12 months after development of a DVT.[28] However, up to 30% of segments will develop reflux without evidence of an initial thrombus, and this phenomenon appears to be related to persistent proximal obstruction.[29] The interval between the development of these defects and symptoms and signs of chronic venous insufficiency may range out to 20 years.[30]

The clinical diagnosis of DVT can be unreliable, as the disease mimics the patterns of many other disorders.[18,31] More than half of the patients who present with the classical symptoms of DVT do not have the disease.[18] Clinical suspicion in combination with diagnostic imaging should be used to confirm the diagnosis.[32] The proportion of patients with clinically suspected DVT, in whom the diagnosis is confirmed by objective testing, increases with the number of risk factors identified. Approximately half of the patients with deep venous thrombosis who develop pulmonary embolism have no symptoms of deep venous disease. This causes a delay in the administration of appropriate prophylactic and therapeutic measures. Duplex ultrasonography is a popular screening method of choice for the noninvasive assessment of blood flow in leg veins and of valve cusp movement.[33] It also can differentiate between acute and chronic venous thrombosis. All major deep veins of the lower limb can be assessed, but it cannot exclude the presence of thrombi in small veins of the calf. With experience, ultrasonography is accurate, repeatable, and inexpensive.[34] Positive tests indicating above-knee DVT do not require further follow-up unless the condition of the leg significantly worsens. Below-knee DVT requires repeat scanning and is recommended to confirm that there is no antegrade propagation on therapy. Duplex ultrasonography sensitivity and specificity are 94% and 96%, respectively. Overall accuracy is considered to be 95%. Cross-sectional imaging with computed tomography (CT) or magnetic resonance imaging (MRI) is a reliable method of diagnosing venous thrombosis, especially in the pelvic veins.[35] Venography is recommended to validate and diagnose a DVT when duplex ultrasonography has failed to rule out a DVT and should be performed prior to iliofemoral thrombolysis or thrombectomy. A recent review of the evidence strongly supports the use of clinical prediction rules, particularly the Wells model, for establishing the pretest probability of DVT or pulmonary embolism in a patient before ordering more definitive testing.[36] Fifteen studies support the conclusion that when a D-dimer assay is negative and a clinical prediction rule suggests a low probability of DVT or pulmonary embolism, the negative predictive value is high enough to justify foregoing imaging studies in many patients. The evidence in 5 systematic reviews regarding the use of D-dimer, in isolation, is strong and demonstrates sensitivities of the enzyme-linked immunosorbent assay (ELISA) and quantitative rapid ELISA, pooled across studies, of approximately 95%.

Eight systematic reviews found that the sensitivity and specificity of ultrasonography for diagnosis of DVT vary by vein; ultrasonography performs best for diagnosis of symptomatic, proximal vein thrombosis, with pooled sensitivities of 89% to 96%. The sensitivity of single-detector helical computed tomography for diagnosis of pulmonary embolism varied widely across studies and was below 90% in 4 of 9 studies; more studies are needed to determine the sensitivity of multidetector scanners.[36]

Management

Prevention

The American College of Chest Physicians (ACCP) has recently provided the following guidelines for DVT prophylaxis.[37] In patients admitted to the hospital with an acute medical illness, major trauma, and spinal cord injury, thromboprophylaxis with a low-molecular-weight heparin (LMWH), low-dose unfractionated heparin (LDUH), or fondaparinux is recommended with grade 1A weighting. For patients undergoing major general, gynecologic, and urological surgery, thromboprophylaxis with LMWH, LDUH, or fondaparinux is recommended. However, for patients undergoing elective hip or knee arthroplasty and hip fracture surgery, an alternative regimen of therapy with a vitamin K antagonist (VKA) with a goal of an international normalized ratio (INR) target of 2.5 (range, 2.0–3.0) is recommended for 10 to 35 days. All major trauma and all spinal cord injury (SCI) patients receive thromboprophylaxis. Mechanical methods of thromboprophylaxis are recommended primarily for patients at high bleeding risk or possibly as an adjunct to anticoagulant thromboprophylaxis.

Lower Extremity DVT

American College of Chest Physicians Evidence-Based Clinical Practice Guidelines (8th edition) on the treatment for venous thromboembolic disease recommend anticoagulant therapy with subcutaneous (SC) low-molecular-weight heparin (LMWH), monitored intravenous or subcutaneous unfractionated heparin (UFH), unmonitored weight-based SC UFH, or SC fondaparinux followed by VKA.[38] For patients with a high clinical suspicion of DVT, treatment with anticoagulants while awaiting the outcome of diagnostic tests is recommended. In acute DVT, initial treatment with LMWH, UFH, or fondaparinux for at least 5 days prior to initiation of VKAs and concomitant administration of LMWH, UFH, or fondaparinux on the first treatment day, and discontinuation of these heparin preparations when the INR is ≥ 2 for at least 24 hours is recommended. For patients with DVT secondary to a transient (reversible) risk factor, it is recommended that treatment with a VKA be for 3 months. For patients with unprovoked DVT, the ACCP recommends treatment with a VKA for at least 3 months and that all patients are then evaluated for the risks to benefits of indefinite therapy. Indefinite anticoagulant therapy is recommended for patients with a first unprovoked proximal DVT or PE and a low risk of bleeding, when this is consistent with the patient's preference, and for most patients with a second unprovoked DVT. The dose of VKA should be adjusted to maintain a target INR of 2.5 (INR range, 2.0–3.0) for all treatment durations. The ACCP recommends at least 3 months of treatment with LMWH for patients with venous thromboembolism (VTE) and cancer, followed by treatment with LMWH or VKA as long as the cancer is active. Treatment with VKA for more than 3 months is indicated for patients with recurrent venous thromboembolism or in patients in whom there is a continuing risk factor for venous thromboembolism. Patients should be followed up for 3 years to ensure that there is no recurrent thromboembolic event. Discontinuation of anticoagulant therapy in patients with recurrent venous thromboembolism is associated with an approximate 20% risk of recurrent venous thromboembolism during the following year and a 5% risk of fatal pulmonary embolism.[39,40] In patients with a continuing risk factor, which is reversible, long-term therapy should usually be continued until the risk factor is reversed. Anticoagulant therapy should be continued indefinitely in patients with an irreversible risk factor. For prevention of postthrombotic syndrome (PTS) after proximal DVT, the use of an elastic compression stocking is recommended. For DVT of the upper extremity, we recommend similar treatment as for DVT of the leg. Selected patients with lower extremity and upper extremity DVT may be considered for thrombus removal, generally using catheter-based thrombolytic techniques. For extensive superficial vein thrombosis, treatment with prophylactic or intermediate doses of LMWH or intermediate doses of UFH for 4 weeks is recommended.

Upper Extremity DVT

For patients with acute upper extremity DVT (UEDVT), treatment is as described for lower extremity DVT including treatment with a VKA for >3 months. If the DVT is due to a central venous catheter and the catheter is removed, then the duration of anticoagulation can be reduced for 3 months. Except in unusual circumstances, routine use of catheter-directed thrombolytic therapy is not recommended.

Decompression of Thoracic Outlet

Acute upper extremity DVT can be due to thoracic outlet syndrome. The frequency of PTS after UEDVT ranges from 7% to 46% (weighted mean 15%). Residual thrombosis and axillosubclavian vein thrombosis appear to be associated with an increased risk of PTS, whereas catheter-associated UEDVT may be associated with a decreased risk. There is currently no validated, standardized scale to assess upper extremity PTS, and little consensus regarding the optimal management of this condition. Quality of life is impaired in patients with upper extremity PTS, especially after DVT of the dominant arm.[41] These patients often present with obstructive symptoms and if acute thrombosis is noted, common practice is to perform catheter-directed thrombolysis followed by resection of the first rib.[42] Decompression of the thoracic outlet requires resection of either the clavicle and/or the first rib with division of the scalene muscle fibers at their insertion; division of the subclavius tendon and local venolysis must supplement each of these procedures.[43] First rib resection has most commonly been accomplished from a transaxillary approach but may be performed by supraclavicular, transclavicular, and infraclavicular approaches.[41] If venous repair is considered a possibility, then either supraclavicular anterior clavicular or infraclavicular approaches are required.

Pulmonary Embolism

For patients with a high clinical suspicion of pulmonary embolism (PE), treatment with anticoagulants while awaiting the outcome of diagnostic tests is recommended. Patients with confirmed PE, and who are hemodynamically compromised, should be considered for a short-course thrombolytic therapy.[38] For those with nonmassive PE, the use of thrombolytic therapy should also be considered. In acute PE, initial treatment with LMWH, UFH, or fondaparinux for at least 5 days is recommended with subsequent initiation of vitamin K antagonists together with LMWH, UFH, or fondaparinux on the first treatment day, and discontinuation of these heparin preparations when the INR is ≥ 2 for at least 24 hours. For patients with PE secondary to a transient (reversible) risk factor, therapy with a VKA should continue for 3 months. For patients with an unprovoked PE, it is recommended that therapy with a VKA should continue for at least 3 months and that all patients are then evaluated for the risks to benefits of indefinite therapy. The dose of VKA should be adjusted to maintain a target INR of 2.5 (INR range, 2.0–3.0) for all treatment durations.

Thrombolysis

Percutaneous clot removal using thrombolysis, mechanical thrombectomy, or a combination of the 2 is fast becoming a treatment of choice for patients presenting with acute iliofemoral and axillosubclavian deep venous thrombosis.[42,44] By restoring venous patency and preserving valvular function, catheter-directed thrombolytic therapy potentially affords an improved long-term outcome in selected patients with DVT. In selected patients with extensive acute proximal DVT (ie, iliofemoral DVT, symptoms for <14 days, good functional status, life expectancy of >1 year) who have a low risk of bleeding, catheter-directed pharmacomechanical thrombolysis is suggested by the ACCP.[38] This percutaneous therapy should include correction of any underlying venous lesions.

Conclusion

Management of DVT has progressed significantly in the last decade with the recognition of the need for aggressive DVT prophylaxis, improvements in diagnosis, and the use of more aggressive standards on initial and chronic therapy for the diagnosis of DVT.

References

1. White RH. The epidemiology of venous thromboembolism. Circulation. 2003;107: I-4-I-8.
2. van Korlaar IM, Vossen CY, Rosendaal FR, Bovill EG, Cushman M, Naud S, et al. The impact of venous thrombosis on quality of life. Thromb Res. 2004;114:11-8.
3. Cushman M, Tsai AW, White RH, Heckbert SR, Rosamond WD, Enright P, et al. Deep vein thrombosis and pulmonary embolism in two cohorts: the longitudinal investigation of thromboembolism etiology. Am J Med. 2004;117:19-25.
4. Heit JA, Silverstein MD, Mohr DN, Petterson TM, O'Fallon WM, Melton LJ. Predictors of survival after deep vein thrombosis and pulmonary embolism: a population-based cohort study. Arch Intern Med. 1999;159: 445-53.
5. Silverstein M, Heit JA, Mohr D, Petterson T, O'Fallon W, Melton L. Trends in the incidence of deep vein thrombosis and pulmonary embolism: a 25-year population-based study. Arch Intern Med. 1998;158:585-93.
6. Tsai AW, Cushman M, Rosamond WD, Heckbert SR, Polak JF, Folsom AR. Cardiovascular risk factors and venous thromboembolism incidence: the longitudinal investigation of thromboembolism etiology. Arch Intern Med. 2002;162:1182-9.
7. Dalen JE, Alpert JS. Natural history of pulmonary embolism. Prog Cardiovasc Dis. 1975;17:257-70.
8. Dismuke SE, Wagner EH. Pulmonary

embolism as a cause of death; the changing mortality in hospitalized patients. JAMA. 1986;255:2039-42.

9. Salzman EW, Hirsh J. The epidemiology, pathogenosis and natural history of venous thromboembolism. In: Colman RW, Hirsh J, Marder VJ, Salzman EW, eds. Hemostasis and Thrombosis. Philadelphia: JP Lippincott; 1994. p1275-96.

10. Clagett GP, Anderson FA Jr, Levine MN, Salzman EW, Wheeler HB. Prevention of venous thromboembolism. Chest. 1992;102:391S-407S.

11. Hill S, Berry R. Subclavian vein thrombosis: a continuing challenge. Surgery. 1990;108:1-9.

12. Smith V, Hallet J. Subclavian vein thrombosis during prolonged catheterization for parenteral nutrition: early management and long term follow-up. South Med J. 1983;76:603-6.

13. Fraschini G, Jadeja J, Lawson M, Holmes FA, Carrasco HC, Wallace S. Local infusion of urokinase for the lysis of thrombosis associated with permanent central venous catheters in cancer patients. J Clin Oncol. 1987;5:672-8.

14. Cosgriff TM, Bishop DT, Hershgold EJ, Skolnick MH, Martin BA, Baty BJ, et al. Familial antithrombin III deficiency: its natural history, genetics, diagnosis and treatment. Medicine. 1983;62:209-20.

15. Comp PC, Esmon CT. Recurrent venous thromboembolism in patients with a partial deficiency of protein S. N Engl J Med. 1984;311:1525-8.

16. Ridkar PM, Hennekens CH, Lindpaintner K, Stampfer MJ, Eisenberg PR, Miletich JP. Mutation of the gene coding for coagulation factor V and the risk of myocardial infarction, stroke and venous thrombosis in apparently healthy men. N Engl J Med. 1995;332:912-7.

17. Tollefsen DM. Antithrombotic deficiency. In: Scriver CR, Beaudet AL, Sly WS, Valle D, eds. The metabolic basis of inherited disease. 6th ed. New York: McGraw-Hill; 1989. p2207-18.

18. Anderson FA Jr, Wheeler HB, Goldberg RJ, Hosmer DW, Patwardhan NA, Jovanovic B, et al. A population-based perspective of the hospital incidence and case fatality rates of deep venous thrombosisand pulmonary embolism. The Worcester DVT Study. Arch Intern Med. 1991;151:933-8.

19. Anderson FAJ, Wheeler HB. Physician practices in the management of venous thromboembolism: a community-wide survey. J Vasc Surg. 1992;15:707-14.

20. Hughes E. Venous obstruction in the upper extremity (Paget Schroetter Syndrome). Int Abst Surg. 1949;88:89-127.

21. Adams J, DeWeese J. "Effort" thrombosis of the axillary and subclavian veins. J Trauma. 1971;11:923-30.

22. Lee S, Neilberger R. Subclavian vein stenosis: complication of subclavian vein catheterization for hemodialysis. Child Nephrol Urol. 1991;11:212-4.

23. Schillinger F, Schillinger D, Montagnac R, Milcent T. Post-catheterization venous stenosis in hemodialysis: comparative angiographic study of 50 subclavian and 50 jugular accesses. Nephrology. 1992;13:127-33.

24. Meissner MH, Caps MT, Bergelin RO, Manzo RA, Strandness DE. Propagation, rethrombosis and new thrombus formation after acute deep venous thrombosis. J Vasc Surg. 1995;22:558-67.

25. VanRamshorst B, VanBemmelen PS, Honeveld H, Faber JAJ, Eikelbloom BC. Thrombus regression in deep venous thrombosis. Quantification of spontaneous thrombolysis with duplex scanning. Circulation. 1992;86:414-9.

26. Killewich LA, Bedford GR, Beach KW, Strandness DE. Spontaneous lysis of deep venous thrombi: rate and outcome. J Vasc Surg. 1989;9:89-97.

27. Meissner MH, Manzo RA, Bergelin RO, Markel A, Strandness DE Jr. Deep venous insufficiency: the relationship between lysis and subsequent reflux. J Vasc Surg. 1993;18:596-608.

28. Markel A, Manzo R, Bergelin RO, Strandness DE Jr. Valvular reflux after deep vein thrombosis: incidence and time of occurance. J Vasc Surg. 1992;15:377-87.

29. Caps MT, Meissner MH, Manzo R, Bergelin RO, Strandness DE. Venous valvular reflux in veins not involved at the time of acute deep vein thrombosis. J Vasc Surg. 1995;22:524-31.

30. Bulger CM, Jacobs C, Patel NH. Epidemiology of acute deep vein thrombosis. Tech Vasc Interv Radiol. 2004;7(2):50-4.

31. Browse N. Deep vein thrombosis. Diagnosis. Brit J Med 1969;4:676-8.

32. Hull R, Hirsh J, Sackett DL, Stoddard G. Cost effectiveness of clinical diagnosis, venography and non-invasive testing in patients with symptomatic deep vein thrombosis. N Engl J Med. 1986;314:823-8.

33. Appleman PT, DeJong TE, Lampmann LE. Deep venous thrombosis of the leg: US findings. Radiology. 1987;163:743-6.

34. Cronan JJ. Venous thromboembolic disease. The role of ultrasound. Radiology. 1993;186:619-30.

35. Erdman WA, Jayson HT, Redman HC, Miller GL, Parkey RW, Peshock RW. Deep venous thrombosis of the extremities: role of MR imaging in the diagnosis. Radiology. 1990;174:425-31.

36. Segal JB, Eng J, Tamariz LJ, Bass EB. Review of the evidence on diagnosis of deep venous thrombosis and pulmonary embolism. Ann Fam Med. 2007;5(1):63-73.

37. Geerts WH, Bergqvist D, Pineo GF, Heit JA, Samama CM, Lassen MR, et al. Prevention of venous thromboembolism: American College of Chest Physicians Evidence-Based Clinical Practice Guidelines (8th ed.). Chest. 2008;133: 381S-453S.

38. Kearon C, Kahn SR, Agnelli G, Goldhaber S, Raskob GE, Comerota AJ. Antithrombotic therapy for venous thromboembolic disease: American College of Chest Physicians Evidence-Based Clinical Practice Guidelines (8th ed.). Chest. 2008;133(6 suppl): 454S-545S.

39. Schulman S, Granqvist S, Holmström M, Carlsson A, Lindmarker P, Nicol P, et al. The duration of oral anticoagulant therapy after a second epsiode of venous thromboembolism. N Engl J Med. 1997;336:393-8.

40. Hyers TM, Hull RD, Weg JG. Antithrombotic therapy for venous thromboembolic disease. Chest. 1995;108(suppl 4):335-51.

41. Elman EE, Kahn SR. The post-thrombotic syndrome after upper extremity deep venous thrombosis in adults: a systematic review. Thromb Res. 2006;117(8):609-14.

42. Molina JE, Hunter DW, Dietz CA. Protocols for Paget-Schroetter syndrome and late treatment of chronic subclavian vein obstruction. Ann Thorac Surg. 2009;87(2):416-22.

43. Melby SJ, Vedantham S, Narra VR, Paletta GAJ, Khoo-Summers L, Driskill M, et al. Comprehensive surgical management of the competitive athlete with effort thrombosis of the subclavian vein (Paget-Schroetter syndrome). J Vasc Surg. 2008;47(4): 809-21.

44. Meissner MH, Wakefield TW, Ascher E, Caprini JA, Comerota AJ, Eklof B, et al. Acute venous disease: venous thrombosis and venous trauma. J Vasc Surg. 2007;46(suppl S): 25S-53S.

Diagnostic Approach to Venous Thromboembolism

L. Bernardo Menajovsky, Patricia Hightower Lambden, and Ruth L. Bush

Venous thromboembolism (VTE) refers to pathologic thrombosis that occurs within the venous circulation. The most common form of VTE is deep venous thrombosis (DVT) of the lower extremities; however, the most life-threatening manifestation of VTE is embolization of venous thrombi resulting in pulmonary embolism (PE).

VTE is often a silent disease that can lead to multiple complications when left undetected or inadequately treated. Potential complications of DVT include PE, death, postthrombotic syndrome (PTS), and pulmonary hypertension. PTS is characterized by signs and symptoms similar to those associated with DVT and is common in patients with VTE (~30%).[1]

While mortality rates due to VTE have declined substantially over the last few decades as a result of advances in diagnostic techniques and treatments and a better understanding of the disease,[2] VTE and its complications remain a common cause of death in the United States. An estimated 200,000 new cases of VTE occur in the United States every year, including 94,000 with PE.[3] This translates into an incidence of 23 newly diagnosed cases per 100,000 patients per year.[3] Without treatment, PE is associated with a mortality rate of approximately 30%, or nearly 300,000 deaths per year.[3]

VTE is generally triggered by a combination of environmental and inherited risk factors. Accurate assessment of clinical symptoms, risk factor stratification, and appropriate use of objective diagnostic tests are pivotal in the accurate diagnosis and treatment of VTE. The reference standard for VTE diagnosis remains clot visualization with contrast venography or pulmonary

Venous Thromboembolic Disease. Contemporary Endovascular Management series. © 2011 Mark G. Davies MD and Alan B. Lumsden MD, eds. Cardiotext Publishing, ISBN 978-1-935395-22-5.

angiography. However, the invasiveness and the risks of these modalities have led to a steady increase in the use of noninvasive or minimally invasive VTE testing. These tests should optimally be used after clinical examinations and risk assessments reveal results highly suggestive of VTE. This chapter discusses the clinical symptoms and signs indicative of possible VTE and provides an overview of the clinical models and diagnostic strategies available to assess for thromboembolic disease.

Pathophysiology and Risk Stratification

VTE can occur as an idiopathic syndrome or may be caused by an underlying condition that predisposes a patient to thrombosis. In a retrospective study of 366 validated cases of VTE, approximately 48% were idiopathic and 52% were secondary to an underlying condition.[4] Rudolf Ludwig Karl Virchow was the first to identify 3 primary clinical factors associated with a substantial risk of thrombosis. Together, these factors are known as Virchow's triad, and include (1) vessel wall damage due to inflammation or trauma; (2) changes in blood flow or volume due to immobility, ischemia, and other conditions; and (3) hypercoagulable factors present in the blood, including inherited and acquired coagulation disorders.[5]

The consideration of risk factors in the assessment and diagnostic evaluation of patients with potential DVT is important; however, it is also important to consider the relative risk for each factor independently. Some reports suggest that hospitalized medical patients subjected to an extended period of immobility may be at risk for VTE, especially if presenting with additional risk factors, including acute infectious disease, previous history of VTE, or advanced age (>75 years).[6]

Endothelial injury has been attributed to both overt as well as subtle insults. Direct trauma such as soft tissue injury or fracture, as well as intravenous infusion of irritating substances, are more obvious factors that cause endothelial injury. Chemical changes, ischemia, anoxia, and inflammation are more subtle factors that may cause endothelial tissue damage.

In theory, during episodes of immobilization or prolonged limb dependency, venous flow becomes sluggish, which may give rise to platelet and fibrin deposit, thereby initiating venous thrombosis development. However, results from some studies suggest that the associated risk may not be as significant.[3,7,8] In one small study, Gatt and colleagues observed no difference in the risk of VTE in immobilized vs. mobile patients.[7] In a retrospective cohort analysis, Gatt and colleagues evaluated 18 mobile and 8 immobile patients with a mean age of 85 for a duration of 10 years. The immobile patients were bedridden for a prolonged period (>3 months). No difference in baseline characteristics, which included the assessment of risk factors, was observed between the 2 groups. The incidence of VTE was similar between the immobile and mobile patient groups (13.9 and 15.8, respectively; $P = 0.77$). While these results are not consistent with previous studies[9,10]—an inconsistency that is due, in part, to a relatively small study population—they do highlight the importance of considering the added threat conferred by each risk factor both independently and in combination with other risk factors.

Similarly, an analysis that was conducted using data from the American College of Surgeons National Trauma Data Bank evaluated the frequency of VTE following trauma. The results demonstrated that incidence of VTE in these patients is also relatively low.[11] Data were collected from 131 trauma centers. The following 6 risk factors were found to be associated with VTE: aged ≥40 years, lower extremity fracture with Abbreviated Injury Score (AIS) ≥3, head injury with AIS ≥3, ventilator delays >3, venous injury, and the performance of a major operative procedure. Of the 450,375 patients who experienced trauma from 1994 to 2001, a total of 1602 experienced DVT, resulting in an incidence of 0.36%.[11]

In contrast to the lower relative risk conferred by immobilization and trauma, a much stronger association exists between VTE and cancer.[12] In one study, 26% of patients presenting with bilateral DVT were diagnosed with cancer after the occurrence of DVT, and metastasis had occurred in 70% of these patients.[12] Other reports cite as much as a 2-fold increase in DVT risk among patients with cancer and suggest that the risk of recurrent thromboembolism is as much as 3.5 times higher in patients with malignancy vs. cancer-free patients.[1,13,14]

Finally, hypercoagulability—especially hypercoagulability due to a genetic predisposition, acquired syndromes, and certain medications, such as oral contraceptives—can increase the risk of thrombosis.[15,16] Hereditary risk factors include factor V Leiden mutation; prothrombin G 20210A gene mutation; and deficiencies of protein C, protein S, and antithrombin III.[17] Hyperhomocysteinemia and elevated levels of factors XIII and V, which may be hereditary and/or acquired, are also risk factors.[17] Additionally, ABO blood type is another VTE risk factor that was recently noted in cancer patients and is believed to be associated with hypercoagulability resulting from influence on the levels of von Willebrand factor (vWF) and factor VIII.[18]

Hypercogulability can be potentiated by any force that creates an imbalance between platelets, clotting factors, and the fibrinolytic system. There are many variables that contribute to hypercoagulability; however, the most common causes are hematologic disorders, malignancy, trauma, estrogen therapy, and surgical events.

Clinical Diagnosis of Venous Thromboembolism

The vast majority of thrombi that originate within the lower extremities resolve spontaneously; however, propagation of fibrin networks may lead to venous thrombosis. Such thromboembolic events are classified based upon the system involved (deep or superficial) as well as by location. Classification of thromboembolic events with regard to location refers to the thrombus in relation to the popliteal vein (distal or proximal).

The deep venous system possesses the ability to encompass a rather large amount of systemic flow. This heightened volume capacity, as well as ease of effective collateralization, allows many thromboembolic events to remain asymptomatic and undiagnosed. Unfortunately, the insidious nature of DVT allows for a great deal of vessel destruction prior to diagnosis. In many cases, the severity of symptomatology ineffectively represents the extent of the disease.

It is important to note that 50% of patients who have VTE do not present with any symptoms.[19] Clinical presentation of DVT most frequently involves unilateral lower extremity edema; however, iliofemoral obstruction may elicit bilateral edema. Increased intravascular blood volume, elevated hydrostatic pressure, and seepage of fluid across the capillary membrane all produce DVT-related edema. Increased tissue turgor and elevated temperature of the affected area are also secondary to edema and dilation of superficial vessels. Mottling or cyanosis of the extremity is often related to venous stasis, increased oxygen consumption, and reduction of hemoglobin.

Most individuals suffering from DVT report limb pain, described as aching or throbbing in nature, which is aggravated by ambulation. Although considered somewhat unreliable, there are 2 techniques utilized to assess limb tenderness. Homan's sign entails the dorsiflexion of the foot of the affected extremity to elicit calf pain. With Lowenberg's sign, calf pain is elicited by cuff inflation over the affected limb. As mentioned previously, each technique possesses a low pretest probability.

Long-term disability related to venous thrombosis involves the destruction of vessel endothelium, which renders venous valves incompetent. Such valvular incompetence allows for reversal of venous flow, stasis, and recurrent thrombosis. Venous thrombosis most frequently involves the vessels within the calf; however, the proximal veins of the lower extremities and the pelvic vessels are the primary etiology of pulmonary embolus, the most common life-threatening complication of deep venous thrombosis. Because of the correlation of life-threatening pulmonary embolus with the presence of DVT, it is of extreme importance to assess for pulmonary embolus in conjunction with DVT evaluation.

Initial evaluation for DVT must include screening for risk factors. There are many common risk factors; however, any event that leads to the elements included within Virchow's triad (venous stasis, endothelial injury, and hypercoagulability) may lead to DVT. The most common risk factors for DVT include immobility, dehydration, malignancy, blood dyscrasias, estrogen therapy, postoperative status, trauma, pregnancy/postpartum state, congestive heart failure, and obesity.

Wells and colleagues developed the first clinical model for the diagnosis of patients presenting with suspected DVT.[20-26] This model includes a thorough clinical examination and identification of any risk factors that predispose patients to have increased risk of thrombosis. In accordance with this model, patients are first divided into 3 risk categories (low, moderate, or high) and are further assessed through ultrasonography.[23] Patients who are stratified to the high-risk category, or who have abnormal ultrasonography results, are further assessed through venography.[23] Clinical practice guidelines for the diagnosis of DVT from the American Thoracic Society concur with this strategy, recommending the use of venography as a follow-up to inconclusive compression ultrasonography results, and the use of serial ultrasonography or impedance plethysmography in patients with normal compression ultrasonography results.[27]

For patients presenting with PE, shortness of breath, with or without leg pain, may be the first symptom; however, a number of specific criteria allow for a more accurate diagnosis. Similar to the clinical model for diagnosis of DVT, Wells and colleagues also defined a clinical algorithm for the diagnosis of PE (Figure 4.1),[26] which when used in conjunction with D-dimer testing, safely reduces the need for expensive imaging diagnostics.[26] This model for assessment of PE uses a point system for calculating the low, moderate, or high pretest probability of PE. Points are assigned based on clinical symptoms of DVT, including heart rate of >100 beats per minute, immobilization for ≥3 days or recent surgery in the past 4 weeks,

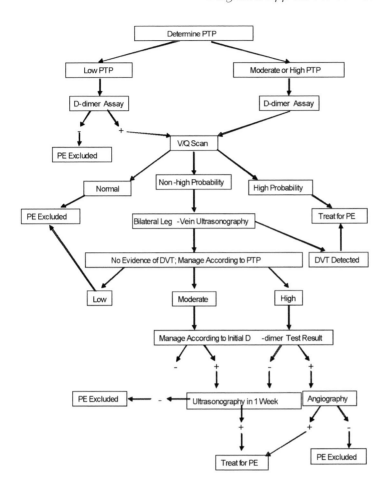

FIGURE 4.1 Clinical algorithm for initial evaluation of patients with suspected pulmonary embolism. DVT = deep venous thrombosis; PTP = pretest probability; V/Q = ventilation-perfusion. Reprinted with permission from Wells PS, Anderson DR, Rodger M, Stiell I, Dreyer JF, Barnes D, et al. Excluding pulmonary embolism at the bedside without diagnostic imaging: management of patients with suspected pulmonary embolism presenting to the emergency department by using a simple clinical model and D-dimer. Ann Intern Med. 2001;135:98-107.

a clinical history of VTE, hemoptysis, malignancy, or the clinician determination that PE is as likely or more likely than another diagnosis.[26]

The patient history and physical examination findings reported in the Prospective Investigation of Pulmonary Embolism Diagnosis (PIOPED) trial illustrate the difficulty in quickly identifying or ruling out a diagnosis of PE. In PIOPED, the most common past and current physical findings included dyspnea, pleuritic chest pain, cough, tachycardia, and tachypnea.[28] These symptoms also can be indicative of heart failure, interstitial lung disease, or pneumonia. For this reason, it is especially important to conduct thorough examinations and risk stratification when examining patients for potential VTE.

Objective Testing for Venous Thromboembolism

Diagnostic evaluation of suspected VTE includes a clear correlation between clinical probability, test selection, and test interpretation.[29] However, a variety of diagnostic approaches are feasible, and availability and familiarity with particular technology may influence the choice of approach. Additionally, the sensitivity of certain diagnostic tests is affected by the location of the thrombus.[27] In addition to traditional tests, such as contrast venography for DVT and pulmonary angiography for PE, newer modalities such as D-dimer assays and magnetic resonance direct thrombus imaging (MRDTI) offer promise for better detection with less invasiveness and have the potential for use in detection of both DVT and PE.

Imaging Modalities for Deep Venous Thrombosis

Contrast Venography Imaging

Contrast venography is no longer appropriate as the initial diagnostic test in patients exhibiting DVT symptoms, although it remains the gold standard for confirmatory diagnosis of DVT. Venography is nearly 100% specific and sensitive, and provides the ability to investigate the distal and proximal venous system for thrombosis. Its use is no longer widespread due to the need for administration of a contrast medium and the increased availability of noninvasive diagnostic strategies.[27] However, venography is still warranted when noninvasive testing is inconclusive or impossible to perform.[27] Additional drawbacks of venography include contraindication in patients with renal insufficiency and lack of accuracy in recurring cases of suspected DVT due to the difficulty of visualizing an intralumenal defect in veins that have been thrombosed previously.[27]

Compression Ultrasonography

Doppler compression ultrasonography with real-time, B-mode imaging is employed at most institutions because of its safety, availability, reliability, and noninvasive nature. Benefits include detection of acute symptomatic proximal DVT, as well as DVT of the upper extremities, and it is also capable of identifying other pathologies.[23,27,29-31] Its 2-dimensional, cross-sectional representation of lower extremity veins is also useful in combination with venous flow detection (duplex ultrasonography).[27] However, compression ultrasonography is not specific or sensitive for the detection of DVT in patients with asymptomatic proximal DVT or in patients with symptomatic or asymptomatic DVT of the calf, and it demonstrates limited accuracy in chronic DVT cases.[27] Its use is also limited in patients who are obese or who have edema.[27] Currently, a number of ongoing large trials are in progress for the assessment of magnetic resonance venography and computerized tomographic venography in the diagnosis of DVT.

Diagnostic Tests for Pulmonary Embolism

Blood Gas Analysis and Electrocardiogram

Arterial blood gas analysis and electrocardiogram (ECG) are routinely used to diagnose PE with varying rates of success. Hypoxemia is a common feature of acute PE but is not present in all cases.[27] Thus, while arterial blood gas levels reveal the blood oxygen saturation level, they are not specific or sensitive for the definitive diagnosis of PE. The use of transcutaneous oximetry will provide

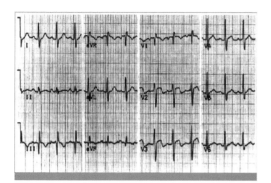

FIGURE 4.2 The S1Q3T3 pattern with concomitant symptoms and signs of pulmonary embolism warrants further investigation.

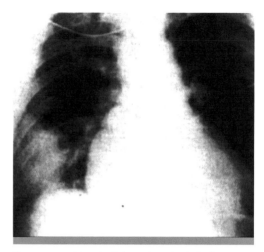

FIGURE 4.3 Hampton's hump is a classic finding caused by a pleural-based abnormality due to pulmonary infarction and visible in some X-rays. Its presence is not common and should not be used to confirm or exclude pulmonary embolism.

information regarding hypoxemia without the need for an arterial puncture, but it is not sensitive or specific for the diagnosis of PE.

Hemodynamically significant PE induces transient ECG abnormalities reflecting right ventricular overload and/or strain[32]; however, it is neither sensitive nor specific to VTE,[33] although a classic S1Q3T3 pattern (Figure 4.2) might warrant consideration of PE in the presence of other signs and symptoms. ECG can also be used to suggest an alternative cardiac diagnosis. Additionally, recent investigations have suggested that a simple scoring system based on ECG might be useful in predicting individuals with the greatest percentage of perfusion defect.[34] Because neither of these methods is suggested as a proven diagnostic tool for the initial screening or exclusion of VTE, they should not be routinely used for definitive diagnosis. Instead, they should be used in conjunction with clinical examinations and other diagnostic studies to reinforce the clinical suspicion of PE.[32]

Imaging Techniques

Chest X-ray
Chest X-ray is often used in combination with ECG to reinforce suspicion of PE.[32]

Although chest X-ray is commonly ordered during the process of differential diagnosis of pulmonary conditions, PE patients most commonly have normal chest X-ray results but sometimes present with nonspecific radiographic findings.[27] A normal chest X-ray in the presence of severe dyspnea or hypoxemia without evidence of bronchospasm or cardiac shunt is strongly suggestive of, but not diagnostic for, PE.[27]

"Hampton's hump" is a classic finding caused by a pleural-based abnormality due to pulmonary infarction and is visible in some X-rays; its presence, however, is not common and cannot be used to confirm or exclude PE (Figure 4.3). Chest X-ray is most useful to rule out other conditions that may mimic PE, such as pneumothorax or pneumomediastinum.[27,35]

Ventilation-Perfusion Scan
The ventilation-perfusion (V/Q) scan is used to detect areas of abnormal perfusion due to PE and has long been considered a

preferred diagnostic modality in suspected PE (Figure 4.4).[27,29] The ventilation component of the test excludes a diagnosis of pneumonia and other respiratory conditions. However, the V/Q scan is only diagnostic of PE in a minority of cases. Moreover, PE frequently occurs in combination with other lung diseases, such as pneumonia or chronic obstructive pulmonary disease. Because most lung diseases affect pulmonary blood flow as well as ventilation, their presence may decrease the scan's specificity.[27] The PIOPED study investigators at the National Heart, Lung, and Blood Institute (NHLBI) reported that a high-probability V/Q scan was sensitive for the diagnosis of PE, and a low-probability scan was sensitive for the absence of PE.[36] The V/Q scan was not useful

in patients with previous VTE.[36] Indeterminate scans require further diagnostic studies to accurately assess disease,[37] and 33% of PIOPED participants with indeterminate scans were later found through angiography to have thromboemboli.[36]

Spiral Computerized Tomographic Pulmonary Arteriography

Spiral (also known as helical) CT has demonstrated a higher degree of sensitivity and interobserver agreement than V/Q scan, making this strategy a less invasive, alternative diagnostic tool in patients with suspected PE (Figure 4.5).[38] Spiral CT has demonstrated a high rate of sensitivity and specificity in detecting PE to segmental levels,[39] but it cannot accurately detect sub-

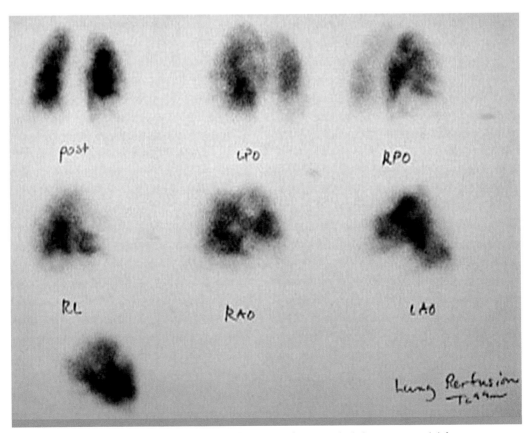

FIGURE 4.4   99m Tc macroaggregated albumin perfusion scan showing multiple large segmental defects.

segmental emboli.[39] Although the clinical significance of these subsegmental emboli has not been established, a negative spiral CT cannot safely rule out thrombosis and must be confirmed with pulmonary angiography.[39] In addition, a low sensitivity rate of 70% has been reported in a previous study, providing additional evidence that confirmatory pulmonary angiography is required in patients with negative spiral CT findings.[40] A 1-year follow-up study in patients with a normal spiral CT scan demonstrated a low 2% rate of clinical PE, suggesting that additional data will be required to characterize the safety of a negative spiral CT without other confirmatory diagnostics.[4]

Pulmonary Angiography

Pulmonary angiography has been considered a gold standard test for PE.[27] It is an invasive test and in some settings used to detect PE in patients with indeterminate V/Q scans. However, it is not necessary for diagnosis of PE in the acute setting when the perfusion scan is normal.[27] One study of pulmonary angiography demonstrated a

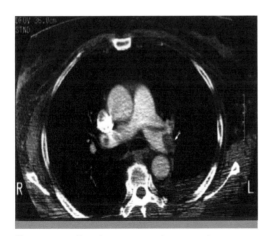

FIGURE 4.5 Spiral computerized tomographic pulmonary arteriography has demonstrated a high rate of sensitivity and specificity in detecting pulmonary embolism.

sensitivity of 85% for the detection of lobar and segmental emboli, with less reliability in detecting peripheral subsegmental emboli (1 in 5).[35] These results are consistent with those of the PIOPED study, in which interobserver agreement was 98% for lobar PE, 90% for segmental PE, and only 66% for subsegmental emboli.[42] However, there has been some debate surrounding the true clinical importance of these peripheral emboli.[35] Some investigators posit that they are caused by isolated calf vein thrombi and do not require treatment, whereas others believe that they are a precursor to larger emboli.[43,44]

Newer Diagnostic Techniques

Indirect CT Venography

Indirect CT venography has been investigated as an adjunct to the pulmonary angiography conducted during the differential diagnosis of PE.[45] This technique results in a high rate of detection of DVT—the underlying cause of many subsequent PE events—and requires no additional contrast material.[46,47]

Magnetic Resonance Direct Thrombus Imaging

MRDTI is a novel technique that has demonstrated accuracy and reproducibility for DVT diagnosis in limited studies.[48] It detects the presence of methemoglobin in clots, allowing visualization of thrombus without using intravenous contrast and making it useful for detection of subacute thrombosis.[49] The major advantages of MRDTI over conventional modalities include (1) early data suggesting that it is highly accurate for the detection of both DVT and PE, providing a single imaging modality for the detection of VTE;[49,50] (2) direct visualization of thrombus, avoiding the pitfalls of conventional techniques that have either identified thrombus as a filling defect or in terms of surrogates; and (3) simultaneous imaging of the legs and chest, allowing a comprehensive assessment of thrombus load, minimizing the importance of overlooked subsegmental PE, and potentially facilitating more titrated treatment. The safety of withholding treatment in suspected DVT and PE on the basis of negative MRDTI alone is being evaluated in ongoing outcome studies.[50] Additionally, because it has proven useful in identifying complicated plaque in the carotid arteries in the setting of transient and permanent cerebral ischemia, MRDTI offers promise as a technique that is capable of detecting high-risk vessel wall disease prior to significant or permanent end-organ damage.[49] As costs for this type of imaging decrease and institutions gain wider access to the technology, it should offer an attractive alternative to the invasive use of contrast venography with application in a wide range of vascular disease settings.

Bedside D-dimer Assays

A number of D-dimer assays have been evaluated as diagnostic markers for VTE and are considered to be inexpensive as well as timely[25]; the predictive value of the assay depends on several attributes, one being the prevalence of VTE in the population being tested. Ruiz-Giménez and colleagues found that the VIDAS and ELISA D-dimers as a first diagnostic tool for the exclusion of DVT are suitable approaches.[22] To the contrary, some data suggest that D-dimer testing of-

fers limited specificity and cannot be solely used to exclude a diagnosis of DVT. Such results have been demonstrated in emergency department patients,[51] patients who are elderly, and those hospitalized for >3 days.[52] Another important issue is that some institutions do not have access to immediate D-dimer results. Nevertheless, D-dimer testing, especially the most specific enzyme-linked immunosorbent assay, still offers an attractive bedside assay that is sensitive for DVT diagnosis if not specific under certain circumstances, and will still result in a reduction in the need for imaging diagnostics when DVT can be diagnosed and treated earlier.[53] A positive D-dimer is not useful for necessarily ruling in the diagnosis of VTE; rather, the value is found in the negative test, which, when it coincides with ultrasonography, can rule out the diagnosis.[25]

While measurement of D-dimers is a recent addition to the diagnostic strategy of PE and has been shown to be a valuable tool with excellent sensitivity, there have been rare reports of patients with PE but negative D-dimer tests. One investigation at an academic health center indicated that D-dimer measurement was of limited utility in patients with suspected PE and nondiagnostic lung scans or negative spiral (helical) CT results.[54] Another study of 150 patients admitted to hospital for PE who underwent D-dimer measurement compared results in patients with negative D-dimers vs. raised D-dimers. The sensitivity of raised D-dimers for PE was high (96%), but the finding of chest pain was statistically greater in the group with negative D-dimers ($P = 0.01$). In these negative D-dimer cases, the emboli were all distal ($P = 0.0003$), and the diagnostic value of ultrasound investigations (echocardiography, ultrasonography of lower limb veins) was less than in patients with higher D-dimers ($P < 0.0001$). The authors suggested that measurement of D-dimers by the ELISA method may be nondiagnostic in distal PE, perhaps because of the less extensive thromboembolic process. They concluded that in cases with negative D-dimers, a strong clinical suspicion of PE should signal a need for further investigation.[55]

Conclusion

Clinical evidence indicates that patients who are at moderate to high risk for developing VTE include those with a history of cancer, prior thrombosis, acquired syndromes, or genetic disorders that predispose them to a hypercoagulative state, among others. Among these patients, VTE should be highly suspected with the presentation of classic symptoms. Such cases require rapid assessment and accurate diagnosis to prevent the progression of DVT, long-term morbidity due to postthrombotic syndrome, and/or the occurrence of potentially fatal PE.

However, clinical presentation for 50% of patients with VTE is often nonspecific, and can be confused with a variety of other conditions, including heart failure, cellulitis, hematoma, or edema due to an unrelated condition.

New additions to the diagnostic battery and increased awareness of risk stratification paradigms have the potential to allow more accurate identification of VTE in some patients, thereby greatly reducing incidence of mortality and morbidity.

References

1. Prandoni P, Lensing AW, Cogo A, Cuppini S, Villalta S, Carta M, et al. The long-term clinical course of acute deep venous thrombosis. Ann Intern Med. 1996;125: 1-7.

2. Horlander KT, Mannino DM, Leeper KV. Pulmonary embolism mortality in the United States, 1979-1998: an analysis using multiple-cause mortality data. Arch Intern Med. 2003;163:1711-7.

3. Kroegel C, Reissig A. Principle mechanisms underlying venous thromboembolism: epidemiology, risk factors, pathophysiology and pathogenesis. Respiration. 2003;70: 7-30.

4. Cushman M, Tsai AW, White RH, Heckbert SR, Rosamond WD, Enright P, et al. Deep vein thrombosis and pulmonary embolism in two cohorts: the longitudinal investigation of thromboembolism etiology. Am J Med. 2004;117:19-25.

5. Nielsen H. Pathophysiology of venous thromboembolism. Semin Thromb Hemost. 1991;17 (suppl 3):250-3.

6. Alikhan R, Cohen AT, Combe S, Samama MM, Desjardins L, Eldor A, et al; MEDENOX Study. Risk factors for venous thromboembolism in hospitalized patients with acute medical illness: analysis of the MEDENOX Study. Arch Intern Med. 2004;10;164:963-8.

7. Gatt M, Paltiel O, Bursztyn M. Is prolonged immobilization a risk factor for symptomatic venous thromboembolism in elderly bedridden patients? Thromb Haemost. 2004;91:538-43.

8. Rosenow E. Concise review for primary-care physicians. Mayo Clin Proc. 1995;70:45-9.

9. Duggan C, Marriott K, Edwards R, Cuzick J. Inherited and acquired risk factors for venous thromboembolic disease among women taking tamoxifen to prevent breast cancer. J Clin Oncol. 2003;21:3588-93.

10. Samama MM, Dahl OE, Qunlan DJ, Mismetti P, Rosencher N. Quantification of risk factors for venous thromboembolism: a preliminary study for the development of a risk assessment tool. Haematologica. 2003;88: 1410-21.

11. Knudson MM, Ikossi DG, Khaw L, Morabito D, Speetzen LS. Thromboembolism after trauma: an analysis of 1602 episodes from the American College of Surgeons National Trauma Data Bank. Ann Surg. 2004;240:490-8.

12. Bura A, Cailleux N, Bienvenu B, Léger P, Bissery A, Boccalon H, Fiessinger JN, Levesque H, Emmerich J. Incidence and prognosis of cancer associated with bilateral venous thrombosis: a prospective study of 103 patients. J Thromb Haemost. 2004;2:441-4.

13. Hansson PO, Sorbo J, Eriksson H. Recurrent venous thromboembolism after deep vein thrombosis: incidence and risk factors. Arch Intern Med. 2000;160:769-74.

14. Schulman S, Lindmarker P, Johnsson H. A comparison of six weeks with six months of oral anticoagulant therapy after a first episode of venous thromboembolism. N Engl J Med. 1995;332:1661-5.

15. Allaart CF, Poort SR, Rosendaal FR, Reitsma PH, Bertina RM, Briët E. Increased risk of venous thrombosis in carriers of hereditary protein C deficiency defect. Lancet. 1993;341:134-8.

16. Hedenmalm K, Samuelsson E, Spigset O. Pulmonary embolism associated with combined oral contraceptives: reporting incidences and potential risk factors for a fatal outcome. Acta Obstet Gyn Scand. 2004;83:576-85.

17. Mazza JJ. Hypercoagulability and venous thromboembolism: a review. WMJ. 2004;103:41-9.

18. Streiff MB, Segal J, Grossman SA, Kickler TS, Weir EG. ABO blood group is a potent risk factor for venous thromboembolism in patients with malignant gliomas. Cancer. 2004;100:1717-23.

19. Gathof BS, Picker SM, Rojo J. Epidemiology, etiology and diagnosis of venous thrombosis. Eur J Med Res. 2004;9:95-103.

20. Cranley JJ, Canos AJ, Sull WJ. The diagnosis of deep venous thrombosis. Fallibility of clinical symptoms and signs. Arch Surg. 1976;111:34-6.

21. Anderson DR, Wells PS, Stiell I, MacLeod B, Simms M, Gray L, et al. Thrombosis in the emergency department: use of a clinical diagnosis model to safely avoid the need for urgent radiological investigation. Arch Intern Med. 1999;159:477-82.

22. Ruiz-Giménez N, Friera A, Artieda P, Caballero P, Sanchez Moliní P, Morales M, et al. for the Thromboembolic Disease Group. Rapid D-dimer test combined a clinical model for deep vein thrombosis. Validation with ultrasonography and clinical follow-up in 383 patients. Thromb Haemost. 2004;91:1237-46.

23. Wells PS, Hirsh J, Anderson DR, Lensing AW, Foster G, Kearon C, et al. Accuracy of clinical assessment of deep-vein thrombosis. Lancet. 1995;345:1326-30.

24. Wells PS, Ginsberg JS, Anderson DR, Kearon C, Gent M, Turpie AG, et al. Use of a clinical model for safe management of patients with suspected pulmonary embolism. Ann Intern Med. 1998;129:997-1005.

25. Wells PS, Anderson DR, Ginsberg J. Assessment of deep vein thrombosis or pulmonary embolism by the combined use of clinical model and noninvasive diagnostic tests. Semin Thromb Hemost. 2000;26:643-56.

26. Wells PS, Anderson DR, Rodger M, Stiell I, Dreyer JF, Barnes D, et al. Excluding pulmonary embolism at the bedside without diagnostic imaging: management of patients with suspected pulmonary embolism presenting to the emergency department by using a simple clinical model and D-dimer. Ann Intern Med. 2001;135:98-107.

27. Tapson VF, Carroll BA, Davidson BL, Elliott CG, Fedullo PF, Hales CA, et al. for the American Thoracic Society. The diagnostic approach to acute venous thromboembolism. Clinical practice guideline. Am J Resp Crit Care Med. 1999;160:1043-66.

28. Stein PD, Terrin ML, Hales CA, Palevsky HI, Saltzman HA, Thompson BT, et al. Clinical, laboratory, roentgenographic, and electrocardiographic findings in patients with acute pulmonary embolism and no pre-existing cardiac or pulmonary disease. Chest. 1991;100:598-603.

29. Baker WF Jr. Diagnosis of deep venous thrombosis and pulmonary embolism. Med Clin North Am. 1998;82(3):459-76.

30. Elias A, Cadène A, Elias M, Puget J, Tricoire JL, Colin C, et al. Extended lower limb venous ultrasound for the diagnosis of proximal and distal vein thrombosis in asymptomatic patients after total hip replacement. Eur J Vasc Endovasc Surg. 2004;27:438-44.

31. Stevens SM, Elliott CG, Chan KJ, Egger MJ, Ahmed KM. Withholding anticoagulation after a negative result on duplex ultrasonography for suspected symptomatic deep venous thrombosis. Ann Intern Med. 2004;140:985-91.

32. Costantini M, Bossone E, Renna R, Sticchi G, Licci E, De Fabrizio G, et al. Electrocardiographic features in critical pulmonary embolism. Results from baseline and continuous electrocardiographic monitoring [in Italian]. Ital Heart J. 2004;5:214-6.

33. Rodger M, Makropoulos D, Turek M, Quevillon J, Raymond F, Rasuli P, et al. Diagnostic value of the electrocardiogram in suspected pulmonary embolism. Am J Cardiol. 2000;86:807-9.

34. Iles S, Le Heron CJ, Davies G, Turner JG, Beckert LE. ECG score predicts those with the greatest percentage of perfusion defects due to acute pulmonary thromboembolic disease. Chest. 2004;125:1651-6.

35. Gupta A, Frazer CK, Ferguson JM, Kumar AB, Davis SJ, Fallon MJ, et al. Acute pulmonary embolism: diagnosis with MR angiography. Radiology. 1999;210:353-9.

36. The PIOPED Investigators. Value of the ventilation/perfusion scan in acute pulmonary embolism. Results of the Prospective Investigation of Pulmonary Embolism Diagnosis (PIOPED). JAMA. 1990;263:2753-9.

37. Kember PG, Euinton HA, Morcos SK. Clinicians' interpretation of the indeterminate ventilation-perfusion scan report. Br J Radiol. 1997;70:1109-11.

38. Mayo JR, Remy-Jardin M, Müller NL, Remy J, Worsley DF, Hossein-Foucher C, et al. Pulmonary embolism: prospective comparison of spiral CT with ventilation-perfusion scintigraphy. Radiology. 1997;205:447-52.

39. Remy-Jardin M, Remy J, Deschildre F, Artaud D, Beregi JP, Hossein-Foucher C, et al. Diagnosis of pulmonary embolism with spiral CT: comparison with pulmonary angiography and scintigraphy. Radiology. 1996;200:699-706.

40. Perrier A, Howarth N, Didier D, Loubeyre P, Unger PF, de Moerloose P, et al. Performance of helical computed tomography in unselected outpatients with suspected pulmonary embolism. Ann Intern Med. 2001;135:88-97.

41. Tillie-Leblond I, Mastora I, Radenne F, Paillard S, Tonnel AB, Remy J, et al. Risk of pulmonary embolism after a negative spiral CT angiogram in patients with pulmonary disease: 1-year clinical follow-up study. Radiology. 2002;223:461-7.

42. Stein PD, Athanasoulis C, Alavi A, Greenspan RH, Hales CA, Saltzman HA, et al. Complications and validity of pulmonary angiography in acute pulmonary embolism. Circulation. 1992;85:462-9.

43. Dalen JE. When can treatment be withheld in patients with suspected pulmonary embolism. Arch Intern Med. 1993;153:1415-8.

44. Moser KM. Venous thromboembolism. Am Rev Respir Dis. 1990;141:235-49.

45. Richman PB, Wood J, Kasper DM, Collins JM, Petri RW, Field AG, et al. Contribution of

indirect computed tomography venography to computed tomography angiography of the chest for the diagnosis of thromboembolic disease in two United States emergency departments. J Thromb Haemost. 2003;1:652-7.

46. Cham MD, Yankelevitz DF, Shaham D, Shah AA, Sherman L, Lewis A, et al. for the Pulmonary Angiography-Indirect CT Venography Cooperative Group. Deep venous thrombosis: detection by using indirect CT venography. Radiology. 2000;216: 744-51.

47. Loud PA, Katz DS, Bruce DA, Klippenstein DL, Grossman ZD. Deep venous thrombosis with suspected pulmonary embolism: detection with combined CT venography and pulmonary angiography. Radiology. 2001;219:498-502.

48. Fraser DGW, Moody AR, Morgan PS, Martel AL, Davidson I. Diagnosis of lower-limb deep venous thrombosis: a prospective blinded study of magnetic resonance direct thrombus imaging. Ann Intern Med. 2002;136:89-98.

49. Moody AR. Magnetic resonance direct thrombus imaging. J Thromb Haemost. 2003;1:1403-9.

50. Kelly J, Hunt BJ, Moody A. Magnetic resonance direct thrombus imaging: a novel technique for imaging venous thromboemboli.

Thromb Haemost. 2003;89:773-82.

51. Farrell S, Hayes T, Shaw M. A negative SimpliRED D-dimer assay result does not exclude the diagnosis of deep vein thrombosis or pulmonary embolus in emergency department patients. Ann Emerg Med. 2000;35:121-5.

52. Brotman DJ, Segal JB, Jani JT, Petty BG, Kickler TS. Limitations of D-dimer testing in unselected inpatients with suspected venous thromboembolism. Am J Med. 2003;114:276-82.

53. Stein PD, Hull RD, Patel KC, Olson RE, Ghali WA, Brant R, Biel RK, Bharadia V, Kalra NK. D-dimer for the exclusion of acute venous thrombosis and pulmonary embolism: a systematic review. Ann Intern Med. 2004;140:589-602.

54. Rathbun SW, Whitsett TL, Vesely SK, Raskob GE. Clinical utility of D-dimer in patients with suspected pulmonary embolism and nondiagnostic lung scans or negative CT findings. Chest. 2004;125:851-5.

55. Mansencal N, Joseph T, Vieillard-Baron A, El Hajjam M, Bendaoud M, Drouin A, Jondeau G, Lacombe P, Jardin F, Dubourg O. Negative D-dimers and peripheral pulmonary embolism [in French]. Arch Mal Coeur Vaiss. 2003;96:1143-8.

Treatment of Acute Deep Venous Thrombosis

What's New in the ACCP Guidelines?

Anthony J. Comerota

Guidelines for patient care offer recommendations to physicians for diagnosis and management of common diseases that generally apply to the typical patient. This chapter addresses the most recent edition of the American College of Chest Physicians (ACCP) guidelines to help clinicians manage patients with acute deep venous thrombosis (DVT). The eighth ACCP consensus conference recently published "Antithrombotic Therapy for Venous Thromboembolic Disease"[1] to help physicians care for patients with venous disease. The authors have made specific changes with recommendations and suggestions linked to objective grades, which form the basis of this discussion.

The method of determining the strength and quality of the recommendations deserves mention. Recommendations are generally accompanied by a number, which refers to the *strength* of the recommendation, and a letter, which refers to the *quality of the evidence* supporting the recommendation. The current ACCP guidelines use 2 levels for the strength of their recommendations: grade 1 for strong and grade 2 for weak.[2] They further indicate that statements accompanied by a grade 1 level are "recommendations" and statements accompanied by a grade 2 level are "suggestions."

The quality of evidence upon which the strength of the recommendation is based ranges from "A" for high quality, which is consistent evidence from multiple randomized trials, to "B" for moderate quality, which is evidence from a single randomized trial or inconsistent evidence from random-

Venous Thromboembolic Disease. Contemporary Endovascular Management series. © 2011 Mark G. Davies MD and Alan B. Lumsden MD, eds. Cardiotext Publishing, ISBN 978-1-935395-22-5.

ized trials. Level "C" is low quality, which is suggestive evidence from nonrandomized trials, observational reports, or expert opinion. Guideline-writing committees are becoming increasingly aware of costs of care and patient values and preferences, as are physicians. It stands to reason that a clear-thinking, well-informed patient will agree with treatment recommendations that follow strong guidelines (grades 1A) whereas when physicians are faced with atypical clinical circumstances or weak guideline recommendations (ie, suggestions), cost of care and patient values and preferences should be considered in addition to the risks and benefits of the treatment.

Magnitude of the Problem

Venous disease is one of the most common disorders afflicting the populations of developed and developing countries. New studies show that acute venous thrombosis resulting in fatal pulmonary embolism kills more people than acute myocardial infarction or acute stroke.[3] Over 1 million people per year will suffer an acute venous thromboembolic event in the United States alone. The postthrombotic morbidity that follows is substantial and is proportional to the extent of venous thrombosis.[4-6]

Acute DVT often leads to chronic postthrombotic morbidity, and the severity of postthrombotic venous disease correlates directly with the extent of the acute DVT. Extensive DVT results in severe chronic morbidity unless patients are treated with a strategy to eliminate the acute clot.

What's New in Guidelines?

The 2008 ACCP recommendations for the management of extensive venous thrombosis and pulmonary embolism are a major departure from previous guideline versions. The authors acknowledged that extensive venous thrombosis is clearly associated with the development of the postthrombotic syndrome. Moreover, they recognized the existing evidence supporting the value of venous thrombectomy (grade 2B) and catheter-directed thrombolysis (grade 2B) as components of a strategy of thrombus removal, especially for patients with iliofemoral DVT.

The morbidity of the postthrombotic syndrome was a driving force for revising the ACCP recommendations as was evidence that early removal of thrombus prevents or reduces postthrombotic morbidity. Studies have shown that patients with postthrombotic venous insufficiency suffer reduced quality of life (QOL),[7,8] and the development of the postthrombotic syndrome is directly related to the severity of acute DVT. This is particularly true in patients with iliofemoral DVT, who appear to be a clinically relevant subset of patients with acute DVT and suffer the most severe postthrombotic morbidity.[6,9,10] The available evidence clearly shows that a strategy of thrombus removal is the preferred management for patients with iliofemoral DVT and offers them the best long-term outcome.[11]

The committee went on to refine anticoagulant therapy for patients with venous thromboembolism, addressing the needs of patients with malignancy and idiopathic venous thromboembolic disease. They also dispelled the myth of bed rest for patients with acute DVT, highlighting the benefit of early anticoagulation, early compressions of the affected leg, and the significant benefit of continued use of 30- to 40-mm Hg compression stockings.

Treatment of Iliofemoral Venous Thrombosis

The writing committee for the 2008 ACCP guidelines recognized the excess morbidity of this particular distribution of disease. It is important to understand the anatomy of lower extremity venous drainage, which functionally resembles a funnel, with distal veins draining into larger but progressively fewer veins as blood moves cephalad. The common femoral and iliac veins represent the spout of the funnel, which is the single common channel of lower extremity venous drainage. If this channel is obstructed, it will affect the entire leg, with adverse functional consequences on all distal veins.

The greatest change in guidelines is the recommendation for consideration of a strategy of thrombus removal in patients with iliofemoral DVT. This is a reversal of the statements from guidelines published in 2004.[12]

Venous Thrombectomy

The 2008 ACCP guidelines recommend considering venous thrombectomy for acute iliofemoral DVT in patients with symptoms for <7 days, good functional status, and a life expectancy ≥1 year (grade 2B).

Rationale This is based upon level 1 data emanating from a large randomized study by Plate et al.[13-15] Patients were followed up and reported at 6 months, 5 years, and 10 years following randomization to venous thrombectomy or anticoagulation. Patients randomized to thrombectomy demonstrated improved patency, lower venous pressures, less leg swelling, and fewer postthrombotic

symptoms compared to patients treated with anticoagulation alone. Other, nonrandomized series also reported favorable outcomes of contemporary venous thrombectomy. Long-term observational results from 10 reports with the mean of 41 months of follow-up demonstrated a 76% patency, with 8 reports demonstrating functional venous valves in the femoropopliteal segment in 63%.[11]

Since venous thrombectomy is infrequently performed, the committee suggested that "catheter-directed thrombolysis is usually preferable to operative venous thrombectomy" (grade 2C).[1]

Catheter-Directed Thrombolysis

The recommendation for catheter-directed thrombolysis (CDT) for acute iliofemoral DVT in patients with a low risk of bleeding, symptoms <14 days, good functional status, and a life expectancy ≥1 year is also proposed to reduce acute symptoms and postthrombotic morbidity (grade 2B).

Rationale A small randomized trial of catheter-directed lytic therapy vs. anticoagulation demonstrated significantly better patency and preservation of valve function in patients treated with CDT vs. anticoagulation.[16] Large single-center series and multicenter venous registries demonstrate an 80% to 90% success rate, with progressively lower bleeding complications over time.[17-19] A case-controlled cohort study, which followed the National Venous Registry, demonstrated significantly improved quality of life (QOL) in patients with iliofemoral DVT treated with CDT compared to those treated with anticoagulation.[20] The improved QOL was directly related to lytic success.

The committee suggests *correction of underlying venous lesions* using balloon angioplasty and stents (grade 2C). While there are no objective data supporting this statement, the collective clinical observations and expert opinion suggest that residual (uncorrected) venous lesions increase the likelihood of rethrombosis. Alternatively, correction of focal lesions in the proximal system is associated with good long-term outcome. This suggestion applies to both venous thrombectomy and CDT.

Another suggestion new to this edition of the guidelines is for the use of *pharmacomechanical thrombolysis to reduce treatment times*, shorten hospital and intensive care unit stays, and reduce costs (grade 2C). Pharmacomechanical techniques complement catheter-directed thrombolysis, often resulting in better patient outcomes in addition to facilitating treatment. Current pharmacomechanical techniques include pulse-spray, isolated segmental, and ultrasound-accelerated thrombolysis. While randomized trials comparing pharmacomechanical techniques with catheter-directed thrombolysis alone are lacking, single-center reports,[21,22] multicenter registries,[23] and expert opinion suggest that thrombus removal can be achieved more rapidly with lower doses of plasminogen activators using pharmacomechanical techniques.

The committee recommends the same intensity and duration of anticoagulation following thrombectomy and CDT as patients who do not undergo these treatments (grade 1C). This is a uniformly strong opinion by the experts that underscores the need to avoid recurrence, although proper trials of intensity and duration of anticoagulation following interventional therapy have not been performed.

Anticoagulation for Acute Venous Thromboembolic Disease

For patients with acute DVT, early therapeutic anticoagulation with intravenous unfractionated heparin (UFH), subcutaneous low-molecular-weight heparin (LMWH), subcutaneous fondaparinux, subcutaneous weight-adjusted UFH, or subcutaneous monitored UFH is recommended (grade 1A).

Rationale The writing committee emphasizes the importance of both early and long-term anticoagulation for the treatment of acute DVT. Early anticoagulation, otherwise termed "initial treatment," is designed to prevent thrombus extension and embolization, and, when patients are treated properly, reduces the risk of early and late recurrence. The objective of long-term anticoagulation is to avoid recurrence. Slow or delayed therapeutic anticoagulation results in a significantly increased risk of recurrent of venous thromboembolism compared to early and immediate therapeutic anticoagulation.[24] If early anticoagulation with UFH falls below a therapeutic level, patients have a 15-fold risk of recurrence.[25]

For isolated distal DVT (calf vein thrombosis), 3 months of anticoagulation is recommended (grade 2B).

Rationale A randomized trial of isolated calf vein thrombosis treated with 5 days of anticoagulation with heparin followed by 3 months of vitamin K antagonists (VKA) vs. 5 days of heparin followed by placebo demonstrated significant benefit to 3 months of oral VKA. Nonrandomized trial observation of thrombus propagation in patients not anticoagulated would support this approach. If a patient with isolated calf DVT were at high risk for bleeding with anticoagulation, calf compression and ambulation with ultrasound surveillance appear to be an appropriate approach.

For patients with proximal DVT, a minimum of 3 months of anticoagulation is recommended over shorter periods (grade 1A). For patients with proximal DVT who are at low risk for bleeding, long-term anticoagulation is recommended (grade 1A).

Rationale Numerous studies evaluating the appropriate duration of anticoagulation for proximal DVT have been performed. As a general observation, studies have demonstrated that the longer the course of therapy, the less risk of recurrence. Levine and colleagues[26] randomized patients with venographically proven proximal DVT to 4 weeks vs. 3 months of anticoagulation. They demonstrated that 3 months of anticoagulation was significantly better than 4 weeks. Schulman et al[27] randomized patients to 6 weeks vs. 6 months of oral anticoagulation for acute DVT and demonstrated significant reduction in recurrence in the patients treated for 6 months. The bleeding complications were no different between the 2 groups. Kearon and colleagues[28] randomized patients to 3 months vs. indefinite anticoagulation and demonstrated significant long-term benefit to indefinite anticoagulation. There was a trend to more major bleeding in patients with long-term anticoagulation vs. the 3-month cohort. Although Ridker et al[29] demonstrated long-term low intensity warfarin to be significantly better than placebo for treatment of idiopathic venous thromboembolism, Kearon and colleagues[30] compared conventional long-term anticoagulation to low-intensity long-term anticoagulation and showed no difference in bleeding complications; the study did show a significant benefit to conventional doses compared to subtherapeutic doses of VKA. Therefore, patients with venous thromboembolic disease who are at low risk for bleeding should be considered for long-term anticoagulation (grade 1A). The patient should be reevaluated at specified time intervals for the ongoing risk-benefit ratio.

In patients with recurrent, unprovoked DVT, long-term, indefinite anticoagulation is recommended (grade 1A). For patients on long-term therapy, reassessment should occur at periodic intervals to evaluate their risks of anticoagulation vs. their benefits.

Rationale A randomized trial has demonstrated that in patients with unprovoked recurrent DVT, indefinite anticoagulation significantly reduced recurrence compared to 6 months of therapy (relative risk [RR], 8.0; P <0.001).[31] There was a trend toward reduced mortality; however, there was an increased risk of a major bleed from indefinite anticoagulation (RR 0.3; P = 0.0084). The above data underscore the benefit of long-term anticoagulation with regard to recurrence. However, reassessment of a patient's bleeding risk over time is crucial to maintain benefit vs. risk.

In patients with malignancy, LMWH is recommended as the treatment of choice for the first 3 to 6 months following diagnosis of acute DVT (grade 1A). Subsequent treatment with VKA or LMWH is recommended for an indefinite period or until the cancer is resolved (grade 1C).

Rationale A randomized trial evaluating the LMWH dalteparin vs. VKA with Coumadin demonstrated a significant reduction in recurrent venous thromboembolism (RR 0.48; P = 0.002). There was no difference in bleeding complications nor was there a difference in mortality. Since cancer is a major thrombotic risk, recurrence rates are high. Therefore, the recommendations are for anticoagulation until cancer is resolved.

Early Ambulation and Compression

Early ambulation in patients with acute DVT is now recommended in preference to initial bed rest (grade 1A).

Rationale Bed rest and immobilization are known risk factors for DVT and thrombus propagation. Randomized trials of early ambulation and leg compression have demonstrated reduced pain, edema, and postthrombotic morbidity compared to patients treated with bed rest and anticoagulation.[32-36] Application of a snug wrap from the base of the toes to the upper thigh at the time of diagnosis of acute DVT combined with ambulation and anticoagulation is the method described by Partsch et al.[37] This has been shown to be effective in the early management of patients with acute proximal DVT.

For patients who have symptomatic proximal DVT, elastic compression stockings of 30 to 40 mm Hg are recommended (grade 1A). Stockings should be applied as soon as available and worn from the time the patient awakens in the morning until going to bed at night.

Rationale Two randomized trials treating patients after a first episode of acute symptomatic proximal DVT demonstrated significant reduction (50% reduction) of postthrombotic symptoms in patients wearing compression stockings compared to those treated without compression.[38,39] A Cochrane review of compression following acute DVT also concluded that compression stockings substantially reduced the incidence of the postthrombotic syndrome after 2 years.[40]

Intermittent Pneumatic Compression

For patients with severe edema of the leg due to postthrombotic syndrome, a course of intermittent pneumatic compression is suggested (grade 2B).

Rationale In a crossover study [41] in patients with severe postthrombotic syndrome, intermittent pneumatic compression (IPC) of 40 mm Hg was proven more effective than placebo pressures. Patients uniformly preferred therapeutic pressures to placebo.

In patients with venous ulcers resistant to healing with wound care and standard

compression, the addition of IPC is suggested (grade 2B).

Rationale IPC has been shown to increase venous velocity, reduce edema, increase TcPO2, increase popliteal artery blood flow, and increase endothelial nitric oxide synthase. These basic effects of IPC have translated into improved healing of venous leg ulcers in clinical trials. Randomized trials in patients with persistent venous ulcers have demonstrated significantly increased healing[42,43] and more rapid healing of venous leg ulcers when IPC was used in addition to standard wound care and compression wraps. Compression pressures and cycles have varied in the studies reported; therefore, IPC prescription for the treatment of postthrombotic syndrome and venous ulcers has not been standardized. With our understanding of the pathophysiology of chronic venous disease (high ambulatory venous pressures) and the improved effectiveness of high-pressure, rapid-inflation devices,[44] it appears that patients would benefit from higher inflation pressures, short inflation time, and cycles of 2 to 3 minutes.

Conclusion

The 2008 ACCP guidelines have suggested new approaches for patients with iliofemoral DVT with their recommendations for a strategy of thrombus removal to avoid postthrombotic morbidity. The data supporting operative venous thrombectomy and catheter-based techniques were used to support such a recommendation. The committee also recognized the need for early therapeutic anticoagulation. Furthermore, they underscored the importance of long-term anticoagulation for patients with unprovoked DVT and for cancer patients who suffer DVT. Finally, the myth of bed rest was dispelled with their recommendations for early ambulation and the importance of good compression from the time of diagnosis and long-term treatment with 30 to 40 mm Hg ankle-gradient compression stockings were highlighted.

References

1. Kearon C, Kahn SR, Agnelli G, Goldhaber SZ, Raskob G, Comerota AJ. Antithrombotic therapy for venous thromboembolic disease: ACCP evidence-based clinical practice guidelines (8th ed). Chest. 2008;133(6):454S-545S.

2. Guyatt G, Gutterman D, Baumann MH, Addrizzo-Harris D, Hylek EM, Phillips B, et al. Grading strength of recommendations and quality of evidence in clinical guidelines: report from an American College of Chest Physicians task force. Chest. 2006;129(1):174-81.

3. Heit JA, Cohen AT, Anderson FA Jr, on behalf of the VTE Impact Assessment Group. Estimated annual number of incident and recurrent, non-fatal and fatal venous thromboembolism (VTE) events in the US. ASH Annual Meeting Abstracts 2005;106(11):910.

4. Strandness DE, Jr., Langlois Y, Cramer M, Randlett A, Thiele BL. Long-term sequelae of acute venous thrombosis. JAMA. 1983;250(10):1289-92.

5. Beyth RJ, Cohen AM, Landefeld CS. Long-term outcomes of deep-vein thrombosis. Arch Intern Med. 1995;155(10):1031-7.

6. Delis KT, Bountouroglou D, Mansfield AO. Venous claudication in iliofemoral thrombosis: long-term effects on venous hemodynamics, clinical status, and quality of life. Ann Surg. 2004;239(1):118-26.

7. Kahn SR, Hirsch A, Shrier I. Effect of postthrombotic syndrome on health-related quality of life after deep venous thrombosis. Arch Intern Med. 2002;162(10):1144-8.

8. Kahn SR, Kearon C, Julian JA, Mackinnon B, Kovacs MJ, Wells P, et al. Extended Low-intensity Anticoagulation for Thromboembolism (ELATE) Investigators. Predictors of the post-thrombotic syndrome during long-term treatment of proximal deep vein thrombosis. J Thromb Haemost. 2005;3(4):718-23.

9. O'Donnell TF, Browse NL, Burnand KG, Thomas ML. The socioeconomic effects of an iliofemoral venous thrombosis. J Surg Res. 1977;22(5):483-8.

10. Akesson H, Brudin L, Dahlstrom JA, Eklof B, Ohlin P, Plate G. Venous function assessed during a 5 year period after acute ilio-femoral venous thrombosis treated with anticoagulation. Eur J Vasc Surg. 1990;4(1):43-8.

11. Comerota AJ, Gravett MH. Iliofemoral venous thrombosis. J Vasc Surg. 2007;46(5):1065-76.

12. Buller HR, Agnelli G, Hull RD, Hyers TM, Prins MH, Raskob GE. Antithrombotic therapy for venous thromboembolic disease: the Seventh ACCP Conference on Antithrombotic and Thrombolytic Therapy. Chest. 2004;126(3 suppl):401S-28S.

13. Plate G, Einarsson E, Ohlin P, Jensen R, Qvarfordt P, Eklof B. Thrombectomy with temporary arteriovenous fistula: the treatment of choice in acute iliofemoral venous thrombosis. J Vasc Surg. 1984;1(6):867-76.

14. Plate G, Akesson H, Einarsson E, Ohlin P, Eklof B. Long-term results of venous thrombectomy combined with a temporary arterio-venous fistula. Eur J Vasc Surg. 1990;4(5):483-9.

15. Plate G, Eklof B, Norgren L, Ohlin P, Dahlstrom JA. Venous thrombectomy for iliofemoral vein thrombosis—10-year results of a prospective randomised study. Eur J Vasc Endovasc Surg. 1997;14(5):367-74.

16. Elsharawy M, Elzayat E. Early results of thrombolysis vs anticoagulation in

iliofemoral venous thrombosis. A randomised clinical trial. Eur J Vasc Endovasc Surg. 2002;24(3):209-14.

17. Bjarnason H, Kruse JR, Asinger DA, Nazarian GK, Dietz CA Jr, Caldwell MD, et al. Iliofemoral deep venous thrombosis: safety and efficacy outcome during 5 years of catheter-directed thrombolytic therapy. J Vasc Interv Radiol. 1997;8(3):405-18.

18. Comerota AJ, Kagan SA. Catheter-directed thrombolysis for the treatment of acute iliofemoral deep venous thrombosis. Phlebology. 2000;15:149-55.

19. Mewissen MW, Seabrook GR, Meissner MH, Cynamon J, Labropoulos N, Haughton SH. Catheter-directed thrombolysis for lower extremity deep venous thrombosis: report of a national multicenter registry. Radiology. 1999;211(1):39-49.

20. Comerota AJ, Throm RC, Mathias SD, Haughton S, Mewissen M. Catheter-directed thrombolysis for iliofemoral deep venous thrombosis improves health-related quality of life. J Vasc Surg. 2000;32(1): 130-7.

21. Martinez J, Comerota AJ, Kazanjian S, DiSalle RS, Sepanski DM, Assi Z. The quantitative benefit of isolated, segmental, pharmacomechanical thrombolysis for iliofemoral DVT. J Vasc Surg. 2008;48(6):1532-7.

22. Lin PH, Zhou W, Dardik A, Mussa F, Kougias P, Hedayati N, et al. Catheter-direct thrombolysis versus pharmacomechanical thrombectomy for treatment of symptomatic lower extremity deep venous thrombosis. Am J Surg. 2006;192(6):782-8.

23. Parikh S, Motarjeme A, McNamara T, Raabe R, Hagspiel K, Benenati JF, et al. Ultrasound-accelerated thrombolysis for the treatment of deep vein thrombosis: initial clinical experience. J Vasc Interv Radiol. 2008;19(4):521-8.

24. Brandjes DP, Heijboer H, Buller HR, de RM, Jagt H, ten Cate JW. Acenocoumarol and heparin compared with acenocoumarol alone in the initial treatment of proximal-vein thrombosis. N Engl J Med. 1992;327(21): 1485-9.

25. Hull RD, Raskob GE, Rosenbloom D, Panju AA, Brill-Edwards P, Ginsberg JS, et al. Heparin for 5 days as compared with 10 days in the initial treatment of proximal venous thrombosis. N Engl J Med. 1990;322(18): 1260-4.

26. Levine MN, Hirsh J, Gent M, Turpie AG, Weitz J, Ginsberg J, et al. Optimal duration of oral anticoagulant therapy: a randomized trial comparing four weeks with three months of warfarin in patients with proximal deep vein thrombosis. Thromb Haemost. 1995;74(2):606-11.

27. Schulman S, Rhedin AS, Lindmarker P, Carlsson A, Larfars G, Nicol P, et al. A comparison of six weeks with six months of oral anticoagulant therapy after a first episode of venous thromboembolism. Duration of Anticoagulation Trial Study Group. N Engl J Med. 1995;332(25):1661-5.

28. Kearon C, Gent M, Hirsh J, Weitz J, Kovacs MJ, Anderson DR, et al. A comparison of three months of anticoagulation with extended anticoagulation for a first episode of idiopathic venous thromboembolism. N Engl J Med. 1999;340(12):901-7.

29. Ridker PM, Goldhaber SZ, Danielson E, Rosenberg Y, Eby CS, Deitcher SR, et al. PREVENT Investigators. Long-term, low-intensity warfarin therapy for the prevention of recurrent venous thromboembolism. N Engl J Med. 2003;348(15):1425-34.

30. Kearon C, Ginsberg JS, Kovacs MJ, Anderson DR, Wells P, Julian JA, et al. Extended Low-Intensity Anticoagulation for Thrombo-Embolism Investigators. Comparison of low-intensity warfarin

therapy with conventional-intensity warfarin therapy for long-term prevention of recurrent venous thromboembolism. N Engl J Med. 2003;349(7):631-9.

31. Schulman S, Granqvist S, Holmstrom M, Carlsson A, Lindmarker P, Nicol P, et al. The duration of oral anticoagulant therapy after a second episode of venous thromboembolism. The Duration of Anticoagulation Trial Study Group. N Engl J Med. 1997;336(6):393-8.

32. Aschwanden M, Labs KH, Engel H, Schwob A, Jeanneret C, et al. Acute deep vein thrombosis: early mobilization does not increase the frequency of pulmonary embolism. Thromb Haemost. 2001;85(1):42-6.

33. Blattler W, Partsch H. Leg compression and ambulation is better than bed rest for the treatment of acute deep venous thrombosis. Int Angiol. 2003;22(4):393-400.

34. Junger M, Diehm C, Storiko H, Hach-Wunderle V, Heidrich H, Karasch T, et al. Mobilization versus immobilization in the treatment of acute proximal deep venous thrombosis: a prospective, randomized, open, multicentre trial. Curr Med Res Opin. 2006;22(3):593-602.

35. Partsch H, Blattler W. Compression and walking versus bed rest in the treatment of proximal deep venous thrombosis with low molecular weight heparin. J Vasc Surg. 2000;32(5):861-9.

36. Schellong SM, Schwarz T, Kropp J, Prescher Y, Beuthien-Baumann B, Daniel WG. Bed rest in deep vein thrombosis and the incidence of scintigraphic pulmonary embolism. Thromb Haemost. 1999;82 suppl 1:127-9.

37. Partsch H. Immediate ambulation and leg compression in the treatment of deep vein thrombosis. Dis Mon. 2005;51(2-3):135-40.

38. Brandjes DP, Buller HR, Heijboer H, Huisman MV, de Rijk M, Jagt H, et al. Randomised trial of effect of compression stockings in patients with symptomatic proximal-vein thrombosis. Lancet. 1997;349(9054):759-62.

39. Prandoni P, Lensing AW, Prins MH, Frulla M, Marchiori A, Bernardi E, et al. Below-knee elastic compression stockings to prevent the post-thrombotic syndrome: a randomized, controlled trial. Ann Intern Med. 2004;141(4):249-56.

40. Kolbach DN, Sandbrink MW, Hamulyak K, Neumann HA, Prins MH. Non-pharmacological measures for prevention of post-thrombotic syndrome. Cochrane Database Syst Rev. 2004;(1):CD004174.

41. Ginsberg JS, Magier D, Mackinnon B, Gent M, Hirsh J. Intermittent compression units for severe post-phlebitic syndrome: a randomized crossover study. CMAJ. 1999;160(9):1303-6.

42. Smith PC, Sarin S, Hasty J, Scurr JH. Sequential gradient pneumatic compression enhances venous ulcer healing: a randomized trial. Surgery. 1990;108(5):871-5.

43. Kumar S, Samraj K, Nirujogi V, Budnik J, Walker MA. Intermittent pneumatic compression as an adjuvant therapy in venous ulcer disease. J Tissue Viability. 2002;12(2): 42-4, 46, 48.

44. Malone MD, Cisek PL, Comerota AJ, Jr., Holland B, Eid IG, Comerota AJ. High-pressure, rapid-inflation pneumatic compression improves venous hemodynamics in healthy volunteers and patients who are post-thrombotic. J Vasc Surg. 1999;29(4):593-9.

Anticoagulation Therapy

Ruth L. Bush, Brandi Huf, and CleAnn Toner

The main aim of venous thromboembolism (VTE) therapy is to prevent extension of thrombosis and embolization to the lungs. Other long-term goals include reduction in the incidence of recurrent VTE, prevention of postthrombotic syndrome, and avoidance of pulmonary hypertension.[1] Anticoagulants have been the mainstay of VTE therapy since Barritt and Jordan demonstrated the efficacy of heparin and warfarin in reducing morbidity and mortality in patients with acute PE.[2] Since then, a vast array of drugs have emerged, including low-molecular-weight heparin (LMWH), direct thrombin inhibitors, and factor Xa inhibitors.

When looking at agents for anticoagulation, an understanding of the coagulation cascade needs to be achieved. There are 2 pathways of the coagulation cascade: the contact activation pathway (intrinsic pathway) and the tissue factor pathway (extrinsic pathway).[3] These 2 pathways meet to form the final common pathway. Of the 2 initial pathways, the tissue factor pathway is the primary pathway. Figure 6.1 gives a simplified diagram of the coagulation cascade and the site of action of the most commonly used commercially available anticoagulant drugs.

Oral Agents

Vitamin K Antagonist—Warfarin

While there are many ongoing studies to find a new anticoagulant medication, warfarin remains the only oral anticoagulant available on the market in the United States. Indications for warfarin include VTE (deep venous thrombosis and pulmonary embolism), atrial fibrillation, mechanical and

Venous Thromboembolic Disease. Contemporary Endovascular Management series. © 2011 Mark G. Davies MD and Alan B. Lumsden MD, eds. Cardiotext Publishing, ISBN 978-1-935395-22-5.

Available Anticoagulants

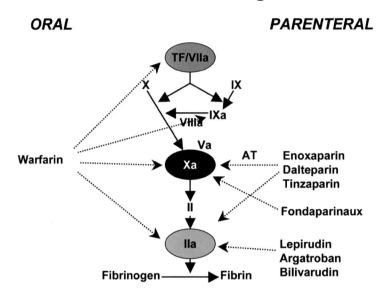

FIGURE 6.1   The coagulation cascade and available anticoagulants. Adapted from Weitz JI, Bates SM. New anticoagulants. J Thromb Haemost. 2005;3:1843-1853. Used with permission.

bioprosthetic heart valve replacement, myocardial infarction (MI), and hypercoagulable conditions.[4]

Vitamin K antagonists (VKAs) exert their anticoagulation effect by inhibiting the enzyme vitamin K oxide reductase, blocking the conversion of vitamin K epoxide to vitamin K. This inhibits the carboxylation and activation of the vitamin K–dependent coagulation factors II, VII, IX, and X, and proteins C and S.[5] Warfarin is a racemic mixture of 2 active isomers, the R and S enantiomers. Of the 2 enantiomers, the S enantiomer is 2.7 to 3.8 times more potent than the R enantiomer. The S enantiomer is metabolized by the CYP2C9 enzyme of the cytochrome P450 system, whereas the R enantiomer is metabolized by CYP 1A2 and 3A4.[5] Therefore, medications that are metabolized through the CYP2C9 enzyme

are more likely to affect the metabolism of warfarin, including amiodarone, azole antifungals, Flagyl, and Bactrim.

Patients should be advised to monitor their diet when initiating warfarin due to the adverse affect it can have on the patient's therapy. Stressing a diet consistent in vitamin K foods can have a considerable impact on stabilizing patients early on in their therapy. See Figure 6.2 for a list of vitamin K foods divided into low, moderate, and high vitamin K content. In our facility, we watch closely for changes in consumption of dark leafy green vegetables, green tea, nutritional supplements, and multivitamin use. On the other side of the spectrum, 2 foods we advise patients to stay away from are cranberries and grapefruit, along with their juices. Grapefruit can inhibit warfarin metabolism, and the mechanism behind the interaction

Vitamin K Content of Selected Foods vers 12/08

It is important to be consistent with your regular dietary Vitamin K intake to avoid fluctuations in your INR. This list provides information on the vitamin K content of certain foods, and it may be helpful in making consistent dietary decisions.

LOW (<50 mcg)	Moderate (50-100mcg)	High (>100mcg)
Vegetables Alfalfa sprouts ($1^1/_2$ cup) Artichoke (1 medium; 1 cup) Beans, green (2 cup) Beans, lima, kidney (>2 cup) Beans, navy (>2 cups) Beans, yellow (2 cup) Beats (>2 cups) Carrots (2 cup) Cauliflower (2 cup) Celery ($2^1/_2$ sticks) Corn ($^2/_3$ cup) Cucumber (2 cup) Egg plant ($1^1/_4$ cup) Garbanzo beans ($^1/_2$ cup) Mushrooms ($1^1/_2$ cup) Okra ($^1/_2$ cup) Onion Peas, blackeyed (1 cup) Peas, green (1 cup) Pepper, green ($^1/_2$ cup) Potato , Pumpkin Sauerkraut ($^1/_3$ cup) Soybeans ($^3/_4$ cup) Tomato, green ($^1/_2$ cup) Tomato, red ($^3/_4$ cup)	Asparagus (7-12 spears) Avocado ($^1/_2$ cup) Cabbage (1 cup) Peas, green ($1^1/_2$ cup) Lettuce (iceberg – ½ head) Pickle, dill (1 medium)	Beet greens ($^1/_4$ cup) Broccoli ($^1/_2$ cup) Brussels sprouts ($^1/_2$ cup) Cabbage ($^3/_4$ cup) Collard greens ($^1/_8$ cup) Endive (1 cup) Green Scallions ($^1/_2$ cup) Kale ($^1/_8$ cup) Mustard greens (1 cup) Parsley ($^1/_2$ cup) Spinach ($^1/_4$ cup) Swiss chard ($^1/_4$ cup) Turnip greens ($^1/_4$ cup) Watercress (raw chopped) – $1^1/_4$ cup
Fruits Apple, Apricot, Banana, Blueberries (<1 cup) Cantaloupe, Grapefruit, Lemon, Orange, Peach, Pear, Plum, Pineapple	Grapes ($2^1/_2$cups)	
Meats Beef, Chicken, Ham, Mackerel Pork, Shrimp, Turkey	Tuna (> 4oz)	
Fats and Oils Canola oil (< 3 Tbspn) Olive oil (< 6 Tbspn) Corn oil, Peanut oil, Safflower oil, Sesame oil, Sunflower oil (all < 7 Tbspn)	Margarine (4 Tbspn) Mayonnaise (>10 Tbspn) Soybean oil (2-4 Tbspn)	Canola oil (>6 Tbspn)
Dairy products Butter ,Cheese, Eggs, Sour cream Yogurt		
Beverages Coffee, Cola, Fruit juices, Milk, Tea (black)		Tea (green): Brewing green tea may alters vitamin K content
Grains, breads Bagel, Breads, Cereal, Flour, Oatmeal, Rice, Spaghetti		
Misc. Honey, Jell-O Gelatin Peanut butter, Sugar, Tofu		

FIGURE 6.2   Vitamin K foods. Adapted from USDA National Nutrient Database, http://www.nal.usda.gov/fnic /foodcomp/Data/SR17/wtrank/sr17a430.pdf.

with cranberries is largely unknown; however, it is thought to also be involved in metabolism.

Contraindications to using this medication are typically based on risk vs. benefit. If the beneficial use of warfarin is outweighed by a higher risk of bleeding, the patient cannot be placed on warfarin. Disease states and processes included in this consideration are certain blood disorders, active bleeding, any disorder causing the patient to be more prone to bleed, and malignant hypertension. If a patient cannot be properly monitored due to personal/psychological issues or noncompliance, it is more often than not safer for the patient to be taken off warfarin. As with all medications, if the patient develops an allergic reaction to warfarin, other options regarding anticoagulation will need to be evaluated. Warfarin is teratogenic and cannot be used during pregnancy. When a patient already on warfarin is scheduled for any type of surgery or procedure where there is a high risk of bleeding, the patient will need to hold warfarin for a sufficient period of time prior to the procedure with or without an alternative anticoagulant.[4]

Warfarin dosing is highly individualized and must take into account comorbid disease states. The recommended initiation dose for warfarin is 5 mg, which was shown to achieve therapeutic INR as fast as the 10-mg loading dose.[6] This was contested in an outpatient study that demonstrated faster achievement of target INR with a 10-mg loading dose.[7] However, the study also demonstrated increased rates of bleeding associated with the higher loading dose. A lower starting dose of 2 to 3 mg daily may be used in patients with disease states or illnesses causing an increased response to warfarin, including the elderly population.[5,8] Table 6.1 is an example of a warfarin dose adjustment protocol used in our facility for initiation of warfarin.[9]

In patients at high risk for developing another event and in need of immediate anticoagulation, heparin/LMWH is used alongside warfarin for at least 4 to 5 days and pending 2 therapeutic INR levels. The therapeutic INR range for most indications continues to be 2.0 to 3.0 (target 2.5) and for high-risk mechanical valves 2.5 to 3.5 (target 3.0).[5,10,11]

Monitoring is usually done within the first few days of therapy initiation and then is spaced out depending on the patient's response and stabilization of warfarin. If a patient develops a sub/supratherapeutic INR due to diet, noncompliance, interacting medication, hold for surgery, or for any other reason, it is prudent to monitor more closely and restart the cycle of monitoring. A patient should never go more than 4 weeks without having an INR drawn.[5] Dose adjustment protocols vary depending on the institution.[12,13]

Parenteral Anticoagulants

Heparins

First discovered in 1916, unfractionated heparin (UFH) exerts its anticoagulant effect by binding to antithrombin.[14] The resulting heparin-antithrombin complex inhibits the activity of factor Xa and thrombin. Only one-third of the molecules of UFH have the required sequence for binding to antithrombin.[15] UFH also contains molecules that bind to other plasma proteins that are present in variable amounts in each individual. Thus, UFH has an unpredictable effect in different people.[16] UFH is metabolized by the liver and has side effects of bleeding, heparin-induced thrombocytopenia (HIT), and osteoporosis.[16] The dosing of UFH is based on 1 of 2 schedules and

TABLE 6.1   **Warfarin Initial Dosing Protocol**

INR	Day 1	Day 2	Day 3	Day 4	Day 5
<1.5	5.0 mg	5.0 mg	7.5 mg	10.0 mg	10.0 mg
1.5–1.99	2.5 mg	2.5 mg	5.0 mg	7.5 mg	7.5 mg
2.0–2.49		1.0 mg	2.5 mg	5.0 mg	5.0 mg
2.5–2.9		0.0 mg	1.0 mg	2.5 mg	2.5 mg
3.0–3.5		0.0 mg	0.0 mg	1.0 mg	1.0 mg
>3.5		0.0 mg	0.0 mg	0.0 mg	0.0 mg

requires intravenous administration and frequent monitoring of the aPTT, or activated partial thromboplastin time, to ensure that a steady therapeutic level of anticoagulation is achieved.

Heparin is indicated in venous and/or arterial thromboembolism for both prevention and treatment. Other indications include disseminated intravascular coagulation and surgeries that carry a high risk of clotting, as well as procedures or laboratory tests requiring anticoagulation. Contraindications to using this medication include thrombocytopenia, heparin-induced thrombocytopenia, and bleeding.[17] Heparin can be given a few different ways when beginning treatment. When used to treat venous thromboembolism (VTE), for example, different routes and dosing administration can be used (Table 6.2).

The activity of heparin is measured by the degree of inhibition of activated factor X (Xa), which can be monitored using the aPTT, with a therapeutic range being 1.5 to 2.5 times the normal (or 0.3–0.7 anti-factor Xa units/mL).[22,23] As with warfarin, the dose of heparin is adjusted based on the institution's nomogram or dose adjustment protocol. The therapeutic aPTT is dependent on the reagent used during testing, as they do vary.[24]

Fractionated heparin, also known as low-molecular-weight heparin (LMWH), is formed by enzymatic cleavage of UFH. LMWH retains the ability to inhibit factor Xa and thrombin, but its smaller size decreases nonspecific binding to other plasma proteins. Compared to UFH, LMWH has increased bioavailability, a longer half-life, and a more predictable dose response. In addition, LMWH is associated with a lower incidence of heparin-induced thrombocytopenia (HIT), potentially lower risk of bleeding, and lower risk of osteoporosis.[16] It has a dose- dependent renal clearance, which needs to be taken into consideration in patients with renal insufficiency. Other considerations include dosing difficulties in obese patients and problems with reversibility in cases of bleeding. There are currently 8 LMWHs available in the market, each with its own molecular weight and dosing regimen. There is insufficient evidence to differentiate among these LMWHs based on efficacy and safety.[16] LMWHs do not require monitoring to ensure therapeutic anticoagulation. The utility of anti-factor Xa assay is controversial, since its correlation with anticoagulant effect and bleeding risk is unclear.[25]

Early studies demonstrated that LMWH had better efficacy and safety when

TABLE 6.2   **Heparin Dosing**

Route	Weight-Based	Non-Weight-Based
IV	80 units/kg bolus + 18 units/kg/h infusion[18]	5,000 units bolus + 32,000 units/day infusion[19]
SQ	333 units/kg bolus + 250 units/kg twice daily[20]	5,000 units bolus + the weight-based daily dose[21]

compared to UFH, particularly for reducing mortality at 3- to 6- month follow-up.[26] The more recent evidence has shown a lower magnitude of benefit of LMWH over UFH.[27] The majority of the evidence is with respect to therapy of DVT, rather than PE. However, a 2004 meta-analysis provided convincing evidence that LMWH is safe and efficacious in patients with noncritical PE.[28] Cost-effectiveness analyses have shown a benefit or at least equivalency for LMWH in comparison to UFH regardless of treatment setting.[29]

The low-molecular-weight heparins available in the United States are enoxaparin (Lovenox), dalteparin (Fragmin), and tinzaparin (Innohep). Since their FDA indications vary, they will be listed separately. Enoxaparin is indicated in the prophylaxis of venous thromboembolism, as well as in the treatment of venous thromboembolism and ST segment elevation myocardial infarction. The medication is also used in patients with unstable angina and non-Q-wave MI for prevention of ischemic embolisms during treatment of these disease states.[30] Dalteparin is not indicated in the treatment of venous thromboembolism unless the patient has cancer and a history of blood clots; however, it can be used for prophylaxis similar to enoxaparin.[31] Tinzaparin is indicated only for therapy in patients with venous thromboembolism.[32]

Contraindications to using LMWHs as a class include hemorrhage, heparin-induced thrombocytopenia when regional anesthesia is needed,[31] and allergies to the drug, heparin, or pork.[30-32] If a patient is allergic to sulfites or benzyl alcohol, tinzaparin therapy is contraindicated.[32]

Enoxaparin is used most often in the hospital setting, and dosing is listed here. For specific dosing on dalteparin and tinzaparin, please refer to their package insert.[31-32] Treatment dosing for enoxaparin is 1 mg/kg twice daily or 1.5 mg/kg daily. In patients with creatinine clearance (CrCl) of less than or equal to 30 mL/min, dosing is decreased to 1 mg/kg daily. Prophylactic dosing for surgeries is normally 40 mg daily or 30 mg twice daily. In renal dysfunction, the dose is decreased to 30 mg daily.[30]

Low-molecular-weight heparin monitoring is usually not performed; however, high-risk patients can be monitored using anti-factor Xa levels. High-risk patients include those who have received heparin within the past 6 months and women who are pregnant.[22]

Fondaparinux is an indirect factor Xa inhibitor. It has a linear pharmacokinetic profile, allowing for weight-based daily dosing and negating the need for continuous monitoring.[33] It does not bind to platelet factor 4 and theoretically does not cause thrombocytopenia, and it has renal clearance. In 2 large, multicenter clinical trials, fondaparinux was as effective and safe as UFH for the treatment of PE, and as effective and safe as enoxaparin for the treatment of DVT.[34,35] The drug is also used for prophylaxis of venous thromboembolism and is contraindicated in patients with CrCl <30 mL/min, hemorrhage, bacterial endocarditis, thrombocytopenia, and allergy to the drug itself, and for prophylaxis in patients weighing less than 50 kg.[36] Fondaparinux is dosed based on body weight for treatment and at a fixed dose for prophylaxis (Table 6.3).

As with LMWHs, fondaparinux is customarily not monitored.[22]

Direct Thrombin Inhibitors

Direct thrombin inhibitors also have the advantages of predictable dose response and reduced incidence of thrombocytopenia. However, they do not have an antidote for cases of severe bleeding. Argatroban and lepirudin are 2 intravenous direct thrombin inhibitors that are FDA approved for the prevention and/or treatment of VTE in patients with heparin-induced thrombocytopenia.[33] Ximelagatran is an oral direct thrombin inhibitor that has been withdrawn from the market because of an increased risk of hepatic toxicity.

These medications bind directly to thrombin to inhibit the activation of fibrin. Lepirudin and argatroban are indicated for patients with HIT.[37,38] Bivalirudin is indicated for patients undergoing percutaneous transluminal coronary angioplasty (PTCA) who have unstable angina.[39] Contraindications to the direct thrombin inhibitors include hypersensitivity to the products[37-39] and major bleeding.[38,39] Antidotes are not available for the direct thrombin inhibitors.[10]

Lepirudin is dosed 0.4 mg/kg body weight (up to 110 kg) IV as a bolus dose, then 0.15 mg/kg body weight/h IV continuous infusion for 2 to 10 days.[37] If a patient's body weight exceeds 110 kg, the maximum

Table 6.3 **Fondaparinux Dosing**

	Weight (kg)	Dose (mg)
Prophylaxis	2.5 mg	2.5
Treatment	<50 kg	5.0
	50–100 kg	7.5
	>100 kg	10.0

initial dose should be 44 kg, and the maximum infusion dose should be 16.5 mg/h.[37] The dose of lepirudin does need to be renally adjusted starting at a CrCl of 60 mL/min.[37] Monitoring of lepirudin is done with the aPTT. A baseline value should be obtained, and lepirudin should not be started if the baseline aPTT is more than 2.5 times the normal aPTT control.[37] Target range for aPTT during lepirudin treatment should be 1.5 to 2.5 times the normal aPTT control, with the value taken 4 hours after the initial dose of lepirudin.[37]

Argatroban is dosed initially at 2 mcg/kg/min, as a continuous infusion. The dose may be adjusted up to 10 mcg/kg/min to an aPTT of 1.5 to 3 times the baseline.[38] The aPTT levels need to be drawn 1 to 3 hours after the dose is given. No dosage adjustment is necessary in renal impairment. However, adjustments are needed in hepatic impairment to 0.5 mcg/kg/min as an initial dose, and then adjusted according to the aPTT.[38]

Initial dose of bivalirudin is an IV bolus of 0.75 mg/kg, followed with an infusion of 1.75 mg/kg/h during the PTCA.[39] An activated clotting time (ACT) should be drawn 5 minutes after the bolus, and an extra 0.3 mg/kg should be given to achieve the target ACT of 300 to 350 seconds if needed. Dose adjustments are necessary in renal impairment. In patients with CrCl of 30 to 59 mL/min, the infusion rate should be 1.75 mg/kg/h; CrCl less than 30 mL/min, reduce rate to 1 mg/kg/h.[39]

New Anticoagulants

Current medications on the market for anticoagulation have many drawbacks. Vitamin K antagonists require intensive monitoring and have multiple drug interactions. Heparin usually requires admission to the hospital, it is administered parenterally, and there is the possibility for the development of heparin-induced thrombocytopenia. Low-molecular-weight heparins are also parenterally administered, have the potential for developing HIT, and cost considerably more than the other alternatives. Several new medications are being

researched to attempt to alleviate some of the current drawbacks.

When looking at developing agents for anticoagulation, another look to the coagulation cascade provides a graphical understanding of their mechanism of action (Figure 6.3).

As mentioned at the beginning of the chapter, there are 2 pathways of the coagulation cascade: the contact activation pathway and the tissue factor pathway.[3] These 2 pathways meet to form the final common pathway. The first step in this pathway to initiate coagulation is the binding of tissue factor to factor VII, which activates factor VIIa/tissue factor complex. New agents that are being studied target this step to inhibit the initiation of coagulation, including Tifacogin and NAPc2, which are both parenteral medica-

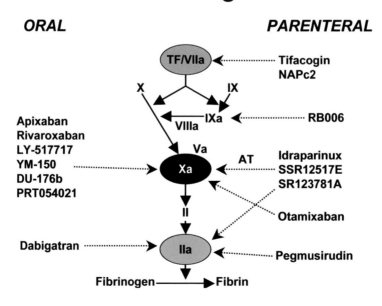

FIGURE 6.3 New anticoagulants. Adapted from Weitz JI, Bates SM. New anticoagulants. J Thromb Haemost. 2005;3:1843-1853. Used with permission.

tions.[10] The propagation step of the coagulation cascade is where the final common pathway begins at factor Xa.[3] With inhibition of factor Xa, propagation is terminated. This can be done indirectly by binding to the plasma cofactors (antithrombin) or directly by binding directly to the enzyme. This can also be achieved by inhibiting factor IXa, thus preventing the activation of X to Xa. The indirect factor Xa inhibitors in development include idraparinux, SSR12517E, and SR123781A, all of which are parenteral.[10] The direct factor Xa inhibitors still under development are otamixaban, apixaban, rivaroxaban, LY-517717, YM-150, DU-176b, and PRT054021.[10] Of these, otamixaban is parenteral, and the rest are oral medications. The only factor IXa inhibitor under development is RB006, which is IV administration. Another target in the coagulation cascade is the final step, the formation of fibrin. Thrombin converts fibrinogen to fibrin and activates platelets.[3] By inhibiting thrombin, the final step of the coagulation cascade is terminated. Again, this inhibition can be done indirectly or directly. The indirect thrombin inhibitors act on the heparin cofactor II. There was an oral indirect thrombin inhibitor in development, odiparcil.[10] However, its development was stopped at phase II. Of the direct thrombin inhibitors being developed, 2 are parenteral: flovagatran and pegmusirudin.[10] The other is oral, dabigatran etexilate.[10] Factor Va is activated by thrombin, which then helps convert more prothrombin into thrombin. Activated protein C degrades factor Va to act as a natural anticoagulant.[3] Two of the new medications being developed act on factor Va. Drotrecogin alfa is a recombinant form of activated protein C, which will degrade factor Va, and ART-123 converts thrombin into an activator of protein C.[10]

References

1. McRae S, Ginsberg J. Initial treatment of venous thromboembolism. Circulation. 2004;110(9 suppl 1):I3-9.

2. Barritt DW, Jordan SC. Anticoagulant drugs in the treatment of pulmonary embolism: a controlled trial. Lancet. 1960;1:1309-12.

3. Haines ST, Zeolla M, Witt DM. Venous thromboembolism. In: DiPiro JT, Talbert RL, Yee GC, Matzke GR, Wells BG, Posey LM, eds. Pharmacotherapy: A Pathophysiologic Approach. 6th ed. New York: McGraw-Hill/ Appleton and Lange; 2005. p373-413.

4. Coumadin [package insert]. Princeton, NJ: Bristol-Myers Squibb Company; 2009. http:// packageinserts.bms.com/pi/pi_coumadin.pdf.

5. Ansell J, Hirsh J, Hylek E, Jacobson A, Crowther M, Palareti G; American College of Chest Physicians. Pharmacology and management of the vitamin K antagonists. Chest. 2008;133:160S-98S.

6. Crowther MA, Ginsberg JB, Kearon C, Harrison L, Johnson J, Massicotte MP, et al. A randomized trial comparing 5-mg and 10-mg warfarin loading doses. Arch Intern Med. 1999;159:46-8.

7. Kovacs MJ, Rodger M, Anderson DR, Morrow B, Kells G, Kovacs J, et al. Comparison of 10-mg and 5-mg warfarin initiation nomograms together with low-molecular-weight heparin for outpatient treatment of acute venous thromboembolism. A randomized, double-blind, controlled trial. Ann Intern Med. 2003;138:714-9.

8. Garcia D, Regan S, Crowther M, Hughes RA, Hylek EM. Warfarin maintenance dosing patterns in clinical practice. Chest. 2005;127;2049-56.

9. Scott and White Healthcare Anticoagulation Guidelines 2009-2010.

10. Antithrombotic and thrombolytic therapy: American College of Chest Physicians Evidenced-Based Clinical Practice Guidelines, 8th ed. Chest. 2008;133(6):67S-968S.

11. Kearon C, Kahn SR, Agnelli G, Goldhaber S, Raskob GE, Comerota AJ; American College of Chest Physicians. Antithrombotic therapy for venous thromboembolic disease: the eighth ACCP conference on antithrombotic and thrombolytic therapy. Chest. 2008;133:454S–545S.

12. Ebell M. A systematic approach to managing warfarin doses. Family Practice Management. 2005:77-83. http://www.aafp.org/fpm /20050500/77asys.html.

13. Franke CA, Dickerson LM, Carek PJ. Improving anticoagulation therapy using point-of-care testing and a standardized protocol. Ann Fam Med. 2008;6 suppl 1:S28-32.

14. McLean J. The thromboplastic action of cephalin. Am J Physiol. 1916;41:250-7.

15. Choay J, Lormeau JC, Petitou M, Sinaÿ P, Fareed J. Structural studies on a biologically active hexasaccharide obtained from heparin. Ann NY Acad Sci. 1981;370:644-9.

16. McRae S, Ginsberg J. Initial treatment of venous thromboembolism. Circulation. 2004; (9 suppl 1):I3-9.

17. Heparin Sodium Injections [package insert]. Schaumburg, IL: APP Pharmaceuticals, LLC, 2008. http://www.apppharma.com /our-products/alphabetical/product-55.html.

18. Raschke RA, Reilly BM, Guidry JR, Fontana JR, Srinivas S. The weight-based heparin dosing nomogram compared with a "standard care" nomogram. A randomized controlled trial. Ann Intern Med. 1993;119(9):874-81.

19. Cruickshank MK, Levine MN, Hirsh J, Roberts R, Siguenza M. A standard heparin nomogram for the management of heparin therapy. Arch Intern Med. 1991;151(2):333-7.

20. Kearon C, Ginsberg JS, Julian JA, Douketis J, Solymoss S, Ockelford P, et al; Fixed-Dose Heparin (FIDO) Investigators. Comparison of fixed-dose weight-adjusted unfractionated heparin and low-molecular-weight heparin for acute treatment of venous thromboembolism. JAMA. 2006;296(8):935-42.

21. Prandoni P, Carnovali M, Marchiori A; Galilei Investigators. Subcutaneous adjusted-dose unfractionated heparin vs fixed-dose low-molecular-weight heparin in the initial treatment of venous thromboembolism. Arch Intern Med. 2004;164(10):1077-83.

22. Hirsh J, Bauer KA, Donati MB, Gould M, Samama MM, Weitz JI; American College of Chest Physicians. Parenteral anticoagulants: American College of Chest Physicians Evidence-Based Clinical Practice Guidelines (8th ed.). Chest. 2008;133(6 suppl): 141S-59S.

23. Basu D, Gallus A, Hirsh J, Cade J. A prospective study of the value of monitoring heparin treatment with the activated partial thromboplastin time. N Engl J Med. 1972;287(7):324-7.

24. Brill-Edwards P, Ginsberg JS, Johnston M, Hirsh J. Establishing a therapeutic range for heparin therapy. Ann Intern Med. 1993;119(2):104-9.

25. Bounameaux H, de Moerloose P. Is laboratory monitoring of low-molecular-weight heparin therapy necessary? No. J Thromb Haemost. 2004;2:551-4.

26. The Columbus Investigators. Low-molecular-weight heparin in the treatment of patients with venous thromboembolism. N Engl J Med. 1997;337:657-62.

27. Mismetti P, Quenet S, Levine M, Merli G, Decousus H, Derobert E, et al. Enoxaparin in the treatment of deep vein thrombosis with or without pulmonary embolism: an individual patient data meta-analysis. Chest. 2005;128:2203-10.

28. Quinlan DJ, Mcquillan A, Eikelboom JW. Low-molecular-weight heparin compared with intravenous unfractionated heparin for treatment of pulmonary embolism: a meta-analysis of randomized, controlled trials. Ann Intern Med. 2004;140:175-83.

29. O'Brien JA, Caro JJ. Direct medical cost of managing deep vein thrombosis according

to the occurrence of complications. Pharmacoeconomics. 2002;20:603-15.

30. Lovenox [package insert]. Greenville, NC: Sanofi-Aventis U.S. LLC, 2008. http://products.sanofi-aventis.us/lovenox/lovenox.html.

31. Fragmin [package insert]. New York, NY: Pfizer Inc, 2007. http://www.eisai.com/package_inserts/Fragmin_PI.pdf.

32. Innohep [package insert]. Summit, NJ: Leo Pharma A/S, 2008.

33. Prandoni P, Lensing AW, Pesavento R. New strategies for the treatment of acute venous thromboembolism. Semin Thromb Hemost. 2006;32(8):787-92.

34. The Matisse Investigators. Subcutaneous fondaparinux versus intravenous unfractionated heparin in the initial treatment of pulmonary embolism. N Engl J Med. 2003;349:1695-702.

35. Buller HR, Davidson BL, Decousus H, Gallus A, Gent M, Piovella F, et al; Matisse Investigators. Fondaparinux or enoxaparin for the initial treatment of symptomatic deep vein thrombosis. Ann Intern Med. 2004;140:867-73.

36. Arixtra [package insert]. Research Triangle Park, NC: GlaxoSmithKline, 2008. http://us.gsk.com/products/assets/us_arixtra.pdf.

37. Refludan [package insert.] Montville, NJ: Berlex, 2004. http://www.bayer.ca/files/REFLUDAN-PM-ENG-29MAY2007-113596.pdf?#.

38. Argatroban [package insert]. Research Triangle Park, NC: GlaxoSmithKline, 2009. http://us.gsk.com/products/assets/us_argatroban.pdf.

39. Angiomax [package insert]. Bedford, OH: BenVenue Laboratories, 2005. http://www.angiomax.com/Files/SalesAidRef/PI.pdf.

Pharmacological Thrombolysis
Indications, Techniques, and Outcomes

Mark G. Davies

Current therapy for extensive deep venous thrombosis (DVT) in both the upper and lower extremities is evolving into a more aggressive lytic-based approach with the goal of rapid clearance of thrombus burden. Lytic therapy can now be achieved by catheter-directed lysis, ultrasound-assisted catheter-directed lysis, mechanical thrombectomy, and pharmacomechanical lysis (power-pulse spray). The single common element in these techniques is a thrombolytic agent. This chapter is focused on thrombolysis and its outcomes in DVT and will complement the subsequent chapters on mechanical thrombolysis, power-pulse spray, and ultrasound-assisted lysis.

Venous Thromboembolic Disease. Contemporary Endovascular Management series. © 2011 Mark G. Davies MD and Alan B. Lumsden MD, eds. Cardiotext Publishing, ISBN 978-1-935395-22-5.

Physiology

"Fibrinolysis" refers to the dissolution of the fibrin network that forms the supporting latticework of a thrombus. Formation of fibrin is a stimulus for activation of fibrinolysis. Plasminogen must be converted to plasmin for fibrinolysis to occur.[1] Plasminogen (glu-plasminogen) binds to endothelial cells and is converted to a form (lys-plasminogen) that is more efficiently activated. Plasmin degrades cross-linked fibrin, non-cross-linked fibrin, and fibrinogen. Degradation of non-cross-linked fibrin and fibrinogen results in the production of fibrin degradation products A, B, D, and E. Degradation of cross-linked fibrin is slower because of the presence of cross-linkages, which results in noncovalently bound fragments (DD and EE, the D-dimers). These latter fragments of fibrin can be considered markers of true fibrin degradation. Endothelial cells synthesize the plasminogen activators as single-chain proteins and then secrete them. These single-chain proteins then assemble into functional complexes and act as serine proteases. There are 2 forms of plasminogen activators (PA): the urokinase type (uPA), which activates plasminogen in the fluid phase, and tissue PA (tPA), which is most active when bound to fibrin.[2,3] Normal endothelial cells express tPA. However, if stimulated by a variety of cytokines and other factors, they preferentially synthesize uPA and down-regulate tPA synthesis. In addition to these 2 fibrinolytic enzymes, endothelial cells also secrete 2 PA inhibitors, PAI-1 and PAI-2. Both are serine protease inhibitors and form equimolar complexes with active uPA or tPA molecules. PAI-1 requires the presence of vitronectin in the extracellular matrix to maintain its active conformation and is therefore inactive outside the matrix. The thrombin-thrombomodulin pathway also is involved in the regulation of fibrinolysis. Thrombin activatable fibrinolysis inhibitor (TAFI), a carboxypeptidase, is a plasma protein that is a substrate, like protein C, for the thrombin thrombomodulin complex. $TAFI_a$ suppresses glu-plasminogen but not lys-plasminogen activation by tPA in the presence of a fibrin analogue that had been exposed to plasmin (clotted fragment X). Through the activation of protein C and TAFI, the thrombin/thrombomodulin complexes can down-regulate coagulation and fibrinolysis. The general schema of fibrinolysis is shown in Figure 7.1. Bleeding, the most serious complication of thrombolytic therapy with tissue-type plasminogen activator (tPA), is thought to result from lysis of fibrin in hemostatic plugs and from the systemic lytic state caused by unopposed plasmin. One mechanism by which systemic plasmin can impair hemostasis is by partially degrading fibrinogen to fragment X, a high-molecular-weight clottable fibrinogen degradation product,

which retains clottability but forms clots with reduced tensile strength that stimulate plasminogen activation by tPA more than fibrin clots.[4] It accumulates after treatment with tPA but not with tPA given with α_2 antiplasmin. It does not accumulate with use of more fibrin-specific agents.[5]

Pharmacology

Thrombolysis is the pharmacological dissolution of fibrin thrombus by exogenously delivered agents. The characteristics of these agents are shown in Table 7.1. These agents form plasmin, which leads to the degradation of fibrin, fibrinogen, factor V, and factor VII. Plasminogen is found free in the circulation and within the thrombus, which allows for activation of plasmin within a thrombus by regional perfusion. Streptokinase binds plasminogen to form an active complex, which then activates another plasminogen to form plasmin. Use of streptokinase is associated with an increased incidence of complications such as allergic reactions or hemorrhages and has fallen out of favor. The success of urokinase was due to its nonantigenic properties and its direct activation of plasminogen without the formation of an intermediate complex. As a nonspecific activator, however, it can, in high doses, induce systemic fibrinolysis. rtPA or alteplase is a recombinant version of the naturally occurring tPA protein; its activity is enhanced by the presence of fibrin. The final product is recombinant plasminogen activator rPA or reteplase. rPA is a recombinantly derived mutant lacking the 3 nonprotease domains of rtPA. A comparison of the efficacy, safety, and costs associated with catheter-directed thrombolysis (CDT) with urokinase (UK) and the recombinant agents alteplase (tissue plasminogen activator [tPA]) and reteplase (recombinant plasminogen activator

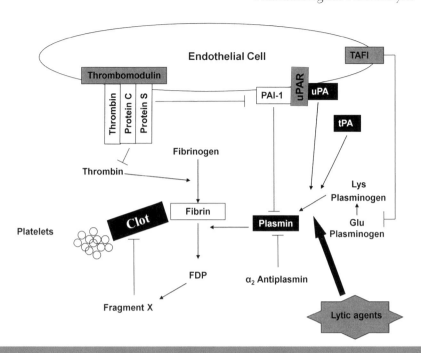

FIGURE 7.1 Control of intravascular coagulation. The endothelium coordinates the procoagulant and anticoagulant pathways to maintain vascular fluidity. It synthesizes several factors: protein S, urokinase-like plasminogen activator (uPA), tissue plasminogen activator (tPA), and plasminogen activator inhibitors (PAI). uPa and PAI are localized on the membrane by uPAR. Several pathways involved in fibrinolysis and anticoagulation reside on the membrane of the endothelial cells (plasminogen activator/inhibitors and the protein C pathway). Clot is formed by the activation of tissue factor, which leads to thrombin activity that cleaves fibrinogen to fibrin and is quickly associated with activated platelets to form a secondary hemostatic plug. At this time the plasmin-activating system is inhibited at various levels by the cells. Once fibrinolysis is activated, plasmin is formed from plasminogen by the actions of tPA and uPA whose activity is in turn modulated by PAI-1 and α_2 antiplasmin. Activated plasmin breaks fibrin into fibrin degradation products, one of which is termed "fragment X" and can lead to clot instability in the presence of long-term infusions of exogenous plasminogen activators.

[RPA]) in the treatment of symptomatic deep venous thrombosis (DVT) reveals that each of the agents is safe and effective, but that the new recombinant agents are significantly less expensive than urokinase.[6] First-generation thrombolytics (streptokinase and urokinase) have no fibrin-binding capabilities and cause systemic plasminogen activation with concomitant destruction of haemostatic proteins.[7] A primary driving force behind the development of the second-generation plasminogen activator tissue plasminogen activator (tPA or alteplase) was its ability to bind to fibrin and target thrombolysis. Several third-generation thrombolytic agents have been developed.[8] They are either conjugates of plasminogen activators with monoclonal antibodies against fibrin, platelets, or thrombomodulin; mutants, variants, and hybrids of alteplase (reteplase, tenecteplase, and pamiteplase) and prourokinase (amediplase); or new molecules of animal (vampire bat) or bacterial (*Staphylococcus aureus*) origin. These variations may lengthen the drug's half-life, increase resistance to plasma protease inhibitors, or cause more selective binding to fibrin. Compared with the second-generation agent (alteplase), third-

TABLE 7.1 **Pharmacology**

	Streptokinase	Urokinase	tPA	rPA
Size (kD)	45,000–50,000	20,000–34,000	63,000–65,000	39,000
Source	β-hemolytic Streptococcus	Fetal renal culture	Recombinant	Recombinant
Activity	SK-plasminogen complex	Direct PA	Direct PA	Direct PA
Metabolism	Liver	Liver	Liver	Liver
1/2 life	18–83 minutes	15 minutes	4 minutes	15 minutes
Fibrin selective	Low	Low	High	Very high
Affinity-free plasminogen	High	High	Low	Very low
Therapeutic window	Wide	Wide	Narrow	Wide
Cost	Low	High	High	High
Availability	Yes	No	Yes	Yes
Advantages	Expense	No allergy	No allergy	No allergy
Disadvantages	Allergy	No available	Expense	Expense

generation thrombolytic agents such as monteplase, tenecteplase, reteplase, lanoteplase, pamiteplase, and staphylokinase result in a greater angiographic patency rate in patients with acute myocardial infarction, although, thus far, mortality rates have been similar for those few drugs that have been studied in large-scale trials. Bleeding risk, however, may be greater.

Indications

Systemic anticoagulation has been the mainstay of therapy to prevent the occurrence of pulmonary embolism. However, the long-term effects of venous thromboembolism have largely gone unnoticed, specifically, the development of postthrombotic syndrome,

which can occur months to years after the initial event.[9] Conventional therapy with heparin has been effective in diminishing and preventing the propagation of thrombus;[10] however, it does not diminish the development of postthrombotic syndrome.[11] In fact, it has been estimated that 30% to 40% of existing thrombi will demonstrate propagation even at therapeutic levels of heparin.[12] A pooled analysis of 13 studies by Comerota[13] showed that 4% of patients who received heparin therapy had significant or complete lysis of thrombus compared with 45% who were randomized to systemic streptokinase therapy. The ideal therapy should dissolve existing thrombus, restore flow, and preserve venous valve function, which will diminish the incidence of venous hypertension. Catheter-directed venous thrombolysis

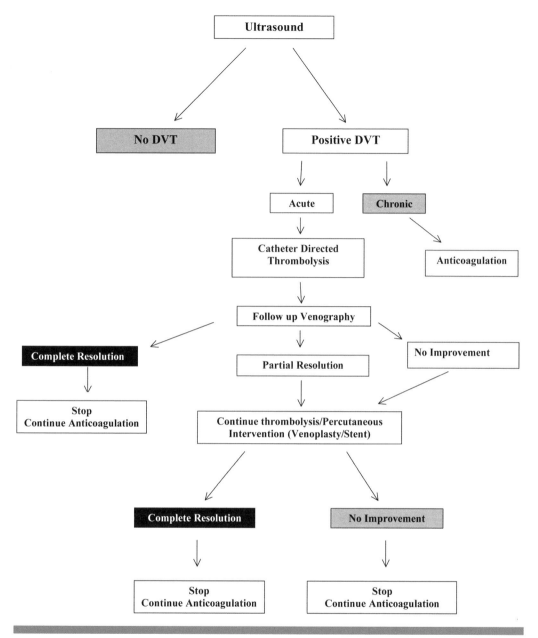

FIGURE 7.2 Algorithm for thrombolysis of venous thrombotic disease. In the patient presenting with a diagnosed deep venous thrombosis in the lower extremity, the acuity of the lesion, the extent of the thrombosis, and the impact of the thrombosis on distal circulation must be considered. In the absence of contraindications, thrombolysis can be instituted. The use of an adjunct inferior vena cava (IVC) filter is institutional-dependent. Lysis of the clot may reveal a lesion that will require intervention, either endoluminally or surgically. With resolution or no documented improvement, thrombolysis may be stopped and a standard heparin/oral anticoagulation protocol instituted.

has the potential to meet these goals—in particular, the retention of venous valvular function, which can prevent the formation of postthrombotic syndrome and its associated complications.

Percutaneous clot removal using thrombolysis, mechanical thrombectomy, or a combination of the 2 is fast becoming a treatment of choice for patients presenting with acute iliofemoral and axillosubclavian deep venous thrombosis.[14,15] By restoring venous patency and preserving valvular function, catheter-directed thrombolytic therapy potentially affords an improved long-term outcome in selected patients with DVT. In selected patients with extensive acute proximal DVT (ie, iliofemoral or axillosubclavian DVT, symptoms for <14 days, good functional status, life expectancy of >1 year) who have a low risk of bleeding, catheter-directed pharmacomechanical thrombolysis is suggested by the American College of Chest Physicians (ACCP).[16] An algorithm for thrombolysis of venous thrombotic disease is shown in Figure 7.2. This percutaneous therapy should include correction of any underlying venous lesions. Patients suitable for catheter-directed thrombolysis would include young, active individuals who have an acute (<14 days) iliofemoral and axillosubclavian deep venous thrombosis. Patients who have signs/symptoms of phlegmasia cerulea dolens, regardless of their clinical condition or age, should be considered for thrombolytic therapy. The contraindications for the use of a thrombolytic agent in any given scenario can be considered to fall into general and disease-specific categories. The general contraindications can be broken down into absolute, relative, and minor.

Contraindications to Thrombolysis

ABSOLUTE
   Active internal bleeding
   Recent cerebrovascular accident
      (<2 months)
   Intracranial pathology

RELATIVE
   Major
      Recent (<10 days) major surgery, obstetric delivery, or organ biopsy
      Active peptic ulcer or GI pathology
      Recent major trauma
      Uncontrolled hypertension
   Minor
      Minor surgery or trauma
      Recent CPR
      High likelihood of left heart thrombus
      Bacterial endocarditis
      Hemostatic defects
      Pregnancy
      Diabetic hemorrhagic retinopathy
AGENT SPECIFIC
   Streptokinase
   Known allergy
   Recent streptococcal infection
   Previous therapy within 6 months

Techniques
Catheter-Directed Thrombolysis

Although a variety of access sites have been utilized, the most common site reported is the popliteal vein.[17] Earlier techniques employed the internal jugular vein or common femoral vein; however, traversal of the occluded vein segment can be difficult due to retrograde passage through the venous valves, which may make further manipulations problematic. Using a popliteal approach, the patient is typically placed in a prone position on the fluoroscopy table, and the popliteal vein is localized using ultrasound guidance. Access is obtained with a small needle under ultrasound guidance and a 4F or 5F sheath is

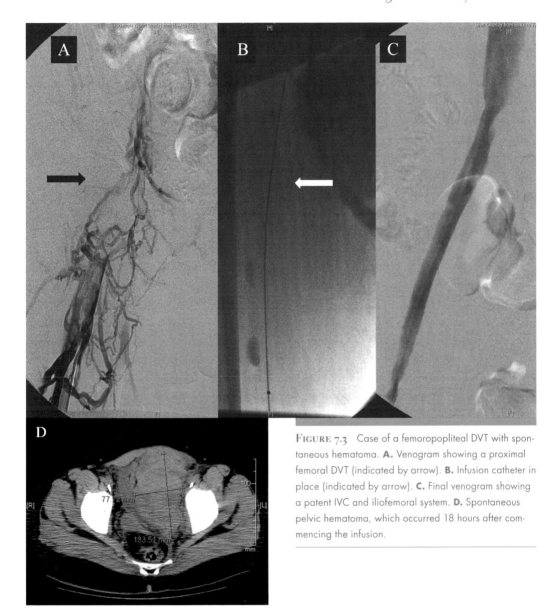

FIGURE 7.3 Case of a femoropopliteal DVT with spontaneous hematoma. **A.** Venogram showing a proximal femoral DVT (indicated by arrow). **B.** Infusion catheter in place (indicated by arrow). **C.** Final venogram showing a patent IVC and iliofemoral system. **D.** Spontaneous pelvic hematoma, which occurred 18 hours after commencing the infusion.

introduced. Baseline venography is then performed. After passage of a 0.035-in guidewire through the occluded venous segment, a diagnostic catheter is advanced past the occluded segment. This catheter is then exchanged for a multiple side hole infusion catheter. It is important that the total volume of thrombus is traversed with an infusible segment of catheter so that the thrombus can come into direct contact with the thrombolytic agent.

Low-dose tPA continuous infusion at 0.5 to 1.0 mg/h is administered through the infusion sheath with intravenous heparin at a rate of 500 U/h. Others recommend giving a lacing bolus of tPA 3 to 5 mg followed by a continuous tPA infusion at 0.05 mg/kg/h. Adding intermittent pneumatic compression to CDT for DVT treatment of the leg resulted in better early and late outcomes compared with CDT alone and was not associated with an increased risk of symptomatic pulmonary emboli.[18]

Monitoring

Currently, there is no need to monitor the changes in coagulation induced by low-dose thrombolytics after the physician has established a baseline coagulation profile. Many centers will follow fibrinogen and seek to maintain a target of >200 mg/dL. The patient does require monitoring of the infusion site to ensure that there is no exit site bleeding or disruption of the thrombolytic delivery system. Progress in thrombolysis may be assessed by interval duplex ultrasonography or more commonly by repeat venography. Repeat imaging is performed at 8- to 12-hour intervals, and infusions may be continued as long as 72 hours, although the mean infusion time is generally 56 hours.[19] The incidence of major clinical hemorrhage after fibrinolysis for DVT is between 6% and 30%, a 3-fold increase compared to standard heparin therapy. Infusion of thrombolysis is associated with increased risk of local hematoma formation at the site of catheter insertion and a lower risk of distant bleeding (Figure 7.3). Hypersensitivity reactions are low with both tPA or rPA.

Outcomes

In the National Multicenter Venous Registry,[17] catheter-directed thrombolysis was performed on acute (66%), chronic (45%), and a mixture of acute and chronic thrombus (19%). The degree of lysis achieved was categorized as grade I (<50% lysis), grade II (50%–90% lysis), and grade III (complete lysis). Continued patency was followed at 3, 6, and 12 months with duplex ultrasonography. Analysis of the registry data demon-strates that a larger proportion of patients with acute deep venous thrombosis (86%) vs. chronic (68%) were able to achieve grade II or III lysis. This is important because the degree of lysis was found to be predictive of early and continued patency. For instance, 75% of limbs with complete lysis remained patent at 1 year compared to 32% of limbs in which there was <50% lysis. A presentation of acute deep venous thrombosis (<10 days) was predictive of a better lysis grade when compared with chronic deep venous thrombosis, although a significant percentage of patients with chronic iliofemoral deep venous thrombosis were found to have significant lysis (grade II–III). The catheter-directed group demonstrated a much higher degree of significant lysis (83% vs. 20%) when compared with the 19% of patients who had a pedal infusion. This point underscores the necessity of having the thrombus in direct contact with the thrombolytic agent. Adjunctive procedures with stent placement and/or venoplasty were performed in 33% of affected limbs, which indicates that an underlying lesion often needs to be treated in conjunction with thrombolysis. Major bleeding complications were noted in 4% of patients enrolled. Subgroup analysis reveals that the best results occurred in patients with acute iliofemoral deep venous thrombosis with no prior history of deep venous thrombosis. Complete lysis occurred in 65% of patients with 96% patency at 1 year. Conversely, the worst results were seen in patients with chronic femoral-popliteal deep venous thrombosis. The groups were not large enough to establish statistical significance, but the investigators believed these results could serve as a guide to patient selection for catheter-directed thrombolysis. Patients most likely to achieve complete lysis and increased patency were those with an acute iliofemoral deep venous thrombosis and no prior history of deep venous thrombosis. Follow-up data are limited because a significant proportion of patients were lost to follow-up at 12 months.[17] Following treatment, patients receiving catheter-directed thrombolysis reported better overall physical functioning, less stigma, less health distress, and fewer postthrombotic symptoms compared to those patients treated with anticoagulation alone.[20] Within the thrombolysis group, successful lysis correlated with health-related quality of life.[20,21]

The results of the current Cochrane database included 12 studies.[22] Complete clot lysis occurred significantly more often in the treatment group in early follow-up (relative risk [RR] 0.24; 95% confidence interval [CI] 0.07–0.82) and in late follow-up (RR 0.37; 95% CI 0.25– 0.54). A similar effect was also seen for any degree of improvement in venous patency. Significantly less postthrombotic syndrome occurred in those receiving thrombolysis (RR 0.66; 95% CI 0.47–0.94). Leg ulceration was reduced, although the data were limited by small numbers (RR 0.53; 95% CI 0.12–2.43). Venous function was improved at late follow-up, but not significantly (RR 0.43; 95% CI 0.06–3.17). Out of 668 patients, those receiving thrombolysis had significantly more bleeding complications (RR 1.73; 95% CI 1.04–2.88). Two strokes occurred in the treatment group (RR 1.70; 95% CI 0.21–13.70). The incidence of bleeding appears to have reduced over time with the introduction of stricter selection criteria. There was no significant effect on mortality detected in either early or late follow-up. Data on occurrence of pulmonary embolism (PE) and recurrent DVT were inconclusive. The conclusions were that thrombolysis appears to offer advantages in terms of reducing postthrombotic syndrome and maintaining venous patency after DVT.[22] Use of strict eligibility criteria has improved the safety and acceptability of this treatment. The optimum drug, dose, and route of administration have yet to be determined. A more recent review of articles on catheter-directed thrombolysis (CDT) from PubMed and the Cochrane library was recently performed.[23] CDT reduced clot burden and DVT recurrence and may prevent the formation of postthrombotic syndrome. Indications for its use include younger individuals with a long life expectancy and few comorbidities, limb-threatening thromboses, and proximal iliofemoral DVTs. These results suggest that the outcomes of CDT in DVT management are encouraging in selected patient cohorts, but further evidence is required to establish longer-term benefits and cost-effectiveness. There is a marked lack of randomized controlled trials comparing CDT-related mortality and long-term outcomes compared to anticoagulation alone. The current ATTRACT trial sponsored by the NIH will hopefully answer many of the questions related to catheter-directed thrombolysis.

References

1. Gertler JP, Abbott WM. Prothrombotic and fibrinolytic functions of normal and perturbed endothelium. J Surg Res. 1992;52:89-95.

2. Henkin K, Marcotte P, Yang H. The plasminogen-plasmin system. Prog Cardiovasc Dis. 1991;34:135-62.

3. Robbins K. The Plasminogen-Plasmin Enzyme System. New York: Lippincott; 1995.

4. Schaeerf AV, Leslie BA, Rischke JA, Stafford AR, Fredenburgh JC, Weitz JI. Incorporation of fragment X into fibrin clots renders them more susceptible to lysis by plasmin. Biochemistry. 2006;45(13):4257-65.

5. Weitz JI. Limited fibrin specificity of tissue-type plasminogen activator and its potential link to bleeding. J Vasc Interv Radiol. 1995;6 (Pt 2 suppl):19S-23S.

6. Grunwald MR, Hofmann LV. Comparison of urokinase, alteplase, and reteplase for catheter-directed thrombolysis of deep venous thrombosis. J Vasc Interv Radiol. 2004;15(4):347-52.

7. Longstaff C, Williams S, Thelwell C. Fibrin binding and the regulation of plasminogen activators during thrombolytic therapy. Cardiovasc Hematol Agents Med Chem. 2008;6(3):212-23.

8. Verstraete M. Third-generation thrombolytic drugs. Am J Med. 2000;109(1):52-8.

9. Strandness DE Jr, Langlois Y, Cramer M, Randlett A, Thiele BL. Long-term sequelae of acute venous thrombosis: a clinical review. JAMA. 1983(250):1289-92.

10. Johnson BF, Manzo RA, Bergelin RO, Strandness DE Jr. Relationship between changes in the deep venous system and the development of the post-thrombotic syndrome after an acute episode of lower limb deep venous thrombosis: a one-to-six year follow-up. J Vasc Surg. 1995;21:307-12.

11. Meissner MH, Manzo RA, Bergelin RO, Markel A, Strandness DE Jr. Deep venous insufficiency: the relationship between lysis and subsequent reflux. J Vasc Surg. 1993;18:596-608.

12. Strandness DE. Thrombus propagation and level of anticoagulation. J Vasc Surg. 1990;12:497-8.

13. Comerota A, Aldridge S. Thrombolytic therapy for deep vein thrombosis: a clinical review. Can J Surg. 1993;36:359-64.

14. Meissner MH, Wakefield TW, Ascher E, Caprini JA, Comerota AJ, Eklof B, et al. Acute venous disease: venous thrombosis and venous trauma. J Vasc Surg. 2007;46 (suppl S):25S-53S.

15. Molina JE, Hunter DW, Dietz CA. Protocols for Paget-Schroetter syndrome and late treatment of chronic subclavian vein obstruction. Ann Thorac Surg. 2009;87(2):416-22.

16. Kearon C, Kahn SR, Agnelli G, Goldhaber S, Raskob GE, Comerota AJ; American College of Chest Physicians. Antithrombotic therapy for venous thromboembolic disease: American College of Chest Physicians Evidence-Based Clinical Practice Guidelines (8th ed.). Chest. 2008;133(6 suppl):454S-545S.

17. Mewissen M, Seabrook G, Meissner M, Cynamon J, Labropoulos N, Haughton S. Catheter-directed thrombolysis for lower extremity deep venous thrombosis: report of a nation multicenter registry. Radiology. 1999;211:39-49.

18. Ogawa T, Hoshino S, Midorikawa H, Sato K. Intermittent pneumatic compression of the foot and calf improves the outcome of catheter-directed thrombolysis using low-dose urokinase in patients with acute proximal venous thrombosis of the leg. J Vasc Surg. 2005;42(5):940-4.

19. Mewissen M, Seabrook GR, Meissner MH, Cynamon J, Labropoulos N, Haughton SH. Catheter-directed thrombolysis for lower extremity deep venous thrombosis: report of a nation multicenter registry. Radiology. 1999;211:39-49.

20. Comerota AJ. Quality-of-life improvement using thrombolytic therapy for iliofemoral deep venous thrombosis. Rev Cardiovasc Med. 2002;3 (suppl 2):S61-7.

21. Comerota AJ, Throm RC, Mathias SD, Haughton S, Mewissen M. Catheter-directed thrombolysis for iliofemoral deep venous thrombosis improves health-related quality of life. J Vasc Surg. 2000;32(1):130-7.

22. Watson LI, Armon MP. Thrombolysis for acute deep vein thrombosis. Cochrane Database Syst Rev. 2004; Oct 18(4):CD002783.

23. Gogalniceanu P, Johnston CJ, Khalid U, Holt PJ, Hincliffe R, Loftus IM, et al. Indications for thrombolysis in deep venous thrombosis. Eur J Vasc Endovasc Surg. 2009;38(2): 192-8.

Pharmacomechanical Thrombolysis for Acute Deep Venous Thrombosis
Indications, Techniques, and Clinical Data

Elina Quiroga and Mark H. Meissner

The primary goals of treatment of acute deep venous thrombosis are the prevention of pulmonary embolism, recurrent deep venous thrombosis (DVT), and postthrombotic syndrome (PTS). Although standard anticoagulation is effective in preventing recurrent venous thromboembolism, it protects imperfectly against postthrombotic syndrome, which may develop in 29.6% of patients by year 5.[1] As an adjunct to anticoagulation, early thrombus removal, including thrombolytic therapy and venous thrombectomy, likely plays a role in reducing the incidence of postthrombotic syndrome.

As venous thrombolytic strategies can rapidly restore venous patency, they have the potential to preserve valve function and theoretically prevent postthrombotic syndrome.

Early strategies focused on the systemic administration of thrombolytic agents, which were 3.7 times more effective in restoring venous patency than anticoagulation alone.[2] Unfortunately, systemic thrombolysis was associated with prolonged infusion times as well as significant rates of bleeding and partial thrombolysis.[3]

Efforts to reduce infusion times, improve thrombolytic efficiency, and reduce bleeding complications led to the development of catheter-directed thrombolytic strategies. Although these strategies were also associated with significant infusion times and bleeding complications, they were critical in establishing the optimal patient population to be considered for thrombolysis and in developing modern interventional techniques for the treatment of acute DVT. Such strategies established the importance of thrombolysis via an ultrasound-guided antegrade puncture of the popliteal artery; the frequency of underlying iliac obstruc-

Venous Thromboembolic Disease. Contemporary Endovascular Management series. © 2011 Mark G. Davies MD and Alan B. Lumsden MD, eds. Cardiotext Publishing, ISBN 978-1-935395-22-5.

tive lesions and need for treatment; and the poor results of lytic therapy for chronic thrombosis.[4]

The limitations of both systemic and catheter-directed thrombolysis have led to a variety of pharmacomechanical strategies directed toward increasing lytic efficiency while reducing procedural times. Theoretically, this would translate into reduced bleeding complications, decreased hospital and intensive care unit stays, and reduced cost.

Pharmacomechanical Thrombolytic Strategies

The isolated use of mechanical devices is rarely successful, and their use in combination with thrombolytic drugs is usually required.[5] However, use of a mechanical device to speed thrombolysis is theoretically attractive since it has the potential to reduce thrombolytic infusion times and thereby decrease bleeding complications, hospital resource utilization, and cost while improving efficacy. Although there is little solid data that this has been achieved, use of such devices would optimally allow the entire venous system to be cleared of thrombus in a single session in the angiography suite.

Amongst several mechanical thrombolytic devices, 3 have been widely utilized in the venous system—the AngioJet power pulse, the Trellis-8 infusion catheter, and the EKOS EndoWave. The mechanical thrombolytic devices share many technical details. If inflow to the popliteal vein is patent, ultrasound-guided puncture of the popliteal vein using a micropuncture set is preferred by many interventionalists, with more distal access via the posterior tibial vein, small saphenous vein, or great saphenous vein (with deep system access through a perforator)

being alternatives. Initial venography is performed to document the extent of thrombus and a wire is advanced across the thrombus. If caval thrombus is suspected, some also recommend a computed tomography (CT) venogram to document thrombus extent prior to bringing the patient to the angiography suite. Further aspects of the procedure are more device-specific.

The AngioJet rheolytic thrombectomy catheter (MEDRAD Inc., Warrendale, PA) is an over-the-wire system using a high-velocity (350/450 km/h) saline jet directed backward from the tip of the catheter. A low-pressure zone is created via a Venturi effect, causing fragmentation of the thrombus, which is aspirated through the effluent lumen (Figure 8.1). In the power-pulse mode, the effluent port is closed with a stopcock and a dilute lytic agent, usually tPA at a dose of 0.4 mg/cc is used in place of the saline jet. After infusion, the lytic agent is allowed to dwell for 20 to 25 minutes prior to aspiration on withdrawal of the catheter with the effluent port open. A variety of catheter sizes are available, allowing treatment of different vessels.[6]

The Trellis-8 infusion catheter (Covidien) has proximal and distal occlusion balloons with a drug-infusion port between the balloons, and a wire that oscillates within the catheter (Figure 8.2). This allows the thrombolytic drug to be isolated between balloons in direct contact with the thrombus. The oscillating wire macerates the thrombus, increasing exposure to the thrombolytic agent and theoretically reducing the dose required for lysis. After treatment, the thrombolytic agent and clot fragments are aspirated. Several thrombolytic agents had been used, including tenecteplase, with doses between 5 and 10 mg and tPA, with a recommend dose of 5 to 10 mg. The current available catheters are 80 and 120 cm in length, and the

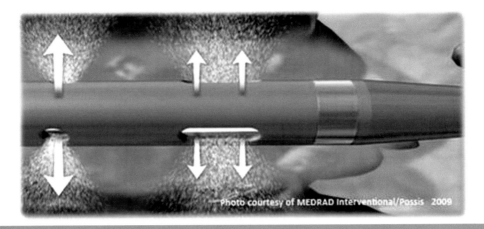

FIGURE 8.1   AngioJet rheolytic thrombectomy catheter. Image Courtesy of MEDRAD Interventional.

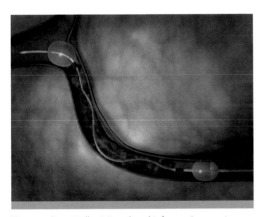

FIGURE 8.2   Trellis-8 Peripheral Infusion System. Image courtesy of Covidien.

treatment zone varies between balloons of 10, 15, and 30 cm.[7]

The EKOS EndoWave (EKOS Corporation, Bothell, WA) device utilizes ultrasound transducers to alter the structure of the thrombus, increasing its permeability and exposing plasminogen receptors (Figure 8.3). The ultrasound forces the drug into the thrombus and may help to "hold" the drug within the thrombosed segment. tPA at a dose of 0.5 to 1.0 mg/h is among the most commonly use thrombolytic agents.[8]

Adjunctive procedures are a critical component of pharmacomechanical thrombolysis. The Venous Registry reported a low incidence (1%) of symptomatic pulmonary embolism with catheter-directed thrombolysis, and it is generally accepted that routine placement of an IVC filter is not required in this setting. However, there is not yet consensus regarding placement and use of IVC filters in pharmacomechanical thrombolysis. Pulmonary embolism has been reported in association with mechanical thrombolytic devices, although the precise incidence is unknown. Some have suggested the routine placement of an IVC filter when using the AngioJet catheter.[9] However, given the relatively short period of risk during the actual use of the mechanical devices, use of a retrievable filter is likely more appropriate than a permanent filter if this is deemed appropriate.

Thrombus maceration using an angioplasty balloon is also used by some to assist with lytic exposure. Thrombolysis will uncover an underlying iliac vein lesion in 45% to 60% of patients presenting with a left-side iliofemoral DVT.[4,10] Such lesions most commonly occur at the crossing of the left com-

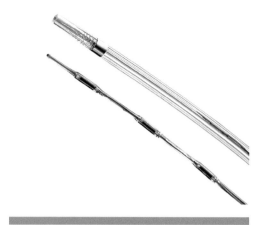

FIGURE 8.3   EKOS EndoWave device. Image Courtesy of EKOS.

mon iliac vein by the right common iliac artery (the May-Thurner or Cockett syndrome), but may occur on the right side as well.[11] Failure to treat such lesions with self-expanding stents is associated with a high rate of recurrent thrombosis and thrombolytic failure.[4] Current studies suggest that when an iliac vein stenosis is uncovered, self-expandable metallic stents improve 1-year venous patency rates from 53% to 74% among limbs treated with metallic stents. Although the data regarding infrainguinal stents are limited, their use is not currently indicated. The Venous Registry reported that 4 of 5 infrainguinal stents occluded early after placement.[4] Although lacking data, it also seems likely that a stented and freely refluxing femoropopliteal venous segment may be more detrimental hemodynamically than a chronically obstructed segment.

The AngioJet and Trellis system theoretically allow treatment in a single setting, although placement of an infusion catheter for completion of thrombolysis is not infrequently required. Although the EndoWave catheter may speed the lytic process, it does not have the potential for single-setting

treatment. If follow-up catheter-directed thrombolysis is required, current guidelines suggest tPA infusion at a rate of 0.5 to 1.0 mg/h. High-volume infusions are generally preferred in the venous system, and follow-up venography is indicated at 12 to 24 hours.[5] Systemic anticoagulation, usually with unfractionated heparin, is utilized during the procedure, usually at a reduced dose to avoid bleeding complications, and conventional anticoagulation therapy is required after the procedure to prevent rethrombosis. The duration of anticoagulation should be based on the patient's underlying risk factors and should follow current ACCP guidelines.[12] As prevention of the postthrombotic syndrome is the primary goal of pharmacomechanical thrombolysis, all patients should be discharged with knee-high 30– to 40–mm Hg compression stockings that should be continued for at least 2 years.[12,13]

Results of Pharmacomechanical Thrombolysis

Unfortunately, the outcomes after pharmacomechanical thrombolysis are entirely derived from case series, and there have been no randomized clinical trials comparing pharmacomechanical thrombolysis with either catheter-directed thrombolysis or conventional anticoagulation. Furthermore, such series tend to focus on surrogate outcomes such as degree of lysis rather than clinically important outcomes such as quality of life or objectively defined postthrombotic syndrome. Many outstanding questions regarding pharmacomechanical thrombolysis are expected to be answered by the ATTRACT trial, which will compare these pharmacomechanical strategies with conventional anticoagulation. The currently available data, although weak, do however show a promising trend favoring pharmacomechanical thrombolysis.

As noted above, degree of lysis and bleeding are the most common outcomes reported in pharmacomechanical series. The percentage of lysis is usually based on the Society of Interventional Radiology classification: grade I, less than 50% thrombus removal; grade II, 50% to 95%; and grade III, >95% to 100% thrombus removal. Grade I or II lysis was achieved in 79% of patients receiving catheter-directed thrombolysis; in 93% of patients using the Trellis-8 device; and in 91% treated with EndoWave. Mean infusion times of 76 ± 34 minutes and 22 ± 11 minutes for the AngioJet and Trellis-8 devices, respectively, have been reported.[10,14] Major bleeding complications were reported in 11.0% of patients treated with catheter-directed thrombolysis and 3.8% of patients treated with EndoWave.[4,8] There were no reports of major bleeding complications in patients treated with either the AngioJet or Trellis-8 devices, although more rigorous methodological evaluations are clearly needed.

Conclusion

Thrombolytic therapy for acute treatment of DVT is an attractive adjunct to conventional anticoagulation, as it has the theoretical ability to rapidly restore venous patency and preserve valvular function. However, early experiences with systemic and catheter-directed thrombolysis were characterized by prolonged infusion times, significant rates of partial lysis, and high rates of bleeding complications. Pharmacomechanical approaches are attractive in that they have

the potential to minimize treatment times, with corresponding decreases in cost and bleeding complications. Unfortunately, such approaches have not yet been evaluated in rigorous randomized trials using clinically relevant, objective measures of quality of life and postthrombotic syndrome. Fortunately, the potential value of this approach is currently being evaluated in the ATTRACT trial, which will evaluate both quality of life and objectively determined postthrombotic syndrome among patients randomized to pharmacomechanical techniques in comparison to conventional anticoagulation.

References

1. Johnson BF, Manzo RA, Bergelin RO, Strandness DE Jr. Relationship between changes in the deep venous system and the development of the postthrombotic syndrome after an acute episode of lower limb deep vein thrombosis: a one- to six-year follow-up. J Vasc Surg. 1995;21:307-13.

2. Goldhaber SZ, Buring JE, Lipnick RJ, Hennekens CH. Pooled analyses of randomized trials of streptokinase and heparin in phlebographically documented acute deep venous thrombosis. Am J Med. 1984;76:393-7.

3. Forster A, Wells P. Tissue plasminogen activator for the treatment of deep venous thrombosis of the lower extremity. Chest. 2001;119:572-9.

4. Mewissen MW, Seabrook GR, Meissner MH, Cynamon J, Labropoulos N, Haughton SH. Catheter-directed thrombolysis of lower extremity deep venous thrombosis: report of a national multicenter registry. Radiology. 1999;211:39-49.

5. Vedantham, Thorpe PE, Cardella JF. Quality improvement guidelines for the treatment of lower extremity deep vein thrombosis with use of endovascular thrombus removal. J Vasc Interv Radiol. 2009;20:S227-39.

6. Kasirajan K, Gray B. Percutaneous angiojet thrombectomy in the management of extensive deep venous thrombosis. J Vasc Interv Radiol. 2001;12:179-85.

7. McLafferty R. Endovascular management of deep venous thrombosis. Perspect Vasc Surg Endovasc Ther. 2008;20;87-91.

8. Parikh S, Motarjeme A. Ultrasound-accelerated thrombolysis for the treatment of deep vein thrombosis: Initial clinical experience. J Vasc Interv Radiol. 2008;19:521-8.

9. Lin PH, Zhou W, Dardik A. Catheter-direct thrombolysis versus pharmacomechanical thrombectomy for treatment of symptomatic lower extremity deep venous thrombosis. Am J Surg. 2006;192:782-8.

10. O'Sullivan GJ, Semba CP, Bittner CA, Kee ST, Razavi MK, Sze DY, et al. Endovascular management of iliac vein compression (May-Thurner) syndrome. J Vasc Interv Radiol. 2000;11:823-36.

11. Raju S, Neglen P. High prevalence of nonthrombotic iliac vein lesions in chronic venous disease: a permissive role in pathogenicity. J Vasc Surg. 2006;44(1): 136-43.

12. Kearon C, Kahn SR, Goldhaber S. Antithrombotic therapy for venous thromboembolic disease: American College of Chest Physicians Evidence-Based Clinical Practice Guidelines (8th ed.). Chest. 2008; 133 (6 suppl):454S-545S.

13. Brandjes D, Büller HR, Heijboer H, Huisman MV, de Rijk M, Jagt H, et al. Randomised trial of effect of compression stockings in patients with symptomatic proximal-vein thrombosis. Lancet. 1997;349:759-62.

14. Hilleman DE, Razavi MK. Clinical and economic evaluation of the Trellis-8 infusion catheter for deep vein thrombosis. J Vasc Interv Radiol. 2008;19:377-83.

Endovascular Intervention for Lower Extremity Deep Venous Thrombosis

Techniques, Devices, and Outcomes

Erin H. Murphy and Frank R. Arko III

Anticoagulation remains the gold standard for calf vein DVT.[1-3] However, strategies of early intervention with clot removal have been advocated for cases of more proximal iliofemoral DVT. These procedures are almost exclusively performed endovascularly, with little downtime for the patient and early clinical improvement. Early clot removal has been shown to dramatically reduce the long-term morbidity of proximal DVT by preventing permanent venous valvular damage and thereby the debilitating sequelae of postthrombotic syndrome.[4-7]

Multiple techniques and devices are available for endovascular DVT intervention. The majority of available treatment options may be separated by mechanism of action and include catheter-directed thrombolysis,

ultrasound-accelerated thrombolysis, and percutaneous mechanical thrombectomy.

Catheter-Directed Thrombolysis

Catheter-directed thrombolysis (CDT) allows infusion of thrombolytics directly into the venous thrombosis, limiting systemic drug exposure. Thrombolytic agents used with CDT include urokinase (ImaRx Therapeutics, Tucson, AZ), tissue plasminogen activator (Activase, Genentech, South San Francisco, CA), recombinant tissue plasminogen activator (Retavase, PDL BioPharma, Fremont, CA), or tenecteplase (Genentech).

Most commonly, patients treated with CDT undergo percutaneous access in the operating room with an initial venogram to determine thrombus extent. A small infusion catheter is placed just proximal to the location of thrombus and secured in place

Venous Thromboembolic Disease. Contemporary Endovascular Management series. © 2011 Mark G. Davies MD and Alan B. Lumsden MD, eds. Cardiotext Publishing, ISBN 978-1-935395-22-5.

externally. Patients are monitored in the intensive care unit, and thrombolytics are slowly administered through the catheter. The patient undergoes repeat venography in the operating room to assess clot lysis once every 24 hours until complete lysis is achieved.

This option has proven effective in proximal DVT, resulting in early clot resolution, prevention of PE, prevention of recurrent DVT, preservation of valve function, and improved quality of life over treatment with isolated anticoagulation. Results have demonstrated 60% to 90% clot resolution in proximal DVT[8-11] with degree of clot removal correlating directly with improvements in long-term patency and reduced incidence of postthrombotic syndrome.[11]

Unfortunately, this therapy is still associated with significant bleeding complications in 11% to 43% of patients.[8-14] Ouriel et al. demonstrated insertion site bleeding in 22% to 44%, transfusion requirements in 12% to 22%, and intracranial hemorrhage in 0.6% to 3.0% of patients undergoing CDT with urokinase and recombinant tissue plasminogen activator, respectively.[14] Further limitations to the widespread use of this technique include prolonged lytic infusion times of 36 to 72 hours, prolonged ICU stay, and expensive drug costs.[8-14]

Ultrasound-Accelerated Thrombolysis

The EKOS EndoWave and EkoSonic systems use low-power, high-frequency ultrasound (2 MHz) in combination with catheter-directed thrombolysis to achieve clot disruption. Ultrasound waves generated by the unit do not directly macerate the clot but rather create microstreams that increase thrombus permeability via alteration of fi-

brin composition. Increased permeability results in augmented lytic dispersion within the thrombus.[15-17] In fact, a 65% increase in the number of fibrin strands exposed to thrombolytic drugs has been demonstrated to occur with a 44% ultrasound-mediated reduction in the diameter of fibrin strands.[16] This translates to increased thrombus uptake of recombinant tissue plasminogen activator by 48%, 84%, and 89% at 1, 2, and 4 hours, respectively.[17] Furthermore, the ultrasound waves penetrate past valves, allowing for thrombus removal behind the valve, which may be inaccessible with other PMT devices.

The device consists of an infusion/aspiration catheter, an ultrasound core wire, and a drive unit. The catheter, available in treatment lengths of 6 to 50 cm, contains a central lumen that accommodates the 0.035-ultrasound core wire and normal saline infusate used for central cooling. In a triangular distribution around the central lumen are 3 separate infusion channels containing microinfusion pores for drug delivery and thermocouples to monitor changes in temperature and flow patterns. The ultrasound core wire has transducers (2.2 MHz) located at 1-cm intervals. When the drive unit is activated, ultrasound waves are delivered to the core wire and transmitted through the catheter, penetrating thrombus and allowing lytic dispersion.

Access is obtained with a 5F introducer sheath and the lesion is crossed with a 0.035-in guidewire. The catheter is positioned such that the treatment zone extends through the length of the thrombosed venous segment. After positioning, the guidewire is exchanged for the ultrasound core wire. The 3 separate drug-infusion lumens are primed with unfractionated heparin. The control unit is activated and delivers ultrasound energy via the core wire while the thrombolytic agent of choice is administered through micropores located throughout the length of the treatment zone on each of the 3 catheters. Normal saline is infused through the central lumen continuously during the procedure to dissipate heat production. The drive unit automatically adjusts power according to changing vessel conditions, reducing power as flow is restored. The procedure is continued until complete lysis is achieved (Figure 9.1).

Early evaluation of the EKOS Endo-Wave system in 53 patients, including 32 patients with lower extremity DVT, demonstrated greater than 90% clot lysis in 70% of patients and at least partial thrombus resolution in 91%. Importantly, at least partial lysis was achieved in 96% of acute DVT (< 14 days), 100% of subacute DVT (15 to 28 days), and 77.8% of chronic (> 28 days) and acute on chronic DVT. Median lytic infusion time was 22 hours, and bleeding complications were low (3.8%). Furthermore, median infusion times and median total drug dosages administered were lower with ultrasound-mediated thrombolysis compared to standard CDT when using UK, tPA, or rtPA. The median dosages and infusion times were similar for CDT and US-mediated thrombolysis when tenecteplase was used.[18] The EKOS EkoSonic Endovascular System with MACH4e is similar to the earlier version but this system allows for faster clot lysis.

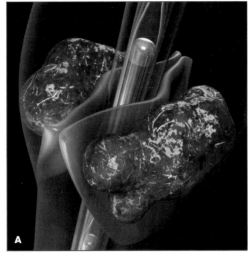

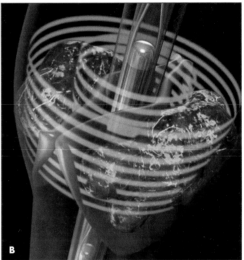

FIGURE 9.1 The EKOS EndoWave and EkoSonic systems. The microstreams alter fibrin composition even behind the valves, as seen in **B**. Image Courtesy of EKOS.

Percutaneous Mechanical Thrombectomy

Percutaneous mechanical thrombectomy (PMT) offers the benefit of early thrombus removal while limiting thrombolytic dosages and bleeding complications. PMT additionally offers a treatment option for patients with absolute contraindications for lytic therapy, as the AngioJet, a PMT device discussed next, is the only device that can be used without the addition of lytics. PMT has further been shown to be more cost effective than alternative treatment regimens when considering the lower thrombolytic dosages administered and decreased length of ICU stay compared to CDT,[19] and the decreased long-term morbidity from postthrombotic syndrome compared to traditional antico-agulation.

AngioJet Rheolytic Thrombectomy System— Power-Pulse Spray Technique

The AngioJet catheter system is comprised of a single-use catheter, a single-use pump set, and a drive unit. The catheter, which is available in working lengths of 60, 100, and 120 cm, contains a central lumen for in-fusate and a larger lumen encompassing the central channel, the guidewire, and aspirate from the thrombus. The drive unit generates 10,000 psi of pulsatile infusion flow, which is released from the catheter in retrograde-directed high-velocity saline jets. These jets create a localized low-pressure zone (Ber-noulli's principle) at the catheter tip, mac-erating thrombus and redirecting flow and debris into outflow channels directed behind the catheter tip for aspiration and removal (see Figure 8.1 on page 91).

Access for the AngioJet system requires a 6F introducer sheath. The AngioJet cath-eter is then advanced over a 0.035 guidewire through the thrombus load. While this sys-tem was originally intended for use without adjunctive thrombolytics, it has been dem-onstrated that the addition of lytics to the infusion solution results in decreased treat-ment time and improved results. We recom-mend that thrombolytics be routinely used except when contraindicated, as is our prac-tice. While thrombolytic choice and dose vary according to surgeon preference, we have experienced good results using 10 mg of tenecteplase in 50 mL of sodium chloride infusing solution.[20]

With the aspiration port clamped, in-fusate is released into the thrombosed ve-nous segment during a slow pull-back of the catheter, effectively lacing the clot with thrombolytic drug. After 10 minutes, the as-piration function of the catheter is turned on. The catheter is then advanced through the thrombosed segment a second time, re-moving macerated thrombus through the aspiration ports as the catheter is advanced. This process may be repeated if there is re-maining thrombus burden at the end of the first pass. Alternatively, as is often our prefer-ence, the patient may then undergo catheter-directed thrombolysis in the intensive care unit (ICU) overnight and return to the oper-ative room the following day for reevaluation with venography and possible repeat throm-bectomy or venous stenting, if indicated.

Success in thrombus removal, restora-tion of venous patency, and preservation of valvular function have been demonstrated with the use of the AngioJet power-pulse spray technique. While Kasirajan reported only 24% of patients had >90% clot resolu-tion, 35% had 50% to 90% resolution, and 41% had less than 50% resolution,[21] im-proved results have been demonstrated with the addition of lytics to the infusate, as dis-cussed previously. Bush et al. reported com-plete thrombus resolution in 65% of patients, with at least partial resolution seen in all of the remaining patients.[22] Lin et al. demon-strated that PMT with the AngioJet system was at least as effective as CDT in treating lower extremity DVT. They showed com-plete clot lysis in 75% of patients treated with AngioJet vs. 70% in patients treated with CDT (P = NS) with similar patency at 1-year follow-up of 64% and 68%, respectively. In addition, they demonstrated reduced ICU stay, reduced total in-hospital length of stay, and reduced costs in the PMT cohort.[19] In our series, we demonstrated a 90% venous patency restoration and maintenance of venous valvular function in 88% at a mean follow-up of 6 months.[20]

This therapy is associated with a low incidence of hemorrhagic complications. Isolated case reports of pancreatitis resulting from massive hemolysis with use of the AngioJet system have been reported but appear to be rare occurences.[23]

Trellis-8 Infusion System— Pharmacomechanical Thrombectomy

The Trellis-8 Periphperal Infusion System incorporates the use of both chemical thrombolysis and mechanical thrombectomy. The Trellis device consists of a single-use catheter, a dispersion wire, and an integral drive unit. The catheter contains proximal and distal occlusion balloons that allow infusion of thrombolytics to an isolated segment of thrombosed vein. Catheters are available in lengths of 80 or 120 cm, with varied distances between occlusion balloons allowing treatment of 10-, 15-, or 30-cm venous segments. Selection of which catheter to use will depend on the location and length of the thrombosed segment determined on ini-

tial venogram, with the goal of minimizing treatment length of nonthrombosed vein. The drive unit is attached to the sinusoidal dispersion wire, which creates catheter oscillatation at 500 to 3500 rpm, causing dispersion of lytics within the thrombus load and mechanical clot disruption. Aspiration of thrombus debris and lytic remaining in the isolated segment completes treatment of the isolated venous segment (Figure 9.2).

Access for the Trellis-8 infusion system requires and 8F introducer sheath. A 0.035 Glidewire (Terumo, Sommerset, NJ) is used to cross the thrombosed venous segment and the Trellis-8 catheter is advanced over the Glidewire. With proximal and distal balloons inflated, 5 to 10 mg of lytics are infused within the thrombus. After 10 minutes, the dispersion wire is inserted into the catheter. Catheter vibration between the occlusion balloons aids in clot maceration and increases the thrombus surface area exposed to the lytics. The dispersion wire may further be advanced and retracted once a minute during the treatment interval to further ensure mixing of the lytics with the thrombus. After 5 to 15 minutes, the distal balloon is deflated and the catheter aspirated via a

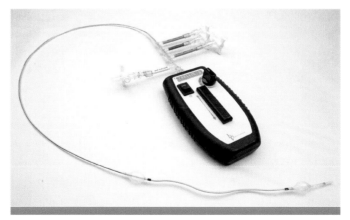

FIGURE 9.2   The Trellis-8 Peripheral Infusion System. Image courtesy of Covidien.

side port to remove macerated thrombus and a substantial portion of the remaining lytics. The proximal balloon is left inflated during aspiration to prevent embolization of clot. After aspiration, with both balloons deflated, the system may be removed or advanced into adjacent thrombosed segments, repeating the procedure until thrombus load is resolved.

Hilleman et al. reported success with the Trellis-8 infusion system for the treatment of proximal lower extremity DVT in 135 patients. They demonstrated superior clot lysis with Trellis-8 compared to conventional catheter-directed thrombolysis with 93% achieving grade II (50%–99% clot resolution) or III lysis (100% clot resolution) verus 79%, respectively. They additionally demonstrated that patients receiving pharmacomechanical lysis required lower lytic dose, was more cost effective and associated with significantly lower rates of hemorrhage (0% vs. 8.5%, P <0.001).[24] Arko et al. further demonstrated 80% of patients experienced complete clot resolution with this technique in a single setting with venous patency maintained in 88% of patients treated with this device at a mean follow-up of 6 months.[20] O'Sullivan demonstrated grade II or III lysis in 96% of patients in a single setting, with 100% assisted primary patency at 30 days.[25]

Adjunctive Procedures

Recalcitrant thrombus after initial treatment with PMT may require further therapy. While small residual thrombus may respond to venoplasty and stenting, larger amounts of residual thrombus may require use of a second PMT device or overnight catheter-directed thrombolysis.[15,20,21,26] Use of an adjunctive device or CDT should not be regarded as a failure of the first device, but

rather as complementary procedures.[26] The initial device achieves significant clot burden reduction, paving an easier path for the second intervention. Use of a second PMT device can be performed in the same setting, often with lower doses of thrombolytics.[20,26] Alternatively, overnight CDT therapy may be sufficient to eliminate residual thrombus after debulking of clot with PMT.[15,20,21] This significantly reduces the time required for effective CDT and thereby reduces the associated bleeding risks with this treatment modality.[15,20,21] Patients should then undergo a second evaluation with intravascular ultrasonography and/or completion venography to evaluate vessel conditions. Underlying venous stenosis may require venoplasty and stenting (Figure 9.3).

Postprocedure Anticoagulation

Patients should be anticoagulated after interventions for DVT with unfractionated heparin or low-molecular-weight heparin and transitioned to oral warfarin for 6 months (goal international normalized ratio 2–3). Patients with recurrent DVT or hypercoagulable disorders may require a longer duration of anticoagulation. Patients with venous stents require lifelong aspirin therapy.

Conclusion

Percutaneous mechanical thrombectomy and ultrasound-accelerated thrombolysis are at least as effective as catheter-directed thrombolysis with reduced ICU and hospital stays and decreased overall costs. Further, use of a second PMT device, adjunctive CDT, and/or stenting of underlying venous stenoses may be needed to achieve optimal clinical results.

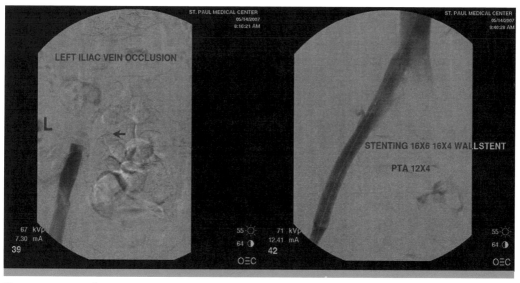

FIGURE 9.3   **A.** Following an IVC filter placement the left iliac vein occlusion is treated with ultrasound-facilitated thrombolysis in the prone position. **B.** PTA and stenting of May-Thurner syndrome results in an excellent venographic result with long-term patency.

With widespread implementation of these advanced treatment options for DVT, we can achieve a significant reduction in long-term morbidity after proximal DVT.

References

1. Kearon C. Natural history of venous thromboembolism. Circulation. 2003;107: I22-30.

2. Buller HR, Sohne M, Middledorp S. Treatment of venous thromboembolism. J Thromb Haemost. 2005;3:1554-60.

3. Fifth ACCP consensus conference on antithrombotic therapy. Chest. 1998;114:439S-769S.

4. Plate G, Einarsson E, Ohlin P, Jensen R, Qvarfordt P, Eklöf B. Thrombectomy with temporary arteriovenous fistula: the treatment of choice in acute iliofemoral venous thrombosis. J Vasc Surg. 1984;1:867-76.

5. Plate G, Akesson H, Einarsson E, Ohlin P, Eklöf B. Long-term results of venous thrombectomy combined with a temporary arterio-venous fistula. Eur J Vasc Sur. 1990;4:483-9.

6. Plate G, Eklöf B, Norgren L, Ohlin P, Dahlström JA. Venous thrombectomy for iliofemoral vein thrombosis—10-year results of a prospective randomized study. Eur J Vasc Endovasc Surg. 1997;14:367-74.

7. Comerota AJ, Aldridge SA. Thrombolytic therapy for acute deep vein thrombosis. Semin Vasc Surg. 1992;5(2):76-84.

8. Blum A, Roche E. Endovascular management of acute deep vein thrombosis. Am J Med. 2005;118 (suppl):31S-36S.

9. Comerota AJ, Throm RC, Mathias SD, Haughton S, Meiwissen M. Catheter-directed thrombolysis for iliofemoral deep venous thrombosis improves health-related quality of life. J Vasc Surg. 2000;32:130-7.

10. Semba CP, Razavi MK, Kee ST, Sze DY, Dake MD. Thrombolysis for lower extremity deep venous thrombosis. Tech Vasc Interv Radiol. 2004;7:68-78.

11. Mewissen MW, Seabrook GR, Meissner MH, Cynamon J, Labropoulos N, Haughton

SH. Catheter-directed thrombolysis for lower extremity deep venous thrombosis: report of a national multicenter registry. Radiology. 1999;211:39-49.

12. Lieberman S, Safadi R, Aner H, Verstandig A, Sasson T, Bloom AI. Local thrombolysis for the treatment of patients with proximal deep vein thrombosis of the leg. Harefuah. 2002;141:424-9.

13. AbuRahma AF, Pekins SE, Wulu JT, Ng HK. Iliofemoral deep vein thrombosis: conventional therapy versus lysis and percutaneous transluminal angioplasty and stenting. Ann Surg. 2001;233:752-60.

14. Ouriel K, Grey B, Clair DG, Olin J. Complications associated with the use of urokinase and recombinant tissue plasminogen activator for catheter directed peripheral aterial and venous thrombolysis. J Vasc Interv Radiol. 2000;11:295-8.

15. McLafferty RB. Endovascular management of deep venous thrombosis. Perspect Vasc Surg Endovasc Ther. 2008;20:87-91.

16. Braaten JV, Goss RA, Francis CW. Ultrasound reversibly disaggregates fibrin fibers. Thromb Haemost. 1997;78:1063-8.

17. Francis CW, Blinc A, Lee S, Cox C. Ultrasound accelerates transport of recombinant tissue plasminogen activator into clots. Ultrasound Med Biol. 1995;21: 419-24.

18. Parikh S, Motarjeme A, McNamara T, Raabe R, Hagspiel K, Benenati JF, et al. Ultrasound-accelerated thrombolysis for the treatment of deep vein thrombosis: initial clinical experience. J Vasc Interv Radiol. 2008;19: 521-8.

19. Lin PH, Zhou W, Dardick A, Mussa F, Kougias P, Hedayati N, et al. Catheter-directed thrombolysis versus pharmacomechanical thrombectomy for treatment of symptomatic lower extremity deep venous thrombosis. Am J Surg. 2006;192:782-8.

20. Arko F, Davis CM, Murphy EH, Smith ST, Timaran CH, Modrall JG, et al. Aggressive percutaneous mechanical thrombosis: Early clinical results. Arch Surg. 2007;142:513-8.

21. Kasirajan K, Grey B, Ouriel K. Percutaneous AngioJet thrombectomy in the management of extensive deep venous thrombosis. J Vasc Interv Radiol. 2001;12(2):179-85.

22. Bush RL, Lin PH, Bates JT, Mureebe L, Zhou W, Lumsden AB. Pharmacomechanical thrombectomy for treatment of symptomatic lower extremity deep venous thrombosis: safety and feasibility study. J Vasc Surg. 2004;40:965-70.

23. Piercy KT, Ayerdi J, Geary RL, Hansen KJ, Edwards MS. Acute pancreatitis: a complication associated with rheolytic mechanical thrombectomy of deep venous thrombosis. J Vasc Surg. 2006;44(5):1110-3.

24. Hilleman DE, Pharm D, Razavi MK. Clinical and economic evaluation of the Trellis-8 infusion catheter for deep vein thrombosis. J Vasc Interv Radiol. 2008;19:377-83.

25. O'Sullivan GJ, Lohan DG, Gough N, Cronin CG, Kee ST. Pharmacomechanical thrombectomy of acute deep vein thrombosis with the Trellis-8 isolated thrombolysis catheter. J Vasc Interv Radiol. 2007;715-24.

26. McLafferty RB. Endovascular management of deep venous thrombosis. Perspect Vasc Surg Endovasc Ther. 2008;20:87-91.

Surgical Thrombectomy

Indications, Techniques, and Outcomes

Bo Eklöf

The options for early removal of an acute thrombus in the proximal veins of the leg are (1) catheter-directed thrombolysis (CDT), (2) percutaneous pharmacomechanical thrombectomy (PMT), and (3) surgical thrombectomy (TE). In this chapter, we propose that if CDT or PMT fails or is contraindicated, surgical TE is a valid alternative, primarily in acute iliofemoral vein thrombosis (IFVT). The techniques and results of this procedure are presented.

Venous Thromboembolic Disease. Contemporary Endovascular Management series. © 2011 Mark G. Davies MD and Alan B. Lumsden MD, eds. Cardiotext Publishing, ISBN 978-1-935395-22-5.

Rationale for Early Thrombus Removal

When deep venous thrombosis (DVT) occurs, the goals of therapy are (1) to prevent the extension or recurrence of the deep venous thrombus and fatal pulmonary embolism (PE) and (2) to minimize the early and late sequelae of DVT. Antithrombotic therapy can accomplish the former goal, but contributes little to the second. Particularly in proximal DVT (ie, IFVT), progressive swelling of the leg can lead to phlegmasia cerulea dolens (literally, painful blue swelling), and to increased compartmental pressure, which can progress to venous gangrene and limb loss. Later, the development of severe post-thrombotic syndrome (PTS) can result from persistent obstruction of the venous outflow and/or loss of valvular competence; and pulmonary embolism can lead to chronic pulmonary hypertension.

Most clinicians seem to focus on the initial treatment (ie, preventing PE, the propagation of the thrombus, or DVT recurrence), with little attention to the limb sequelae, possibly swayed by the medical literature, which demonstrates, in randomized clinical trials (RCTs), that antithrombotic therapy, particularly low molecular weight heparin (LMWH), can achieve these goals. There is a lack of appreciation that the endpoints of these RCTs have not been prevention of postthrombotic sequelae. However, 2 RCTs have compared the late outcome several years after acute, symptomatic proximal DVT in patients who wore compression stockings with those who did not.[1,2]

Both studies, one performed with custom-made thigh-length stockings and one using calf-length ready-made stockings, showed that consequent wearing of stockings could reduce the frequency of a postthrombotic syndrome to one-half. Partsch et al. performed an RCT in 53 patients with proximal DVT, comparing bed rest without compression with walking exercises using either compression stockings or bandages, all undergoing anticoagulation with LMWH.[3] At follow-up after 2 years, a significantly better outcome could be found in the mobile group than in the bed rest group, as judged by the Prandoni scale (median score 5.0 vs. 8.0, $P < 0.01$).

Furthermore, there is apparently also a lack of appreciation of the different natural history of IFVT compared to more distal DVT, as well as a lack of understanding of the different pathophysiologic changes that occur with time following DVT, and their relative contribution to the pathogenesis and severity of the postthrombotic sequelae. These are reviewed in this chapter to provide a selective basis for the decision to opt for early thrombus removal.

Pathophysiological Changes Associated with DVT

The clinical outcome after DVT can be categorized into 4 basic patient subgroups: (1) those with neither detectable obstruction nor valvular incompetence, (2) those with obstruction alone, (3) those with valvular incompetence alone, and (4) those with both outflow obstruction and distal valvular incompetence. Noninvasive testing[4] has shown that less than 20% of those with documented DVT have neither significant obstruction nor reflux. In a 5-year follow-up of 20 patients treated with anticoagulation alone in a Swedish prospective, randomized study in acute IFVT[5] there was residual iliac vein obstruction in 70% of patients and valvular incompetence and pathological muscle pump function in all patients, creating severe venous hypertension and contributing to the severity of the postthrombotic sequelae. However, the overall outcome of DVT, in terms of disturbed venous physiology, depends to a great degree on the location of the thrombosed segments and the extent of involvement (ie, single or multiple segments). The former relates to the likelihood of recanalization of the thrombosed segment, which, in the lower extremity, decreases as one moves proximally. Venographic studies, which were only commonly performed in the 1950s and 1960s, showed that close to 95% of popliteal or tibial thromboses recanalize completely,[6] and at least 50% of femoral venous thromboses recanalize.[7]

In contrast, the minority of iliofemoral thromboses (less than 20%) completely recanalize and form a normal, unobstructed lumen.[8] However, while it is true that only 20% of the iliac vein segments involved in IFVT completely recanalize spontaneously, another 60% partly recanalize, or at least develop adequate enough collaterals that they do not test positive for obstruction on non-invasive study. Thus, in reality, only about 20% remain significantly occluded enough or have such poor collaterals to produce symptomatic venous outflow obstruction detectable on noninvasive physiologic testing, if time (3 to 6 months) is allowed for complete resolution. Nevertheless, a significant degree of obstruction persists for these 3 to 6 months in the majority of patients with iliofemoral venous thrombosis. What is not well appreciated is that persisting proximal obstruction, even if it is ultimately relieved by partial recanalization or collateral development, can lead to progressive breakdown of distal valves, resulting in reflux. This is important because, if the distal venous valves (and particularly those in the popliteal vein) remain competent, the postthrombotic sequelae are relatively modest and controllable by conservative measures.[9] The severity of postthrombotic sequelae correlates with the level of ambulatory venous pressure (AVP), as shown by Nicolaides et al.[10] It is impressive how steadily the frequency of ulceration climbs with increasing levels of AVP. It suggests that anything that significantly reduces AVP will reduce the severity of the PTS, and vice versa. Nicolaides and Sumner[11] have also shown that the highest levels of AVP are found in patients with both obstruction and reflux.

These 2 observations underscore a major point to be made in regard to the disturbed pathophysiology associated with iliofemoral venous thrombosis and the pathogenesis of postthrombotic sequelae. Obstruction alone is rarely sufficient enough to cause venous claudication and mostly causes increased swelling with activity. Valvular incompetence alone causes most of the "stasis sequelae" (pigmentation, lipoder-matosclerosis, and ulceration), but these too can be managed, in the compliant patient, with elastic stockings and elevation. However, those with both obstruction and valvular incompetence have severe postthrombotic sequelae, so severe, in fact, that conservative management is difficult even in a compliant patient.

The importance of the proximal obstruction for the development of distal valvular incompetence has been carefully studied by D. Eugene Strandness Jr. and his group. In a series of articles, they have shown the following: from 20% to 50% of initially uninvolved distal veins become incompetent by 2 years; the combination of reflux and obstruction, as opposed to either alone, correlated with the severity of symptoms and was present in 55% of symptomatic patients; 25% of all venous segments developed reflux in time, of which 32% were documented to not have been previously involved with thrombosis; and finally, in a study of the posterior tibial veins located below a popliteal segment involved with thrombosis, 55% of the distal veins became incompetent if the segment remained obstructed, compared to 7.5% of those below a popliteal vein that recanalized.[12] These changes in the distal veins occur early enough that they cannot be blamed on proximal valvular reflux, although this also comes into play with time. Thus, it would appear that the early relief of obstructing thrombus by thrombolysis or thrombectomy should prevent more extensive postthrombotic sequelae if only by protecting the distal veins against progressive valvular incompetence. This is a point that has not been well recognized not only in terms of basic pathogenesis but in judging the results of thrombolysis and thrombectomy, where critics have largely ignored the restoration of proximal patency while focusing on the presence or absence of valve reflux.

Another aspect of the importance of early thrombus removal is the new data appearing on the inflammatory response to DVT. Thomas Wakefield and his group in Ann Arbor have shown that the leukocyte adhesion molecule—P-selectin—activates the leukocytes emigrating into the venous wall, creating an inflammation that destroys the venous wall and the valves. John Harris and his group from Stanford[13] showed, in another experimental model, that if the thrombus was removed early, the inflammatory changes were reversible.

Finally, while modern venous reconstructive valvuloplasty can achieve good long-term results in primary venous disease with severe reflux, the results of vein segment transfer and autologous vein transplantation in secondary (ie, postthrombotic) venous disease are much less promising.[14] Therefore, there are less suitable late interventions for the venous derangements typically seen in patients with severe PTS. The common mistake is for clinicians to treat all DVT patients with anticoagulation only, and belatedly refer those who complain of severe pain and swelling during follow-up for consideration of thrombolysis or thrombectomy—too late for them to achieve their goals.

The conclusions from this and all the other studies cited are clear: early removal of the thrombus conveys significant benefits, and the earlier the removal, the better the outcome.

Diagnosis

Whether DVT is suspected on the basis of pain, on the basis of discoloration or swelling of one leg, or in search of a source for pulmonary embolism, the diagnosis can be confirmed with accuracy by duplex scanning using color flow imaging. Clinical signs are more likely to be present in proximal DVT (ie, IFVT), but in bedridden patients there may be no apparent swelling and the first signs may be those of PE (pleuritic chest pain, shortness of breath, and/or hemoptysis). Duplex scanning should interrogate not only the femoral and popliteal veins, but the iliac and calf veins as well; otherwise, 30% of DVT will be missed.

Venography is mainly used now when catheter-directed interventions or surgical TE are indicated, to guide and monitor them. Standard ascending venography using foot vein injection may miss isolated iliac vein thrombosis unless an adequate contrast load is infused. In cases of IFVT, with extension into the iliac vein without visualization of the upper end of the thrombus, a femoral venogram from the contralateral side is performed to visualize the inferior vena cava (IVC) and determine the upper extent of thrombus extension. An alternative to the conventional venogram is a CT venogram, particularly if this is indicated for diagnosis of PE.

Indications for Intervention

Early clot removal has clear benefit in 2 categories of patients, with IFVT falling at the 2 ends of the clinical spectrum: (1) in active healthy patients with good longevity in order to prevent or mitigate potentially severe late postthrombotic sequelae and (2) in those with massive swelling and phlegmasia cerulea dolens in order to mitigate early morbidity and prevent progression to venous gangrene. Older patients with significant intercurrent disease and serious comorbidities who are unlikely to be active and live a long life, or those with distal thrombosis, should be treated by anticoagulant therapy. Late PTS is not likely to be an issue with them.

However, even these patients, if faced with the threat of venous gangrene, may deserve prompt clot removal.

In terms of the choice of method of clot removal, CDT is an appropriate choice for removing obstructing thrombus and thereby preserving valve function, although the latter has been presumed rather than proven. If CDT cannot be achieved, the clot removal or dissolution is unsuccessful or does not progress satisfactorily, or the concomitant anticoagulation is contraindicated (eg, IFVT in young women in the peripartum period, or in certain postoperative or trauma patients), then surgical TE or PMT is an appropriate choice.

Historical Background of Venous Thrombectomy in the United States

The history of venous TE in the United States is quite interesting and reveals misconceptions that underscore its current infrequent use. John Homans, an advocate for division of the femoral vein to prevent PE, first suggested thrombectomy in a paper entitled "Exploration and division of the femoral and iliac veins in the treatment of thrombophlebitis of the leg,"[15] presented at the New England Surgical Society in 1940. In this paper, Homans discussed indications for TE with or without ligation of the femoral vein, the technique, the complications, and the importance to prevent reflux.

However, the modern era of TE in the United States started with Howard Mahorner's paper "New management for thrombosis of deep veins of extremities" in 1954,[16] where he advocated TE followed by restoration of vein lumen and regional heparinization. He presented 6 patients, 5 of whom had an excellent result with rapid disappearance of leg swelling, very little late morbidity, and minimum leg edema. There was no PE prior or subsequent to surgery. Mahorner claimed that this method restores vein function with preservation of the vein lumen and vein valves. In a follow-up paper in 1957,[17] he reported 16 patients where TE was performed in 14 legs and 2 arms with excellent results in 12, good in 2, and poor in 2 patients. The enthusiasm for TE created by Mahorner received strong support by the report by Haller and Abrams in 1963.[18] They presented 45 patients with IFVT who underwent TE. In 34 patients with short history (<10 days), excellent bidirectional flow was established in 31 patients (91%). At follow-up after an average of 18 months, 26 out of these 31 patients (84%) had normal legs, and where ascending venography was permitted in 13 patients, normal patency of the deep venous system was demonstrated in 11 (85%).

However, enthusiasm quickly subsided after Lansing and Davis presented their 5-year follow-up of Haller and Abrams's patients in 1968.[19] Of Haller and Abrams 34 patients with short history, only 17 patients (50%) were interviewed, but 16 patients were found to have swelling of the leg requiring stockings and one patient had developed an ulcer. Ascending venography in the supine position was performed in 15 patients, showing patent veins but "the involved area of the deep venous system was found to be incompetent in all cases and there were no functioning valves." Unfortunately, the flaws in Lansing and Davis's study were not recognized and discussed widely enough: (1) they studied only half of the original cohort, and likely those with symptoms bringing them back to the vascular clinic; (2) the outstanding late patency of the thrombectomized veins was completely ignored; and

(3) incompetence of the valves in the femoral and popliteal veins cannot reliably be assessed from an ascending venographic study in the supine position.

In a 1969 paper, "Iliofemoral venous thrombosis: reappraisal of thrombectomy,"[20] William Edwards argued with Lansing's results and concluded that "venous TE offers an effective and safe method of restoring flow in the deep venous system; when the thrombus is less than 10 days in duration and is of the iliofemoral segment, TE is recommended; venograms at operation to determine the patency of the deep venous system will aid in complete removal of the thrombus and give a basis for later comparison and evaluation of long-term patency." In the discussion, Lansing repeated his findings from the 5-year follow-up, still questioning the value of TE, but Haller, who was never consulted about the follow-up report, stated that, at a recent visit to Louisville, he had studied 17 patients in whom total removal of the thrombus had been possible and none had significant residual edema. Despite this rebuttal, the impact of Lansing's study, combined with Karp and Wylie's subsequent 1-page report[21] in the *Surgical Forum* of 10 patients in whom 8 had reocclusion of the femoral vein before discharge (even though all had phlegmasia cerulea dolens and extensive thrombosis) was profound: only a few series on TE were subsequently published from the United States, in spite of the fact that they all showed very good clinical results in >75% of patients.

Surgical Thrombectomy

The first TE for IFVT was performed by Läwen, in Germany in 1937.[22] Surgery today is performed under general intubation anesthesia with 10-cm positive end-expiratory pressure (PEEP) added during manipulation of the thrombus to prevent perioperative PE. The involved leg, contralateral groin, and abdomen are prepared. A cell saver is used to minimize blood loss. A longitudinal incision is made in the groin to expose the great saphenous vein (GSV), which is followed to its confluence with the common femoral vein (CFV), which is dissected up to the inguinal ligament. The superficial femoral artery is cleared off 3 to 4 cm below the femoral bifurcation for construction of the arteriovenous fistula (AVF). In primary IFVT, where the thrombus originates in the iliac vein with subsequent distal progression of the thrombus, a longitudinal venotomy is made in the CFV, and a venous Fogarty TE catheter is passed upward through the thrombus into the IVC. The balloon is inflated and withdrawn, these maneuvers being repeated until no more thrombotic material can be extracted. With the balloon left inflated in the common iliac vein, a suction catheter is introduced to the level of the internal iliac vein to evacuate thrombi from this vein.

Backflow is not a reliable sign of thrombus clearance since a proximal valve in the external iliac vein may be present in 25% of cases, preventing retrograde flow in a cleared vein. On the other hand, backflow can be excellent from the internal iliac vein and its tributaries despite a remaining occlusion of the common iliac vein. Therefore, an intraoperative completion venogram is mandatory. An alternative is the use of an angioscope, which enables removal of residual thrombus material under direct vision, or intravascular ultrasound (IVUS). In early cases, the distal thrombus is usually readily extruded through the venotomy by manual massage of the leg distally, starting at the foot. The Fogarty venous catheter, with a soft flexible tip, can sometimes be advanced in retrograde fashion without significant trauma. The aim is to remove all fresh thrombi from the leg. The venotomy is closed with continuous suture and an AVF created using the saphenous vein, anastomosing it end-to-side to the superficial femoral artery (for illustrations, see Elköf et al[12]). An intraoperative venogram is performed through a catheter inserted in a branch of the AVF. After a satisfactory completion venogram the wound is closed in layers and a closed suction drain is placed in the wound to evacuate blood and lymphatic fluid that may accumulate after the operation.

In IFVT secondary to ascending thrombosis from the calf, the thrombus in the femoral vein may be old and adherent to the venous wall. In such cases, the chance of preserving valve function has already been lost and the opportunity to restore patency significantly diminished. A femoral segment without functioning valves will lead to distal valve dysfunction in time, much as will failure to achieve proximal patency. However, a patent iliac venous outflow plus a competent profunda collateral system will most of the time achieve normal venous function. Therefore, if iliac patency is established but the thrombus in the femoral vein is too old to remove, it is preferable to ligate the femoral vein. If normal flow in the femoral vein cannot be reestablished, we recommend extending the incision distally and exploring the orifices of the deep femoral branches. These are isolated, and venous flow is restored with a small Fogarty catheter. The femoral vein is then ligated distal to the profunda branches. In a 13-year follow-up after femoral vein ligation in this setting, Masuda et al[23] found excellent clinical and physiological results without PTS. Finally, if there is evidence of iliac vein compression on the completion venogram, which can occur in about 50% of left-sided IFVT, we recommend intraoperative endovenous iliac angioplasty and stenting.

If phlegmasia cerulea dolens is the indication, because of the threat of impending venous gangrene, we start the operation with fasciotomy of the calf compartments to release the pressure and improve the circulation immediately. If there is extension of the thrombus into the IVC, the cava is approached transperitoneally through a subcostal incision. The IVC is exposed by deflecting the ascending colon and duodenum medially. Depending on the venographic findings relative to the top of the thrombus, the IVC is controlled, usually just below the renal veins. The IVC is opened and the thrombus is removed by massage, especially of the iliac venous system; then if the femoral segment is involved, the operation is continued in the groin as described previously. As an alternative, a retrievable caval filter can be introduced before the TE to protect against fatal PE. Heparin is continued at least 5 days postoperatively, and warfarin is started the first postop day and continued routinely for 6 months. The patient is ambulated the day after the operation wearing a compression stocking and is usually discharged after a week, to return after 6 weeks for closure of the fistula.

The objectives of a temporary AVF are to increase blood flow in the thrombectomized iliac segment to prevent immediate rethrombosis, to allow time for healing of the endothelium, and to promote development of collaterals in case of incomplete clearance or immediate rethrombosis of the iliac segment. Usually the AVF is performed between the saphenous vein and the superficial femoral artery. More distally placed AVFs have not been functional, in our experience.

A new percutaneous technique for fistula closure was developed by Endrys in Kuwait.[24] Through a puncture of the femoral artery on the opposite, surgically untouched side, a catheter is inserted and positioned at the fistula level. Prior to release of a coil, an arteriovenogram can be performed to evaluate the patency of the iliac and caval veins, which is of prognostic value. More than 10% of patients have been shown to have remaining significant stenosis of the iliac vein despite initial successful surgery. A percutaneous, transvenous angioplasty and stenting can be performed under the protection of the AVF, which is closed 4 weeks later.

Complications and Results of Surgical Thrombectomy

One reason that induced surgeons to abandon thrombectomy in the 1960s was the high mortality associated with early thombectomy. In our series of more than 200 patients, mortality was less than 1%. There was no case of fatal PE in the perioperative period. In an RCT from Sweden,[25] perfusion lung scans were positive on admission in 45% of all patients, with additional defects seen after 1 and 4 weeks in the conservatively treated group, in 11% and 12% respectively, and in the thrombectomized group in 20% and 0%, respectively. Tables with results from the literature are available in Rutherford's sixth edition of *Vascular Surgery*.[12] In the RCT from Sweden where TE was combined with a temporary AVF, 13% of patients had early rethrombosis of the iliac vein.[26] In the Swedish RCT, iliac vein patency at 6 months was 76% in the surgical group compared with 35% in the conservative group, as demonstrated by venography.[26] This significant difference was upheld after 5 and 10 years, with 77% and 83% patency in the surgical group, respectively, vs. 30% and 41% in the conser-

vative group, respectively.[27,28] Femoropopliteal valvular competence at 6 months was 52% in the surgical group compared with 26% in the conservatively treated group, as monitored by descending venography with Valsalva—a significant difference.[26] After 5 years, combining the results of all functional tests, 36% of the surgical patients had normal venous function compared with 11% of the conservatively treated group.[27] These differences were not statistically significant due to loss of patients. At 10 years, using duplex scanning, popliteal reflux was found in 32% in the surgical group compared with 67% in the conservative group.[28]

New Developments to Improve TE

There has been a significant improvement of the results of surgical TE with the understanding to immediately restore iliac vein outflow in patients with iliac vein obstruction as the major cause of their DVT. Control of iliac vein outflow immediately after TE can be achieved by intraoperative venogram, angioscopy, or IVUS. In remaining obstructions, intraoperative endovenous angioplasty and stenting are recommended. Schwarzbach et al. report excellent results in 18 of 20 patients who maintained patency after 21 months of followup.[29] To improve patency and preservation of the valves in the deep veins of the leg Blättler et al. has combined TE of the iliac vein with thrombolysis applied under ischemic conditions to the leg veins.[30] None of the 33 patients experienced clinically apparent recurrence within the first year. Clinical signs of the postthrombotic syndrome were absent in all but 1 patient.

With improved outflow through the iliac system by angioplasty and stenting and increased inflow from the improved distal patency by regional thrombolysis, the temporary AVF may not be necessary. An excellent review of contemporary venous thrombectomy is published by Comerota and Gale 2006.[31]

Evidence-Based Recommendations

The ACCP recommendations from 2004 (Büller, Agnelli, Hull, Hyers, Prins, Raskob)[32] for treatment of acute venous thromboembolism concerning early thrombus removal are the following:

- In patients with DVT or PE the routine use of systemic thrombolytic treatment is not recommended (grade 1A).
- In selected DVT patients, such as those with massive iliofemoral DVT at risk of limb gangrene secondary to venous occlusion, IV thrombolysis is suggested (grade 2C).
- In patients with DVT, we recommend against the routine use of catheter-directed thrombolysis (grade 1C).
- In DVT patients confining catheter-directed thrombolysis to selected patients, such as those requiring limb salvage is suggested (grade 2C).
- In patients with DVT, we recommend against the routine use of venous thrombectomy (grade 1C).
- In selected patients, such as patients with massive iliofemoral DVT at risk of limb gangrene secondary to venous occlusion, venous thrombectomy is suggested (grade 2C).

In the international consensus statement— guidelines according to scientific evidence 2006[33]—the following recommendations are suggested:

- Catheter-directed thrombolysis should be considered for proximal DVT, especially iliofemoral thrombosis in active patients at low risk for bleeding, where the risk of the postthrombotic syndrome is higher than for more distal DVT (grade B). Systemic thrombolysis should be avoided because it is less effective, and because the longer duration of therapeutic infusion required increases the risk of hemorrhagic complications.
- Surgical venous thrombectomy should be considered for patients with symptomatic iliofemoral DVT who are not candidates for catheter-directed thrombolysis (grade C).
- Data concerning the short- and long-term effects of catheter-based mechanical intervention on the vessel wall, venous valve, and pulmonary vasculature are lacking and are required before its role can be clearly defined. This technique needs further short- and long-term evaluation and eventually randomized controlled trials before any recommendations can be made.

The ACCP recommendations from 2008 (Kearon, Kahn, Agnelli, Goldhaber, Raskob, Comerota)[34] are more in favor of early thrombus removal:

- In selected patients with extensive acute proximal DVT (eg, iliofemoral DVT, symptoms for <14 days, good functional status, life expectancy >1 year) who have a low risk of bleeding, we suggest that CDT may be used to reduce acute symptoms and postthrombotic morbidity if appropriate expertise and resources are available.

- After successful CDT in patients with acute DVT, we suggest correction of underlying venous lesions using balloon angioplasty and stents (grade 2C).

- We suggest pharmacomechanical thrombolysis (eg, with inclusion of thrombus fragmentation and/ or aspiration) in preference to CDT alone to shorten treatment time if appropriate expertise and resources are available (grade 2C).

- We suggest that they should not be treated with PMT alone (grade 2C).

- In selected patients with acute iliofemoral DVT (eg, symptoms for <7 days, good functional status, and life expectancy >1 year), we suggest that operative venous thrombectomy may be used to reduce acute symptoms and postthrombotic morbidity if appropriate expertise and resources are available (grade 2B). If such patients do not have a high risk of bleeding, we suggest that CDT is usually preferable to operative venous thrombectomy (grade 2C).

- In patients who undergo any of these interventions, we recommend the same intensity and duration of anticoagulant therapy afterwards as for comparable patients who do not undergo intervention (grade 1C).

Conclusion

Acute iliofemoral deep venous thrombosis remains a severely debilitating problem. Prevention of extension of thrombus, pulmonary embolism, and postthrombotic syndrome remain the primary objectives in treating these patients. More and more data now show that early removal of thrombus provides a better outcome for patients compared to anticoagulation alone. Multiple treatment modalities such as catheter-directed thrombolysis and percutaneous mechanical thrombectomy are now available in addition to surgical thrombectomy. In proper hands, percutaneous techniques for thrombus removal are becoming the first-line treatment with durable outcomes being reported. More clinical trials are needed to assist in determining optimal patient selection to improve immediate success, limit complications, and provide long-term freedom from disease. Figure 10.1 suggests a treatment algorithm for acute iliofemoral thrombosis.

Addendum

Acute Venous Thrombosis: Thrombus Removal with Adjunctive Catheter-Directed Thrombolysis: The ATTRACT Trial This is the NIH-sponsored prospective randomized trial with the primary objective to determine if the initial adjunctive use of pharmacomechanical catheter-directed thrombolysis in symptomatic patients with acute proximal DVT reduces the occurrence of the postthrombotic syndrome (PTS) over 24-month's follow-up. Three methods of initial rtPA will be used: (1) Trellis-8 peripheral infusion system; (2) AngioJet rheolytic thrombectomy system; or (3) catheter-directed rtPA infusion. The control arm will be treated with conventional anticoagulation and compression stockings. The primary efficacy outcome is cumulative incidence of PTS within 24 months, using the Villalta PTS scale. Six hundred ninety-two patients will be included in 30 to 50 centers in the United States, and the study, which started in October 2008, is scheduled to finish in March 2013.

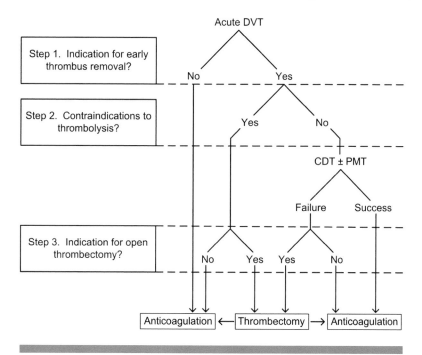

FIGURE 10.1   Treatment algorithm for acute iliofemoral thrombosis. CDT = catheter-directed thrombolysis; PMT = percutaneous mechanical thrombectomy.

References

1. Brandjes DP, Büller HR, Heijboer H, Huisman MV, de Rijk M, Jagt H, et al. Incidence of the postthrombotic syndrome and the effects of compression stockings in patients with proximal venous thrombosis. Lancet. 1997;349:759-62.

2. Prandoni P, Lensing AW, Prins MH, Frulla M, Marchiori A, Bernardi E, et al. Below-knee elastic stockings to prevent the post-thrombotic syndrome. Ann Intern Med. 2004;141:249-56.

3. Partsch H, Kaulich M, Mayer W. Immediate mobilisation in acute venous thrombosis reduces postthrombotic syndrome. Int Angiology. 2004;23:206-12.

4. Lindner DJ, Edwards JM, Phinney ES, Taylor LM Jr, Porter JM. Long-term hemodynamic and clinical sequelae of lower extremity deep vein thrombosis. J Vasc Surg. 1986;4:436-42.

5. Åkesson H, Brundin L, Dahlström JA, et al. Venous function assessed during a 5 year period after acute iliofemoral venous thrombosis treated with anticoagulation. Euro J Vasc Surg. 1990;4:43-48.

6. Arenander E. Varicosity and ulceration of the lower limb: a clinical follow-up study of 247 patients examined phlebographically. Acta Chir Scand. 1957;12:135-44.

7. Thomas ML, McAllister V. The radiological progression of deep venous thrombosis. Radiology. 1971;99:37-40.

8. Mavor GE, Galloway JMD. Iliofemoral venous thrombosis: pathological considerations and surgical management. Br J Surg. 1969;56:45-59.

9. Shull KC, Nicolaides AN, Fernandes é Fernandes J, Miles C, Horner J, et al. Significance of popliteal reflux in relation to ambulatory venous pressure and ulceration. Arch Surg. 1979;114:1304-6.

10. Nicolaides AN, Hussein MK, Szendro G, Christopoulos D, Vasdekis S, Clarke H. The relation of venous ulceration with ambulatory venous pressure measurements. J Vasc Surg. 1993;17:414-9.

11. Nicolaides AN, Sumner DS, eds. Investigation of Patients with Deep Vein Thrombosis and Chronic Venous Insufficiency. Los Angeles: Med-Orion Publishing Company; 1991.

12. Eklöf B, Rutherford RB. Surgical thrombectomy for acute deep venous thrombosis. In: Rutherford RB, ed. Vascular Surgery. 6th ed. Elsevier, Saunders; 2005. p2188-98.

13. See-Tho K, Harris EJ Jr. Thrombosis with outflow obstruction delays thrombolysis and results in chronic wall thickening of rat veins. J Vasc Surg. 1998;28:115-22.

14. Kistner RL. Valve repair and segment transposition in primary valvular insufficiency. In: Bergan JJ, Yao JST, eds. Venous Disorders. Philadelphia: WB Saunders; 1991. p261-72.

15. Homans J. Exploration and division of the femoral and iliac veins in the treatment of thrombophlebitits of the leg. JAMA. 1941;224:179-86.

16. Mahorner H. New management for thrombosis of deep veins of extremities. Am Surg. 1954;20:487-98.

17. Mahorner H, Castleberry JW, Coleman WO. Attempts to restore function in major veins which are the site of massive thrombosis. Ann Surg. 1957;146:510-22.

18. Haller JAJ, Abrams BL. Use of thrombectomy in the treatment of acute iliofemoral venous thrombosis in forty-five patients. Ann Surg. 1963;158:561-9.

19. Lansing AM, Davis WM. Five-year follow-up study of iliofemoral venous thrombectomy. Ann Surg. 1968;168:620-8.

20. Edwards WH, Sawyers JL, Foster JH. Iliofemoral venous thrombosis: reappraisal of thrombectomy. Ann Surg. 1970;171: 961-70.

21. Karp RB, Wylie EJ. Recurrent thrombosis after iliofemoral venous thrombectomy. Surg Forum. 1966;17:147-9.

22. Läwen A. Uber thrombectomie bei Venenthrombose und Arteriespasmus. Zentralbl Chir. 1937;64:961-8.

23. Masuda EM, Kistner RL, Ferris EB. Long-term effects of superficial femoral vein ligation: thirteen-year follow-up. J Vasc Surg. 1992;16:741-9.

24. Endrys J, Eklöf B, Neglén P, Zýka I, Peregrin J. Percutaneous balloon occlusion of surgical arteriovenous fistulae following venous thrombectomy. Cardiovasc Inter Rad. 1989;12:226-9.

25. Plate G, Ohlin P, Eklöf B. Pulmonary embolism in acute iliofemoral venous thrombosis. Br J Surg. 1985;72:912.

26. Plate G, Einarsson E, Ohlin P, Jensen R, Qvarfordt P, Eklöf B. Thrombectomy with temporary arteriovenous fistula: the treatment of choice in acute iliofemoral venous thrombosis. J Vasc Surg. 1984;1:867-76.

27. Plate G, Akesson H, Einarsson E, Ohlin P, Eklöf B. Long-term results of venous thrombectomy combined with a temporary arterio-venous fistula. Eur J Vasc Surg. 1990;4:483-9.

28. Plate G, Eklöf B, Norgren L, Ohlin P, Dahlström JA. Venous thrombectomy for iliofemoral vein thrombosis: 10-year results of a prospective randomized study. Eur J Endovasc Surg. 1997;14:367-74.

29. Schwarzbach MH, Schumacher H, Böckler D, Fürstenberger S, Thomas F, Seelos R, et al. Surgical thrombectomy followed by intraoperative endovascular reconstruction for symptomatic iliofemoral venous thrombosis. Eur J Vasc Endovasc Surg. 2005;29:58-66.

30. Blättler W, Heller G, Largiadèr J, Savolainen H, Gloor B, Schmidli J. Combined regional thrombolysis and surgical thrombectomy for treatment of iliofemoral vein thrombosis. J Vasc Surg. 2004;40:620-5.

31. Comerota AJ, Gale SS. Technique of contemporary iliofemoral and infrainguinal venous thrombectomy. J Vasc Surg. 2006;43:185-91.

32. Büller HR, Agnelli G, Hull RD, Hyers TM, Prins MH, Raskob GE. Antithrombotic therapy for venous thromboembolic disease: the seventh ACCP conference on antithrombotic and thrombolytic therapy. Chest. 2004;126:401S-28S.

33. Nicolaides AN, Fareed J, Kakkar AK, Breddin HK, Goldhaber SZ, Hull R, et al. Prevention and treatment of venous thromboembolism: international consensus statement. (guidelines according to scientific evidence). Int Angiol. 2006;25:101-61.

34. Kearon C, Kahn SR, Agnelli G, Goldhaber S, Raskob GE, Comerota AJ. Antithrombotic therapy for venous thromboembolic disease. Chest. 2008;133:454S-545S.

IVC Filters

Indications, Techniques, and Outcomes

Joseph P. Hart and Claudio J. Schönholz

The inferior vena cava (IVC) filter is implanted with the primary intent to prevent fatal pulmonary embolism. The most basic indications for placement of IVC filters are: contraindication to anticoagulation, a failure of anticoagulation to prevent pulmonary embolism (PE), a deep venous thrombosis (DVT) occurring while on anticoagulation, or an anticoagulated patient for DVT or PE developing a complication from anticoagulation, requiring cessation of therapy. Prophylactic indications are evolving but controversial and are somewhat variable from author to author and from institution to institution. Development of the vena cava filter is attributed to a vascular surgeon, Lazar Greenfield, and a petroleum engineer, Garman Kimmell. Greenfield was motivated by the death of a trauma patient with multiple orthopedic injuries that could not be salvaged from fatal pulmonary embolism. They borrowed from technology used in oil pipelines in which retained sludge and debris are trapped by a cone-shaped filter. Such a filter allows oil to continue to flow around its peripheral edges while allowing debris to slowly erode from the midportion of the filter. Likewise, Greenfield's intent was to create a filter that would trap thromboembolic debris in its central portion and allow continued venous flow around it. This system permits the resolution of the clot over time, prevention of pulmonary embolism, and eventual clearance of the clot from the filter in most cases, so that another episode could be resolved in a similar fashion, all while maintaining caval patency.

The device and the procedure have become increasingly common due to the general escalation of enthusiasm for endovascular procedures, relatively straightforward nature

Venous Thromboembolic Disease. Contemporary Endovascular Management series. © 2011 Mark G. Davies MD and Alan B. Lumsden MD, eds. Cardiotext Publishing, ISBN 978-1-935395-22-5.

of placement, increased patient and practitioner awareness due to educational efforts, and medicolegal concerns about thromboembolism. However, relatively strict adherence to conservative indications for filter placement is advised. Evolving indications such as PE prophylaxis in trauma or bariatric surgery patients are of great interest since venous thromboembolic disease is a significant complication in the management of these patients. However, prospective randomized data in these subgroups are, in general, lacking, and while interest exists in studying these indications, they are not without controversy within the pulmonary, hematologic, general medical, surgical, and endovascular communities. Retrievable filters have further lowered our threshold to utilize IVC filters, especially in these subgroups where the indications are less clear. Retrievability does not equate with actual retrieval. It is thought that since they can be retrieved and are "temporary," most complications due to the filter can be reduced or eliminated with the use of retrievable filters.

The retrievable filters have unique liabilities and these devices do not yet have long-term follow up data. With the recognition of the fact that patients fail to follow up and undergo retrieval, and the technical inability to retrieve the filter either due to placement exceeding the indicated dwell time or to simply technical inability to remove the filter, a relative minority of filters are ever actually retrieved. Thus, although retrievability lends a new and exciting dimension to IVC filter placement and creates the opportunity to do so in a temporary fashion, these devices will require further study to define their exact long-term role in the treatment of patients with venous thromboembolism and/ or prevention of complications from venous thromboembolism. Previous chapters have discussed the pathophysiology and medical treatment of DVT and PE, and in this chapter, we discuss the indications, techniques, and outcomes for placement of IVC filters.

IVC Filter Indications

Only one trial, by Decousus and colleagues, published in the *New England Journal of Medicine* in 1998, has been performed that established the role of inferior vena cava filter use.[1-3] This trial demonstrated that IVC filters are effective in preventing pulmonary embolism in patients with proximal deep venous thrombosis. Four hundred patients with proximal DVT were randomly assigned to placement of IVC filter or no placement of IVC filter, with 200 patients in each group. They found significant differences in incidence of all PE between the 2 groups at day 12. In the filter group, 2 patients, or 1.1%, had either a symptomatic or asymptomatic PE, whereas 9 patients in the no-filter group, or 4.8%, had a symptomatic or asymptomatic PE. Four types of permanent IVC filters were placed, and the authors concluded that in high-risk patients with proximal DVT, there was a significant early beneficial effect of vena cava filter placement for the prevention of PE. However, this was in part offset by an increased rate for recurrent DVT in the filter group and an absence of any difference in mortality between the groups. To this day, this remains the only prospective randomized controlled trial regarding the use of IVC filters to prevent PE.

Despite this, the use of IVC filters has increased dramatically, especially in the United States. This increase is due partially to greater awareness of venous thromboembolic disease (VTE) in general. However, it is clear that further work to evaluate the rational role of IVC filter placement in the treatment of patients with VTE or of patients in need of VTE prophylaxis is necessary. The clearest indications for IVC filter placement are recurrent acute or chronic VTE on adequate therapeutic anticoagulation, contraindication to or complication of anticoagulation in the presence of VTE, and an inability to achieve or maintain therapeutic anticoagulation in the presence of documented VTE. Relative indications include the following: chronic PE treated with thromboendarterectomy; massive PE treated with thrombolysis and/or thrombectomy, filter placement for thrombolysis for iliocaval DVT (controversial); large, free-floating proximal or caval DVT; VTE with limited cardiopulmonary reserve; recurrent PE with a filter in place; difficulty establishing therapeutic anticoagulation; and poor compliance with anticoagulation or high risk for anticoagulation such as unsteady gait or frequent falls. Prophylactic indications for IVC filters are usually cited when primary prophylaxis is not feasible but PE prevention is deemed necessary. Examples of this are a trauma patient with a high risk for VTE, a patient with a high risk for VTE undergoing a surgical procedure, or a medical condition in a patient with a high risk for VTE.[4]

Surgery for morbid obesity is an area in which prophylactic IVC filters are often entertained and placed. Recent data indicate that the fatal PE rate with morbid obesity surgery within 60 days may be as high as 0.85%. Risk factors that contribute to this are underlying venous insufficiency, sleep apnea, and the patient's baseline body mass index (BMI).[5] Abou-Nukta and colleagues compared age and BMI of morbidly obese patients in a randomly selected Roux-en-Y gastric bypass patient control group. Patients were broken down into BMI >55 kg/m^2 and BMI <55 kg/m^2. In super-obese men with BMI >55 kg/m^2 the incidence of PE was 4%. Nine of the 11 patients developed PE after

discharge from the hospital within an average of 10 days. These authors concluded that the super-obese male patient is at a very high risk of developing PE and that their relative risk significantly exceeds that of other Roux-en-Y gastric bypass patients. It was also noteworthy that they found that the PE risk lasted several weeks after discharge, therefore extending PE prophylaxis for several weeks after surgery may be warranted. In the group that had a BMI >55 kg/m^2, patients were assigned to either receive or not receive an IVC filter. In the group with the BMI >55 kg/m^2 that had no IVC filter placed, the PE rate was 28% and the mortality was 11%. In the BMI >55 kg/m^2 group who received filters, there was a 0% incidence of PE and a 0% PE mortality rate. Their conclusion was that there was a significant reduction in the perioperative PE rate when the patient with a BMI >55 kg/m^2 had an IVC filter placed. IVC filters were used in addition to subcutaneous heparin and sequential compression devices (SCD). In the morbidly obese, technical issues for IVC filter placement can arise related to imaging table weight restrictions, inadequate imaging due to body mass, and x-ray penetration issues. Alternative imaging techniques such as intravascular ultrasonography may be useful in this setting. Reports exist of the use of carbon dioxide cavography in these patients. However, published evidence documenting this practice so far is limited.

IVC filter placement in the hands of an experienced practitioner is an extremely safe and low-risk procedure; however, there are contraindications to placement that include the following: an IVC that is either occluded or completely filled with thrombus with no safe region to deploy a filter below the right atrium; active septicemia or bacteremia, which may provide an opportunity to colonize the filter with active infection; and a thrombus presenting between the proposed access site and site of deployment of the filter. Sepsis or bacteremia is often considered a relative contraindication only, and it is controversial as to whether infection should interfere with IVC filter placement.

In patients who have a retrievable filter in place, and if during the course of treatment it is concluded that the filter will no longer be required or is no longer effective, there are several considerations for removal of retrievable filters. If the patient's baseline low risk for PE has returned after resolution of other conditions or if the patient can return to routine anticoagulation, consideration should be given to filter removal. Retrievable filters allow the option for removal if it has become ineffective from migration, excessive angulation, or fracture. If a continued need for the filter exists, these filters could be replaced in a more optimal position or location. Active bacteremia or septicemia is cited by some as a reason not to place a filter; however, if a patient is actively bacteremic at the time filter placement becomes necessary, a retrievable filter may be a good choice in such a patient. Another contraindication to filter retrieval is a filter that is largely or fully laden with clot that cannot be remedied by endovascular means. This filter cannot be removed since it presents an undue risk of PE during the retrieval procedure. For this and various other reasons, many retrievable filters that are initially placed with the intent of future removal will become permanent. An additional contraindication to filter removal is persistence of clot in the pelvic or lower extremity veins unless the patient becomes a candidate for anticoagulation therapy. Until the patient with the retrievable filter has their risk for PE returned to normal baseline, or if the patient becomes a candidate for anticoagulation, filters likely will not be removed. Retrievable filters, although they have a shorter track record for safety and durability than other, better known familiar permanent filter designs, can and often do at this point remain as "permanent" filters. Consequently, additional studies to document their long-term safety, durability, and functionality still need to be done.

Suprarenal IVC filter placements may need to be considered in some cases. Situations in which this might be considered are renal vein thrombus, pregnancy, IVC clots either above the renal veins or above an IVC filter, duplicated IVC, PE that has been documented to occur from a gonadal vein, or an excessively short infrarenal IVC.[6]

Occasionally, superior vena cava (SVC) filters are entertained. In our experience, these are rarely, if ever, necessary, and even proponents of this treatment acknowledge the controversy surrounding it.[7] However, some literature does exist that documents their use in certain cases and the interventionalist or surgeon should be aware of these reports, if only to address the concerns of consulting physicians who request their placement. Upper extremity DVT is in the vast minority, comprising less than 10% of all DVTs. However, upper extremity and major central thoracic vein thromboses are becoming more common with the increased use of vascular access devices. Although its incidence is uncommon, upper limb DVT is more likely to lead to PE, but these emboli are smaller and less likely to be symptomatic or fatal. Considerable controversy continues to surround these questions with regard to management of upper extremity DVT. Placement of a vena cava filter in the reverse orientation in the SVC is conceptually a potential method of managing these thromboses in patients who have a contraindication to anticoagulation or have higher fall risk, which is not uncommon in these populations. Filter placement in this location and in reverse orientation is technically challenging. There is a very short landing zone for placement of these filters in the SVC below the confluence of the major thoracic veins and above the right atrium. Any complications, such as inadvertent deployment even slightly beyond the intended landing area for the filter, could result in embolization to the right atrium, and any perforations that occur would likely be more serious. A femoral insertion kit is used if the filter is to be placed from the jugular position, and a jugular insertion kit is used if the filter is to be placed from the femoral approach.

IVC Filter Techniques

IVC filter implantation is a relatively straightforward procedure that ought to be well studied and mastered by the vascular interventionalist or endovascular surgeon. Patient preparation, intraprocedural imaging, and meticulous technique are required. Most implants are performed either via the common femoral or the jugular vein approaches. Additional approaches can be via the antecubital or the subclavian veins, as well as other veins in unique situations. Extremely careful technique should be utilized when obtaining percutaneous access since many patients are either on anticoagulation, have had one venous thrombosis, or have had a bleeding complication. The location and side of any DVT should be determined before access is obtained. Ultrasound-guided access to the vein is recommended. An initial cavogram is obtained using a pigtail catheter, another multiside hole catheter, or the kit's delivery sheath, which is optimally placed in the confluence of the iliac veins either from the femoral or jugular vein approach; or alternatively, with a catheter tip placed in the left iliac vein since opacification of the cava

from the left iliac vein excludes a duplicated cava. The width of the vena cava should be documented. After documenting caval anatomy and excluding caval thrombosis, duplication, megacava, renal vein anomalies, and/or the presence of a left-sided vena cava, filter placement can proceed. While the individual types of IVC anomalies and conditions are rare, the incidence of an anatomic variation of the IVC, taken all together, approaches 15%. The filter is typically placed with its apex at or just below the level of the lowest renal vein. Some manufacturer instructions for use (IFU) indicate placement of the upper portion of the cone of the filter within the outwash of the renal veins to aid the resolution of thrombi captured by the filter. Placement above the renal veins should be reserved for the indications stated earlier. Deployment protocols for specific filters are per the IFU for the individual filters. Table 11.1 contains filter device details, and fluoroscopic images of several types appear in Figure 11.1. The practitioner should be familiar with the manufacturer's IFU of the various filters available at their institution that they routinely use. Successful deployment is considered routine once the above conditions have been assessed and should occur 95% to 99% of the time in appropriately selected patients.

In the event that any of the abovementioned anomalies of the vena cava are present, significant alterations of filter placement are required. In duplicated cava, a filter in each cava should be considered. Alternatively, a filter in the suprarenal IVC is an option. If megacava is encountered, options include the use of a Bird's Nest Filter (Cook) or placing 2 filters with 1 filter in each common iliac vein. With a left-sided vena cava, the filter can be placed in the solitary left-sided vena cava. Careful documentation of the presence of the aorta to the right of the

TABLE 11.1　**Available IVC Filter Device Details**

Filter	Manufacturer	Retrievable (Route)	Material	Sheath Outer Diameter (Fr) [Jugular]	Maximum IVC Diameter (mm)	Jugular Placement
Greenfield (24 Fr)	Boston Scientific	No	Stainless-steel wire	28.0	28	Yes
Titanium Greenfield	Boston Scientific	No	Titanium wire	14.3	28	Yes
Greenfield (12 Fr)	Boston Scientific	No	Stainless-steel wire	14.0	28	Yes
Bird's Nest	Cook	No	Stainless-steel wire	13.8	40	Yes
Günther Tulip	Cook	Yes (Jugular)	Elgiloy wire	10.0	30	Yes
Celect	Cook	Yes (Jugular)	Conichrome	7.0 [8.5]	30	Yes
Vena Tech LP	B. Braun	No	Phynox wire	9.0	35	Yes
Simon Nitinol	CR Bard	No	Nitinol wire	9.0	28	Yes
G2 X	CR Bard	Yes (Jugular)	Nitinol wire	7.0 [10.0]	28	Yes
Trap Ease	Cordis Endovascular	No	Nitinol hypotube	8.5	30	Yes
Opt Ease	Cordis Endovascular	Yes (4 weeks) (Femoral)	Nitinol hypotube	8.5	30	Yes
Option	Angiotech	Yes (Jugular)	Nitinol	6.0	30	Yes

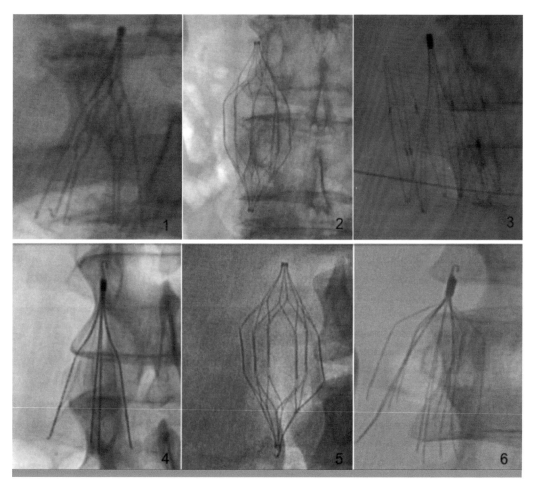

FIGURE 11.1   Fluoroscopic imaging of 6 common IVC filter designs in use today. **1.** Greenfield Titanium (Boston Scientific). **2.** Trap Ease (Cordis). **3.** VenaTech LP (VenaTech). **4.** Günther Tulip (Cook). **5.** Opt Ease (Cordis). **6.** G2 X (CR Bard). The first 3 are examples of permanent filter designs. The latter 3 are retrievable and have hooks at the top or bottom (for either transjugular or transfemoral access for retrieval, respectively) via dedicated retrieval systems or interventional sheath/loop snare combinations.

left-sided vena cava is needed before deployment of the filter. For renal vein anomalies, such as a circumaortic left renal vein or the presence of multiple renal veins on one side, the filter should be placed below the level of the lowest renal vein.

A marker pigtail catheter or sizing pigtail specifically designed to measure the size of the vena cava can be used if it was not clearly documented prior to the procedure. Typically, a cavogram is performed with an injection of contrast at 20 mL/s for a total of 40 mL. Another less established technique is to document the major vena caval branches with selective catheterization without contrast administration.

Many practitioners have chosen to utilize retrievable filters on a fairly regular basis given their apparent reliability as long-term filters from early experience.[8,9] Retrieval procedures are reviewed in Figures 11.2 and 11.3. The Bard recovery filter has been updated,

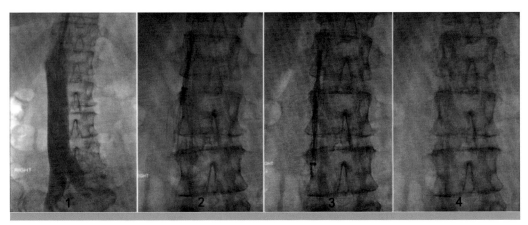

FIGURE 11.2   Recovery sequence of G2 X (CR Bard) IVC filter using a recovery cone (Bard): **1.** Initial cavagram and positioning of recovery cone at apex of filter. The filter is seen to be free of embolic debris or thrombus. **2.** After positioning of the cone over the filter, the sheath is advanced to close the cone. **3.** Retraction of the filter into the cone. **4.** After withdrawal of the filter and sheath removal, a final cavagram demonstrates complete removal of the filter.

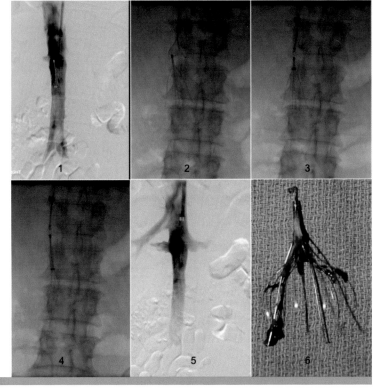

FIGURE 11.3   Recovery sequence of Günther Tulip (Cook) IVC filter using a loop snare and sheath: **1.** Initial cavagram is performed. The filter is free of embolic debris or thrombus. **2.** Positioning of snare at apex of filter. **3.** After positioning of the snare over the filter and capture of the hook, the sheath is advanced to close the filter and begin recovery. **4.** Retraction of the filter into the sheath by the snare. **5.** After withdrawal of the filter, final cavagram is performed to demonstrate absence of spasm, thrombus, or extravasation. **6.** Recovered filter with mix of chronic fibrinous material at the apex and acute thrombotic material that is typically seen at retrieval and probably forms while filter is in sheath with static blood.

which is now the Bard G2 X, and it can be recovered with either a recovery cone or with a snare from a jugular approach. Likewise, the Günther Tulip and the Cook Celect filters can be recovered with a snare from a jugular approach. The Cordis Opt Ease is recovered from a femoral approach also using a snare. Anecdotal evidence indicates that the Cordis Opt Ease has a shorter recovery window (Figure 11.4). For this reason, we would typically prefer any of the other retrievable filters, as there is accumulating evidence that they can often be safely retrieved well beyond the manufacturers' IFU. This may extend the opportunity for filter retrieval in a number of patients whose risk for PE does not return to baseline early, who are initially lost to follow-up, or whose ability to tolerate anticoagulation does not return for a longer period of time. However, this needs to be done on an individualized basis, with great care and attention to signs that retrievability may not be possible at the time of removal.

These retrieval procedures are performed with the patient under anticoagulation in many cases.[10] The patient is ideally accessed under sedation via the right internal jugular vein with ultrasound guidance starting with a micropuncture technique and then upsizing to a short, interventional sheath. Using standard techniques, the inferior vena cava is accessed, and a catheter or sheath is placed at or below the level of the filter. A cavogram is obtained, and documentation of patency of the filter or determination of clot burden is performed. In cases of small clots within the filter cone (25% or less cone volume), retrieval may be performed safely. However, when there is large clot burden (>25%), filters are usually not removed, and patients are typically anticoagulated and brought back at a later time for interval reassessment for possible later retrieval. If a patent filter is documented, a recovery cone in the case of the Bard G2, a loop snare in the case of the Bard G2 X, or a loop snare or

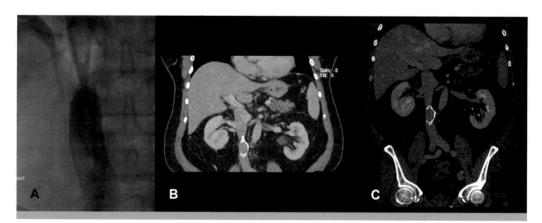

FIGURE 11.4 Opt Ease (Cordis Endovascular) IVC filter retrieval attempted with resulting caval stenosis and inability to remove filter. The patient presented late for retrieval but strongly wished to undergo attempted retrieval despite counseling about decreased potential for successful filter removal and increased risk of stenosis or injury. **A.** Caval stenosis and retained IVC filter. The patient was maintained on warfarin, in accordance with his history of recent PE and DVT. **B.** Three-week CT venogram confirming resulting stenosis (rather than spasm) and continued filter patency. **C.** Four-month CT venogram again documenting continued filter patency and some favorable remodeling of the IVC. It was planned to continue warfarin in this patient (who suffered DVT and PE perioperatively after oncologic surgery) for at least a full 12 months and follow the IVC morphology on subsequent CT scans during oncologic followup.

the respective recovery systems for the Cook Celect or Tulip filters, is brought into place. A snare is brought around the hook and the sheath is advanced over the recovery cone or the snare to collapse the filter within the device. The filter is then withdrawn carefully under fluoroscopy to document that it is not dislodged from the sheath. The catheter or sheath is then reinserted into the abdominal vena cava and a cavogram is obtained to rule out perforation, stenosis, or thrombus formation in the cava following the procedure. Careful attention to both meticulous access technique and hemostasis of the internal jugular vein, particularly if the patient is anticoagulated, is of course critical.

Rosenthal and others have identified techniques to place inferior vena cava filters using intravascular ultrasonography (IVUS) at the bedside of patients in the ICU, providing a way to insert an IVC filter in patients who cannot be easily transported. The IVUS bedside ICU technique has been adopted at other institutions as well.[11-14] Typically, this requires a 2-vein access—via both the right and left common femoral veins—and specialized standing protocols to bring IVUS and filter deployment equipment to the ICU.[11] More recently, beyond the initial IVUS studies done by Rosenthal, other workers have documented a single-vein access technique using markings and dimensions obtained by using IVUS and using this length data to guide deployment. Another use for IVUS is in a procedure suite with fluoroscopy in cases where avoidance of contrast administration, such as in cases of contrast allergy or renal insufficiency, is required. Vascular landmarks are assessed using IVUS—hepatic veins, left renal artery, renal veins, and iliac veins. Then, these landmarks, fluoroscopy of the IVUS catheter in the planned filter landing zone can identify a bony landmark, which then serves to guide

filter placement under fluoroscopy alone. Follow-up IVUS imaging can also provide an additional confirmation of correct filter deployment and the relative position to renal veins following deployment. This combined IVUS and fluoroscopic approach can be a single-access site technique. Ashley and colleagues have argued that IVUS more accurately localizes the renal veins and measures the diameter of the vena cava than contrast venography.[15] Transabdominal ultrasonography can fail to identify proper anatomical landmarks in up to 10% of patients, but in centers that have made a committed effort to this approach, transabdominal ultrasonography can be utilized to document anatomy and adequate filter positioning.[16] If technical support and expertise exist to obtain quality transabdominal venous images, and body habitus, bowel gas, or ileus does not preclude adequate visualization, this is a valuable alternative technique.

IVC Filter Outcomes

Complications of IVC filter placement along with their incidence are important data to incorporate into the decision to place, the placement procedure, and follow-up of these devices. Migration and access site thrombosis are 2 frequent and potentially highly significant adverse events. Conservative estimates place access site thrombosis at a rate of 0% to 6% of placements. Other reports cite access site thrombosis occurring at 2% to 35%. Access site thrombosis appears to be greater with the femoral route. Ultrasound guidance, use of careful micropuncture needle technique, and the smallest-diameter delivery system appropriate to a given patient may limit such thromboses. Access site thrombosis is a particularly worrisome outcome when placement was for a purely prophylactic indication. Filter migration is also a worrisome problem with an uncertain incidence. Estimates of migration occurrence vary from 0%–18% to 3%–69%. Migration may be limited to some extent by careful IVC sizing and meticulous filter deployment procedure in accordance with each device's instructions for use. Reports aiming to quantify both access site thrombosis and filter migration are heavily influenced by follow-up protocol and imaging modality as well as whether or not asymptomatic patients are screened for these adverse outcomes.

Numerous other complications occur related to these devices: death may occur, but well under 1% of cases; recurrent clinical PE may occur in 2% to 5%; filter embolization may occur in 2% to 5%; IVC occlusion may occur in 2% to 30%; depending on the series examined, IVC penetration can occur in 0% to 41%; and filter fracture can occur in 2% to 10% (Table 11.2). IVC penetration is a controversial issue. A computed tomography (CT) scan may poorly identify a collapsed vena cava around the limbs of an IVC filter and present the image of caval penetration, when in fact, this is an underfilled cava collapsed around an IVC filter. It may be more reasonable to be concerned with caval penetration when clear evidence of this exists and/or a complication of such penetration occurs, such as a visceral perforation or bleeding complication. Filter misplacement or migration may occur despite meticulous technique and careful deployment. Rapid and precise deployment of the filter reduces the incidence of strut asymmetry, incomplete opening (Figure 11.5), and tilting. Misplacement of the filter at insertion may occur through a number of mechanisms, and these filters are at an increased risk for migration. Migration of either fractured components or the entire device may occur. Central migration of a filter into the right atrium or further

into the cardiac chambers, although rare, is a dreaded complication of filter placement. Injury to adjacent retroperitoneal structures, which fortunately is extremely rare, is also compelling evidence of a perforation related to filter placement. Occasionally, a filter strut has been seen to migrate through the caval wall and into adjacent vessels, vertebrae, or viscera. In the absence of bleeding or gastrointestinal complications, this probably can best be managed by serial monitoring. Gastrointestinal complications of filter placement may include bleeding or perforation of the adjacent viscera, particularly the duodenum. These rare cases may present either as abnormalities on CT scanning for related or other reasons or upper gastrointestinal bleeding when visceral ulcers are created by local strut trauma. Central venous guidewire manipulation or central line insertions have also contributed to the dislodgement of previously placed IVC filters. Guidewires may become entangled in the vena cava filter during other venous interventional procedures with a J or other wire advanced well into the vena cava and/or during central line placement. It is possible that many of these may be unrecognized by the operator and manifest only as mild to moderate difficulty removing the wire at some point during the procedure. If such a wire becomes impossible to remove or filter entanglement is suspected, intervention to remove it using catheter techniques may be necessary. Such conditions are likely underrecognized and probably underreported. PE or recurrent PE despite the presence of a filter can occur. Anticoagulation should be maintained whenever possible to minimize recurrent PE. Renal complications include renal vein thrombosis related to suprarenal filter placement. Rarely, obstructive uropathy due to a pelvic obstruction of the ureter related to vena cava wall strut perforation

Venous Thromboembolic Disease

TABLE 11.2 **IVC Filter Placement Complications from Selected Authors**

	Major Procedural	Postfilter Recurrent PE	Access Site Thrombosis (Symptomatic)	Caval Thrombosis
Becker et al.,[17] 1992		0.0%–6.8%	2%	0.0%–15.1%
Mohan et al.,[18] 1995	0.0%–6.3%[b]	2.0%–4.4%		0.0%–14.6%
Athanasoulis et al.,[19] 2000	<1%	5%	2%	5%
Sharafuddin et al.,[20] 2001		1.9%–3.4%	2%	0%–19%
Patel,[21] 2004		2%–5%	0%–6%	2%–30%
Hann et al.,[22] 2005		0%–9%	0.0%–13.1%	0.0%–9.5%
Hoppe et al.,[23] 2007		5%	2%	5%
Georgiades et al.,[6] 2008		1%[g]		2%–19%

Abbreviations: PE = pulmonary embolism; DVT = deep venous thrombosis.

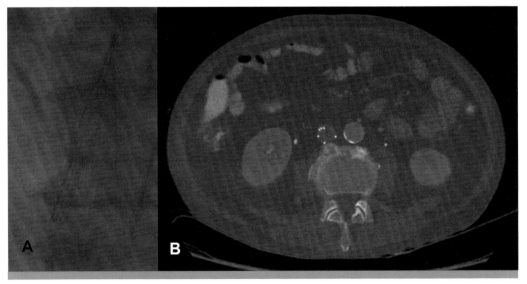

FIGURE 11.5 Fluoroscopic **(A)** and CT **(B)** imaging of partial incomplete opening seen with a Greenfield IVC filter (Boston Scientific). Asking the patient to cough or individual strut manipulation with an angled tipped catheter are options to try to correct this during the initial deployment procedure, but strut tips are usually firmly placed in the IVC wall immediately after release. This deployment configuration will afford some protection from large PE. However, if PE occurs in this situation or more optimal filter protection from PE is needed, a second IVC filter below (if cava and filter are patent) or a suprarenal IVC filter (if the filter itself is shown to be a possible source or caval thrombus is present) may be considered.

TABLE 11.2 (cont.) **IVC Filter Placement Complications from Selected Authors**

Filter Fracture	Filter Migration (Major)	Filter Infection	30 day Mortality (due to filter)	30 day Mortality (overall)	Recurrent DVT
	0.0%–59.3%[a]		<<1%		
			0.0%–10.9%[c]		
<1%	<1%	<<1%	<1%	17%	
	6%–8%[d]	("Rare")			
2%–10%	0%–18%[e]		<1%		
					0%–32%
<1%[f]	<1%				20%
	2%–6%[h]				

[a]All migration, includes single-device series. [b]Filter misplacement. [c]Not limited to 30 days. [d]Single, early device data cited here. [e]All migration. [f]With clinical consequences. [g]Iatrogenic PE. [h]Combined migration and malposition.

may occur. This may manifest as either hematuria or hydronephrosis. Careful imaging and active questioning of position during deployment will avoid other such highly unusual mishaps such as placement in the mesenteric vein via the portal system and/or aortic placement, both of which have been documented to occur in extremely rare cases.[24] Frank phlegmasia complicating prophylactic filter placement is a real, though uncommon, entity.[25] Concern regarding this is one of the factors driving increased consideration for retrievable filters. Fortunately, in patients who can undergo either mechanical or pharmacomechanical thrombolysis with the filter in place, phlegmasia from a filter occlusion can be treated with a minimally invasive approach to attempt to resolve the thrombus and then anticoagulation can be resumed (Figure 11.6).

The IVC filter with the longest clinical experience is the Greenfield filter.[26] Extensive experience has been gained through multiple models of the Greenfield filter. The Greenfield filter is widely regarded as a filter with an excellent long-term safety and efficacy record. Greenfield and colleagues have maintained large registries of filters that they have placed, and their 20-year experience with these filters documented an incidence rate of recurrent PE at 4% and a caval patency rate of 96%, and caval movement of little or no clinical significance was seen in 8% of their cases. They reported minimal procedural morbidity and mortality, and they concluded in their analysis that insertion of the stainless steel Greenfield vena cava filter provides protection from PE while maintaining patency of the IVC over long-term follow-up.

Reports about experience with retrievable filters that have been removed after extended dwell times past the manufacturer's IFU is beginning to become available.[27] When retrieval is attempted and the patient

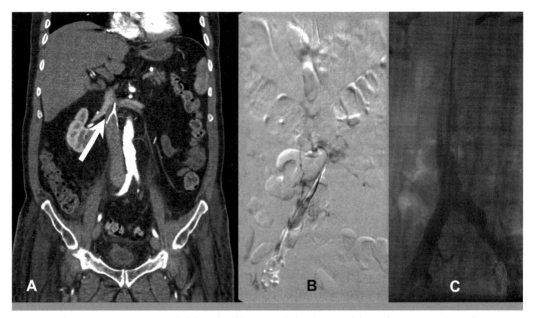

FIGURE 11.6   A patient presenting with bilateral sudden onset limb edema and discomfort occurring late after a filter placed for VTE immediately after spine surgery. There was no frank phlegmasia or compromised lower extremity viability. A CT venogram was the initial study obtained (**A**) and was to some extent equivocal as is often the case due to venous contrast opacification patterns on CT. Correlation with catheter venography did show that the filling defect below the outflow of the right renal vein was in fact filter-associated thrombus (marked by arrow in **A**). Initial catheter venogram (**B**) confirms massive illiocaval thrombosis. Extensive pharmacomechanical debulking of clot was performed with iliofemoral and lower IVC improvement (**C**) in an effort to avoid long-term complications related to lower extremity venous insufficiency. Due to contrast volume and sedation time, it was elected to bring the patient back for a staged second procedure to complete thrombus removal. He was maintained on anticoagulation and had symptomatic improvement but required coronary angiography and intervention. Due to this and transient renal impairment, it was elected not to reintervene on his cava and IVC filter. He was discharged on warfarin anticoagulation with continued symptomatic improvement.

was not lost to follow-up or had secondarily requested to keep the filter in place, technical success approaches 85% or greater. Factors correlating with failure of filter retrieval were due to device angulation, tilt, or canting within the IVC. Most clinical series of retrievable filters are reported to be free or relatively free of symptomatic PE, bleeding, thrombosis, or caval stenosis. These procedure times should be short when retrieval is straightforward. It is reasonable to conclude that when filter retrieval is attempted, it is performed successfully in a large proportion of cases, despite growing evidence that many

patients are either lost to follow-up, the decision to leave the filter in place is made, or the patients themselves decline to undergo the removal procedure.

Filter placement and its use in trauma patients have been assessed by Quirke and colleagues by questionnaire.[28] They queried respondents that were largely at level I trauma centers that have over 1000 trauma admissions per year. These centers reported a low complication rate, with most of these centers reporting one or fewer complications per year despite their relatively high volume. Interesting trends were observed in these respondents. There seemed to be relative agreement on absolute indications such as PE, while on therapeutic anticoagulation, the presence of a DVT with contraindication to anticoagulation, and free-floating iliofemoral thrombosis by venogram or duplex imaging. Relative indications were met with somewhat less agreement such as any DVT documentation, spinal cord injury, pelvic fracture, multiple lower extremity fractures, concurrent cancer, prolonged bed rest, or obesity. Having the potential for removability through use of a retrievable filter, many centers reported that they increased the use of IVC filters for prophylactic use, and this was found to be highly significant in their study. Although the study documented few complications, it was a retrospective questionnaire-based analysis, which limits its reliability.

PE is one of the most feared complications in trauma and neurosurgical trauma practice. Such patients with multisystem injuries, extremity or pelvic fractures, and head or spinal cord injuries often pose a significant dilemma for the surgeon or intensivist due to potential inability to use conventional anticoagulation therapy or at times even sequential compression devices. The incidence of DVT is high among trauma and neurosurgical trauma patients, and the attendant risk of PE is an important cause of morbidity and mortality. IVC filter placement has evolved and escalated in these groups over the past 3 decades. However, as discussed, significant rates of complications are reported from their use in all groups.[29] The available data on IVC filter placement in trauma and neurosurgery patients remain incomplete, and the potential complications of IVC filters must be carefully considered to optimally select patients who will benefit from their use.

Becker and colleagues reviewed multiple large series of IVC filters.[17] Numerous methodological inconsistencies were identified within many of these studies. These authors concluded in their review that recurrent clinical PE was rare after filter placement and that only 8 deaths were reported in the over 2500 cases that they reviewed. Filter complications were common but rarely life threatening, and an extremely low rate of death from filter complications was noted among the reviewed studies. These authors concluded that IVC filters appeared to be effective in preventing PE but not eliminating it completely. Despite the large published experience with IVC filters, many questions remain about their indications, safety, and effectiveness. Anticoagulation therapy, if no contraindication exists, ought to be continued in conjunction with IVC filters whenever possible.

Mohan and colleagues conducted a comparative analysis of multiple filter types (including various Greenfield type filters such as the titanium and stainless steel, Venatech, Bird's Nest, and Simon Nitinol filters) and their complications.[18] They concluded that there is a higher rate of IVC thrombosis with the Bird's Nest filter vs. the various other filter types studied in their analysis. They also found a higher mortality rate with the use of the Bird's Nest filter when compared to other types in this study. However, this is a limited finding given the size of their study.

Guidelines for the use of retrievable IVC is an area of considerable attention at this point in time.[8,9,11,30] The practices of many interventionalists have evolved toward placement of retrievable filters as their first choice when there was any possibility or need for future retrieval. Kaufman and colleagues[31] have endeavored to establish guidelines for the use of retrievable filters through the

Society of Interventional Radiology (SIR). Their consensus document emphasized that the primary means for treatment and prophylaxis of VTE are and should remain pharmacologic. A few unique indications for primary placement of retrievable vena cava filters exist and they are not distinct from the indications for permanent vena cava filters. Some patients with indications for placement of a retrievable vena cava filter have limited periods of risk for clinically significant PE or contraindication to anticoagulation and thus may not require permanent protection from PE with a vena cava filter. Patients with filters in place should be managed by pharmacologic methods according to their VTE status and risk of anticoagulation as soon as anticoagulation is feasible and safe in their case. They concluded that there is no absolute indication for discontinuation of filtration unless the filter itself is documented as a source of major morbidity that would be relieved by retrieval or conversion. They also noted that discontinuation of filtration should occur only when the risk of clinically significant PE is reduced to an acceptable or baseline level and is estimated to be less than the risk of leaving the filter in place. Finally, they further concluded that there is not sufficient evidence in the literature to support true evidence-based recommendations for the use of retrievable filters in patients with VTE or for prophylaxis of VTE at this time. Nonetheless, many practitioners are choosing to use temporary filters as their filter of choice even in patients who are likely to require permanent filter placement. The choice of retrievability, timing, and eventual final decision for removal is individualized in nearly all cases. Careful communication with either the patient's primary physician or surgeon may lead to more IVC filters removed within the window of retrievability. Retrievable filters and the evidence for their use, especially in prophylactic scenarios, will continue to undergo further study and evolution. In particular, these devices need to undergo cost effectiveness evaluation and it is likely that practices surrounding their use will evolve significantly in the short and medium term.

More aggressive percutaneous catheter-directed thrombolysis (CDT) of venous thrombosis is on the increase. Many authorities report a very low threshold to place, or even *routine* placement of, a temporary IVC filter to protect against periprocedural PE during CDT; however, such a strategy is controversial. There remains a question as to whether IVC filter deployment conveys benefit to CDT patients. Protack and colleagues have sought to define the outcomes of CDT with and without prophylactic IVC filter placement for lower extremity DVT.[32] Average follow-up was 2 years. No patients developed PE during therapy, even though only 20% had IVC filter placement prior to or during CDT. They concluded that CDT without protective IVC filter placement is safe and effective in treating acute DVT and that selective rather than routine IVC filter placement is a safe and appropriate approach in such patients.

References

1. Decousus H, Leizorovicz A, Parent F, Page Y, Tardy B, Girard P, et al. A clinical trial of vena caval filters in the prevention of pulmonary embolism in patients with proximal deep-vein thrombosis. Prévention du Risque d'Embolie Pulmonaire par Interruption Cave Study Group. N Engl J Med. 1998;338(7):409-15.

2. Geerts WH, Bergqvist D, Pineo GF, Heit JA, Samama CM, Lassen MR, et al. Prevention of venous thromboembolism. Chest. 2008;133:381S-453S.

3. Young T, Tang H, Aukes J, Hughes R. Vena

caval filters for the prevention of pulmonary embolism. Cochrane Database Syst Rev. 2007;17(4):CD006212.

4. Kaufman JA. Development of a research agenda for IVC Filters. Endovascular Today. 2007;6(10):67-70.

5. Abou-Nukta F, Alkhoury F, Arroyo K, Bakhos C, Gutweiler J, Reinhold R, et al. Clinical pulmonary embolus after gastric bypass surgery. Surg Obes Relat Dis. 2006;2(1): 24-8.

6. Georgiades CS, Hong K. Inferior vena cava filters. In: Cameron JL, ed. Current Surgical Therapy. 9th ed. Philadelphia: Mosby; 2008. p908-13.

7. Usoh F, Hingorani A, Ascher E, Shiferson A, Tran V, Patel N, et al. Superior vena cava perforation following the placement of a superior vena cava filter in males less than 60 years of age. Vascular. 2009;17(1):44-50.

8. Berczi V, Bottomley JR, Thomas SM, Taneja S, Gaines PA, Cleveland TJ. Long-term retrievability of IVC filters: should we abandon permanent devices? Cardiovasc Intervent Radiol. 2007;30(5):820-7.

9. Comerota AJ. Retrievable IVC filters: a decision matrix for appropriate utilization. Perspect Vasc Surg Endovasc Ther. 2006;18(1):11-7.

10. Hoppe H, Kaufman JA, Barton RE, Petersen BD, Lakin PC, Deloughery TG, et al. Safety of inferior vena cava filter retrieval in anticoagulated patients. Chest. 2007;132(1): 31-6.

11. Rosenthal D, Wellons ED, Levitt AB, Shuler FW, O'Conner RE, Henderson VJ. Role of prophylactic temporary inferior vena cava filters placed at the ICU bedside under intravascular ultrasound guidance in patients with multiple trauma. J Vasc Surg. 2004;40(5):958-64.

12. Aidinian G, Fox CJ, White PW, Cox MW, Adams ED, Gillespie DL. Intravascular ultrasound-guided inferior vena cava filter placement in the military multitrauma patients: a single center experience. Vasc EndovascSurg. 2009;43(5):497-501.

13. Wellons ED, Rosenthal D, Shuler FW, Levitt AB, Matsuura J, Henderson VJ. Real-time intravascular ultrasound-guided placement of a removable inferior vena cava filter. J Trauma. 2004;57(1):20-5.

14. Ebaugh JL, Chiou AC, Morasch MD, Matsumura JS, Pearce WH. Bedside vena cava filter placement guided with intravascular ultrasound. J Vasc Surg. 2001;34(1):21-6.

15. Ashley DW, Gamblin TC, Burch ST, Solis MM. Accurate deployment of vena cava filters: comparison of intravascular ultrasound and contrast venography. J Trauma. 2001;50(6): 975-81.

16. Amankwah KS, Seymour K, Costanza M, Berger J, Gahtan V. Transabdominal duplex ultrasonography for bedside inferior vena cava filter placement: examples, technique, and review. Vasc Endovascular Surg. 2009;43(4):379-84.

17. Becker DM, Philbrick JT, Selby JB. Inferior vena cava filters: indications, safety, and effectiveness. Arch Intern Med. 1992;152(10):1985-94.

18. Mohan CR, Hoballah JJ, Sharp WJ, Kresowik TF, Lu CT, Corson JD. Comparative efficacy and complications of vena caval filters. J Vasc Surg. 1995;21(2):235-45.

19. Athanasoulis CA, Kaufman JA, Halpern EF, Waltman AC, Geller SC, Fan CM. Inferior vena caval filters: review of a 26-year single-center clinical experience. Radiology. 2000;216(1):54-66.

20. Sharafuddin MJ, Corson JD. Percutaneous devices for vena cava filtration. In: Ernst CB, Stanley JC, eds. Current Therapy in Vascular Surgery. 4th ed. St. Louis: Mosby; 2001. p884-91.

21. Patel NC. Inferior vena cava interruption. In: Waldman DL, Saad WEA, Patel NC, eds. Interventional Radiology Secrets.

Philadelphia: Hanley & Belfus; 2004. p206-15.

22. Hann CL, Streiff MB. The role of vena caval filters in the management of venous thromboembolism. Blood Reviews. 2005;19(4):179-202.

23. Hoppe H, Kaufman JA. Inferior vena cava filters. In: Kandarpa K, ed. Peripheral Vascular Interventions. Philadelphia: Lippincott Williams & Wilkins; 2007. p401-15.

24. Ascher E, Hingorani A, Yorkovich WR. Complications of vena cava filters. In: Towne JB, Hollier L, eds. Complications in Vascular Surgery. 2nd ed. New York: Marcel Dekker; 2004. p. 569-79.

25. Harris EJ Jr, Kinney EV, Harris EJ Sr, Olcott C 4th, Zarins CK. Phlegmasia complicating prophylactic percutaneous inferior vena caval interruption: a word of caution. J Vasc Surg. 1995;22(5):606-11.

26. Greenfield LJ, Proctor MC. Twenty-year clinical experience with the Greenfield filter. Cardiovasc Surg. 1995;3(2):199-205.

27. Cantwell CP, Pennypacker J, Singh H, Scorza LB, Waybill PN, Lynch FC. Comparison of the recovery and G2 filter as retrievable inferior vena cava filters. J Vasc Interv Radiol. 2009;20(9):1193-9.

28. Quirke TE, Ritota PC, Swan KG. Inferior vena caval filter use in U.S. trauma centers: a practitioner survey. J Trauma. 1997;43(2):333-7.

29. Giannoudis PV, Pountos I, Pape HC, Patel JV. Safety and efficacy of vena cava filters in trauma patients. Injury. 2007;38(1):7-18.

30. Girard P, Stern J-B, Parent F. Medical literature and vena cava filters: so far so weak. Chest. 2002;122:963-7.

31. Kaufman JA, Kinney TB, Streiff MB, Sing RF, Proctor MC, Becker D, Cipolle M, Comerota AJ, Millward SF, Rogers FB, Sacks D, Venbrux AC. Guidelines for the use of retrievable and convertible vena cava filters: report from the Society of Interventional Radiology multidisciplinary consensus conference. J Vasc Interv Radiol. 2006;17(3):449-59.

32. Protack CD, Bakken AM, Patel N, Saad WE, Waldman DL, Davies MG. Long-term outcomes of catheter directed thrombolysis for lower extremity deep venous thrombosis without prophylactic inferior vena cava filter placement. J Vasc Surg. 2007;45(5):992-7.

Percutaneous Pulmonary Embolectomy
Indications, Techniques, and Outcomes

Saher Sabri, Wael E. A. Saad, and Alan H. Matsumoto

Venous thromboembolic disease remains the third most common cardiovascular disease and one of the leading causes of sudden death in the United States. The true incidence of pulmonary embolism (PE) is unknown, but based on historic projections, it is estimated that more than 600,000 cases of PE occur every year in the United States.[1] Approximately 10% of patients with PE do not survive their initial event. Of those who do survive, approximately 70% fail to have the diagnosis made and experience a mortality rate of 30%. If the diagnosis of PE is made promptly and appropriate therapy initiated, the mortality rate can be reduced to less than 10%.[1,2,3]

Once the diagnosis of acute PE is made, treatment should be initiated as soon

as possible. The therapeutic options that are available should be tailored to each patient and clinical scenario. In this chapter, we discuss the management of patients with acute PE using catheter-directed thrombolysis, percutaneous embolectomy and embolus fragmentation techniques, and/or surgical embolectomy. The role of anticoagulation is not addressed in this chapter.

Endovascular and Surgical Interventions

Indications

When obstruction of 70% of the pulmonary arterial circulation occurs, the right ventricle needs to be able to generate a systolic pressure in excess of 50 mm Hg and a mean pulmonary artery pressure greater than 40 mm Hg to maintain pulmonary perfusion.

Venous Thromboembolic Disease. Contemporary Endovascular Management series. © 2011 Mark G. Davies MD and Alan B. Lumsden MD, eds. Cardiotext Publishing, ISBN 978-1-935395-22-5.

A previously normal right ventricle is incapable of generating a systolic pressure exceeding 50 mm Hg, so any incremental embolic obstruction to the vasculature beyond this point results in right ventricular failure.[4] The degree of obstruction of the pulmonary arterial circulation required to cause a change in the pulmonary arterial hemodynamics also depends upon the amount of underlying cardiopulmonary disease prior to an embolic event. Therefore, a patient with massive PE obstructing the majority of the pulmonary circulation or a submassive PE superposed on underlying cardiopulmonary disease may present with right ventricular dysfunction or compromised hemodynamics. In this subset of patients, anticoagulation therapy alone may not be adequate and more aggressive intervention with thrombolysis and/or pulmonary embolectomy and clot fragmentation techniques should be considered.

The most validated risk-assessment tool is echocardiography. Right ventricular hypokinesis on echocardiography predicts a doubling of mortality within the next 30 days, even among initially normotensive patients.[5] Right ventricular enlargement on chest computed tomography (CT) also portends a greater likelihood of death or major in-hospital complication.[6] Accepted indications for catheter-directed therapy are:

- Hemodynamic instability, defined as a SBP of <90 mm Hg, a drop in SBP of >40 mm Hg, or ongoing administration of catecholamines for systemic arterial hypotension or persistent hypoxemia despite appropriate anticoagulation and oxygen therapy
- Subtotal or total occlusion by embolus of the left and/or right main pulmonary artery by chest computed tomography (CT) or by conventional pulmonary angiography

- Echocardiographic findings indicating right ventricular dysfunction as manifested by RV dilation and afterload stress with pulmonary hypertension
- Failure of or contraindication to anticoagulation and thrombolysis in a patient with compromised hemodynamics or persistent hypoxemia

Surgical embolectomy rather than catheter thrombectomy should be considered in the presence of free-floating cardiac thrombi or in patients with paradoxical embolism from a large atrial septal defect.[7,8]

Intravenous Thrombolytic Therapy

The Consensus Development Conference recommended that 2-hour bolus intravenous (IV) thrombolytic therapy be considered in any patient who has a perfusion defect involving equivalent to one or more lobes and hemodynamic compromise.[9,10] Despite the numerous randomized trials demonstrating faster improvement in pulmonary perfusion and hemodynamics and better lung diffusing capacities and pulmonary capillary blood volumes in patients receiving thrombolytic therapy, when symptoms and mortality rates at 6 and 12 months are analyzed, there is no statistical benefit in outcomes between patients who received IV thrombolytic vs. heparin therapy.[11,12] In addition, bleeding complications were more frequent in patients undergoing 2-hour IV bolus thrombolysis. Therefore, screening patients with a careful history and physical examination and a review of old medical records is extremely important to exclude contraindications for thrombolysis (which were discussed in detail in earlier chapters). The argument that most patients with acute PE will have a contraindication for thrombolytic therapy is not supported by a large patient survey that revealed that 50% of patients with high-probability lung scans or pulmonary angiographic evidence for PE are acceptable candidates for treatment with IV thrombolysis.[13]

Catheter-Directed Thrombolysis

Catheter-directed thrombolytic therapy with intrapulmonary administration of a thrombolytic agent has been described by several investigators with encouraging results.[14,15] Catheter-directed techniques aim to accelerate clot lysis and achieve rapid reperfusion of the pulmonary arteries and lung parenchyma. In one study, 13 patients were treated with urokinase (Abbott Labs, Abbott Park, IL) for angiographically proven PE within 14 days of major surgery.[14] The catheter was positioned in the pulmonary artery clot and 2200 IU/kg of urokinase were injected directly into the clot. Continuous infusion of urokinase at 2200 IU/kg/h until the clot lysed or up to a maximum of 24 hours was then performed. Follow-up pulmonary angiography at 24 hours revealed that 98% of the clots had completely disappeared from the pulmonary vasculature. No deaths or bleeding complications occurred. In another series, 16 patients with massive PE were given a bolus of 50,000 IU of urokinase directly into the clot.[15] An infusion of 1,000,000 IU of urokinase was then given into the right atrium over a 12-hour period. Cardiac output, total pulmonary vascular resistance, and mean pulmonary artery pressures all improved following the thrombolytic therapy. One patient did suffer a severe bleeding complication.

In 1988, Verstraete et al[16] published the results of a multicenter comparative study of intravenous vs. intrapulmonary infusion of rtPA (100 mg over a 7-hour period) (Al-teplase, Genetech, South San Francisco, CA) for the treatment of acute massive PE. The findings of this study suggested that the intrapulmonary infusion of rtPA does not offer significant benefit compared to intravenous administration. However, this study did not use the standard catheter-directed technique currently used by most interventionalists, which includes embedding the infusion catheter directly into the thrombus, while attempting to fragment the clot. Since rtPA must cleave clot-bound plasminogen to create the active enzyme plasmin, infusion of rtPA in the main pulmonary artery confers minimum benefit to simple IV infusion as most of the drug does not penetrate the clot, but rather, flows in the path of least resistance (the patent pulmonary arterial segments). In addition, experience with peripheral arterial bypass grafts and thrombosed dialysis fistulas has demonstrated that catheter-directed thrombolysis is associated with better rates of lysis, more rapid lysis, the need for lower doses of the lytic agent, and fewer complications.[17] Ultrasound-enhanced catheter-directed thrombolysis using the EndoWave system (EKOS, Bothell, WA) has been used by some investigators to accelerate the thrombolysis. In one study the median infusion time was 24 hours with 76% complete resolution of clot burden.[18]

Surgical Embolectomy

For patients with massive central PE with marked compromised hemodynamics who are too unstable to undergo or have a contraindication to thrombolytic therapy, the only remaining therapeutic options are percutaneous techniques with clot fragmentation or surgical embolectomy. Traditionally, surgical embolectomy has been associated with a high perioperative mortality rate. With improvements in anesthesia and cardiopulmonary bypass technology, 30-day survival rates after surgical pulmonary artery embolectomy have been reported to be as high as 75% at centers specializing in the treatment of thromboembolic disease. In one study, 20 patients who presented with acute PE and cardiogenic shock had a 5-year survival of 100% following surgical embolectomy. In this study, patients undergoing surgical embolectomy had a more favorable New York Heart Association classification level and a lower incidence of chronic pulmonary arterial hypertension at follow-up when compared to a similar cohort of patients receiving medical therapy.[19] In a more recent study, 47 patients underwent surgical thrombectomy at a single center with 6% perioperative mortality and 83% 3-year survival.[20]

Yet, very few centers in the United States have widespread experience with this type of surgery. Therefore, various percutaneous transvenous devices designed to remove or fragment centrally obstructing PE have been developed.

Percutaneous Embolectomy

Technique

We advocate that all patients undergoing percutaneous embolectomy be intubated and on mechanical ventilation, preferably under heavy sedation or general anesthesia. Meticulous attention is also required for ongoing vasopressor, fluid, electrolyte, and ventilator management. Patient management includes continuous assessment of volume status, urine output, end-organ perfusion, and ECG monitoring during the procedure. Most often, a computed tomographic (CT) or magnetic resonance (MR) pulmonary arterial study or an echocardiogram demonstrates the clot distribution and burden and the presence of compromised right ventricular function. In the absence of one of these noninvasive imaging studies (ie, a ventilation/perfusion nuclear medicine lung scan), a pulmonary angiogram is performed using a minimum amount of contrast to document the presence and distribution of PE and to measure pulmonary arterial and right heart pressures. However, pulmonary arterial pressures (PAP) should be measured prior to the injection of any contrast and prior to any intervention. Most operators agree that the injection of 10 mL of contrast is sufficient to obtain a baseline pulmonary angiogram, especially since the diagnosis of a massive PE has often already been made with another imaging modality. The use of a large amount of contrast (ie, >20 mL with one injection) may be dangerous due to the risk of worsening right ventricular failure and cardiogenic shock from acute volume overload.[7]

If the patient is unable to lay supine, the pulmonary angiogram and catheter-directed intervention can be performed from a basilic or brachial vein approach. Otherwise, the study is usually performed from the femoral vein or less commonly, the internal jugular vein approach. The diagnostic pulmonary arterial catheter is removed over a guidewire, maintaining access in the pulmonary artery. An appropriate-sized 70- or 90-cm introducer sheath (usually 6F–11F depending on the device used) is inserted into access vein and positioned with its tip in the main pulmonary artery. The sheath can be used to perform suction embolectomy, but more importantly, it is used to minimize trauma to the heart and stabilize the various mechanical thrombectomy devices during their use in the pulmonary arterial segments. The sheath is connected to a heparinized saline flush (4000 IU heparin/1000 cc normal saline) and infused at 30 cc/hr. The sheath side port can also be connected to a pressure transducer to allow real-time monitoring of the main pulmonary artery during the intervention.

Performing catheter-directed interventions in the segmental arteries is discouraged due to the risk of arterial perforation. Unless strongly contraindicated, the use of intraclot infusion of thrombolytic agents with the appropriate embolectomy device is recommended. A 5 or 6 F pigtail catheter can be embedded directly into the clot, manually rotating the catheter with hopes of fragmenting the clot and creating more surface area for the lytic agent. A pigtail catheter is used for this application since it has multiple side holes, and its rounded configuration is less likely to traumatize the pulmonary artery.

Typically, 4 to 10 mg of rtPA is vigorously injected in small aliquots (pulse-sprayed) using the pigtail catheter or power-pulsed using a dedicated mechanical device such as the AngioJet Xpeedior catheter (MEDRAD, Inc., Warrendale, PA) directly into the clot (Figure 12.1). Alternatively, a multi-side hole infusion catheter (AngioDynamics, Glen Falls, NY or EV3, Minneapolis, MN) can be used to pulse-spray a bolus of the lytic agent into the clot to effect better drug distribution; however, use of an end-hole catheter that could erode through a pulmonary artery branch during cardiac pulsations obviates against its use for infusion therapy. For intraclot infusion of a lytic agent, a pigtail catheter that has been embedded into the clot is recommended.

The available literature on the use of the various percutaneous embolectomy devices is summarized in Table 12.1. The published experience with the use of these devices is limited to small case series and case reports from single institutions. In addition, many of the catheter-directed studies for the treatment of acute PE described the use of a combination of techniques in which local or systemic thrombolytics were applied in a very heterogeneous patient population, which makes it difficult to compare the efficacy and outcomes related to the use of these devices. Given these limitations, the summary of the re-

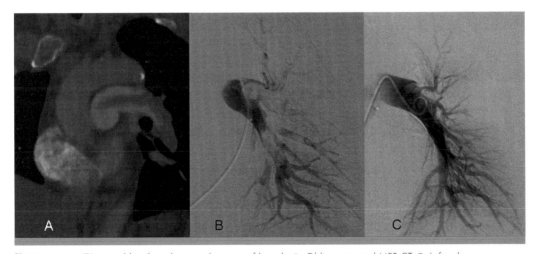

FIGURE 12.1. 71-year-old male with acute shortness of breath. **A**. Oblique coronal MPR CT. **B**. Left pulmonary angiogram demonstrates left PA embolus. Mean PAP was 42 mm Hg. **C**. Angiogram post AngioJet and catheter-directed thrombolysis with tPA over 12 hours. Mean PAP decreased to 30 mm Hg.

TABLE 12.1. **Summary of Published Articles on Catheter-Directed Interventions for Acute Pulmonary Embolism**

Technique	Patient no.	Mean BP pre (mm Hg)	Mean BP post (mm Hg)	Mean PAP pre (mm Hg)	Mean PAP post (mm Hg)	Clinical Success (%)	Mortality (%)
Aspiration (Greenfield embolectomy device or guiding catheters)							
No lytics	89	60	81	33	21	81	25
Systemic lytics	9	50	87	31	20	100	10
Local lytics	9			31	24	100	0
Fragmentation (balloons, rotating pigtail, or standard catheters)							
No lytics	3	28	63	38	29	67	0
Systemic lytics	21	70	93	25	21	71	5
Local lytics	121	67	81	33	22	95	4
Amplatzer thrombectomy device (ATD)							
No lytics	8	86	106	49	53	88	12
Local lytics	6	85	93			100	0
Hydrodynamic thrombectomy devices							
Hydrolizer							
Local lytics	12	47	97	46	30	92	8
Systemic plus local	8			43	36	100	12
AngioJet							
No lytics	25			42	30	75	0
Local lytics	21					87	13
Combination of techniques							
Fragmentation plus Apirex	18	74	88	37	31	89	11
Fragmentation, aspiration, hydrodynamic devices plus lytics	12					83	17

Adapted from Kucher N. Catheter embolectomy for acute pulmonary embolism. Chest. 2007;132:657-63. With permission.

sults from these series reveals an overall clinical success rate with catheter-directed therapy for acute PE of >80% (Table 12.1), with clinical success being defined as immediate hemodynamic improvement. The reported mortality rates range from 0% to 25%, again reflecting the wide variations in the patients being treated.

The ideal thrombectomy device should: (1) be easy to use and position within the pulmonary artery clots, (2) be highly maneuverable to allow rapid right heart passage and advancement into major pulmonary arteries, (3) be able to promote complete removal of clots or fragmentation of clots into very small particles, and (4) have a low profile and be safe to use in the pulmonary circulation.[7,8] A review of the most commonly used devices is detailed below. None of the currently available devices described below are FDA-approved for application in the pulmonary arterial system, and their use for acute PE represents an off-label use of these devices.

Greenfield Embolectomy Device

The Greenfield device (Boston Scientific, Natick, MA) (Figure 12.2) is a 10F braided catheter designed for pulmonary artery embolectomy. The catheter is maneuvered by using a large control handle and is designed for insertion via a femoral or jugular venotomy. The tip of the catheter has threads on it that allow the use of either a 5-mm or 7-mm diameter plastic cup. Once the cup on the catheter tip comes into contact with the embolic material, manual suction is generated via a side port on the control handle. The catheter and the clot are then removed as a unit through the venotomy site or a vascular sheath. Multiple passes with the catheter may be required. Dr. Greenfield and his colleagues have re-

ported on their experience using this device in 46 patients over a 22-year period.[21] Emboli were extracted in 35 (76%) of 46 patients. There was an average reduction in mean pulmonary artery pressure of 8 mm Hg and a significant increase in mean cardiac output after embolectomy. The 30-day mortality rate was 30%. When subgroups of patients were analyzed, embolectomy was most successful for major and submassive PE, and least likely to be helpful in patients with chronic, recurrent PE. Experience with the Greenfield suction embolectomy catheter has been relatively small. The device is somewhat bulky, requires familiarity with the control handle, and is designed for insertion via a surgical venotomy, since it requires insertion through a 22F sheath. The device was not widely used, so it is no longer manufactured.

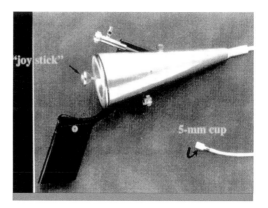

FIGURE 12.2. The Greenfield suction embolectomy device consists of a large handle with a "joy stick" (straight arrow) that is used to control the steerable catheter. A 5-mm cup (curved arrow) is seen on the end of the catheter. From Uflacker R. Interventional therapy for pulmonary embolism. *J Vasc Interv Radiol.* 2001;12:147-64. Used with permission from Elsevier.

Amplatz Thrombectomy Device

The Amplatz Thrombectomy Device (ATD) (EV3) consists of a 120-cm-long, 8F, polyurethane catheter with an impeller mounted on a drive shaft inside a metal cap 5 mm in length. The metal cap has 3 side ports that are used for recirculation of clot particles (Figure 12.3). An air turbine can generate up to 150 rpm at 50 psi. The high speed of the impeller creates a vortex that recirculates and pulverizes acute clot, creating a fluid with very small, suspended particles. There are 2 side ports in the distal catheter that allow for high-pressure infusion of saline to reduce friction and cool the system or to inject contrast medium to facilitate visualization during fluoroscopic manipulation.[22]

The device is advanced through a multipurpose 10F guiding catheter positioned into the clot. To avoid bends and kinks, the device should be introduced and advanced very carefully through the guiding catheter. The device is advanced in a slow, back-and-forth motion. The multipurpose configuration of the guiding catheter allows for some degree of steerability of the device inside the pulmonary artery. After thrombectomy with the ATD, some of the resulting fluid may be aspirated through the guiding catheter. Contrast medium can be injected through the guiding catheter to visualize the amount of residual clot (Figure 12.4).

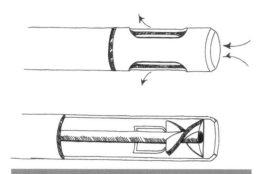

FIGURE 12.3. A drawing of the distal tip of the ATD shows a recessed impeller within a 5-mm metal capsule. Thrombus is aspirated, liquefied, and then expelled through the side ports (curved arrows). The authors would like to acknowledge Leanne Lessley for her expert help in image illustration.

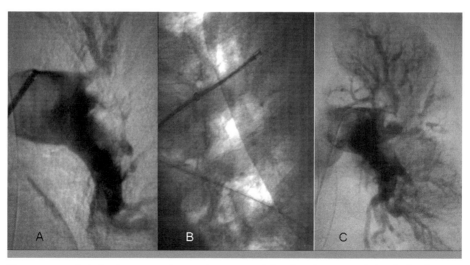

FIGURE 12.4. **A.** Left pulmonary angiogram demonstrates left main pulmonary embolus. **B.** Amplatz Thrombectomy Device (ATD) was used for 7 minutes. **C.** Post-angiogram demonstrates decrease in clot burden.

Initial experience with the ATD showed clinical improvement in a limited group of patients, with reduction of the respiratory symptoms and improvement of hypotension.[22,23] Transient hemoptysis and arrhythmias have been described as complications associated with the use of the ATD. Hemolysis also occurs commonly with the use of the ATD, but there are no reported cases of associated renal failure. The use of the ATD has been limited recently due to its bulkiness and lack of steerability.

Arrow-Trerotola Percutaneous Thrombolytic Device

The Arrow-Trerotola device (Arrow, Reading, PA) is a low-speed (3000 rpm) rotational basket designed for thrombectomy in dialysis grafts. It scrapes the walls of the vessel and fragments the thrombus. The device was modified for the treatment of PE in an animal model and was shown to be effective in fragmenting the clots and relatively safe for treating large acute central pulmonary emboli. A modified 8F, 120-cm-long device was redesigned with a nitinol wire basket that measures 9 to 15-mm in diameter when expanded. When this device was applied in a porcine pulmonary artery, histologic specimens showed that there was moderate acute intimal injury, but no evidence of pulmonary artery disruption. In a case report on the use of the Trerotola device (7F 80-cm-long over-the-wire device) for mechanical thrombectomy of massive pulmonary embolism,[24] the device was found to be difficult to direct into some of the vessels being treated. In this case report, there was no improvement in pulmonary pressures and large portions of clot remained untreated, although clinical improvement was observed. We have performed 2 procedures at our institution combining the use of the over-the-wire Trerotola device with local thrombolytic therapy and achieved clinical success in one patient with no complications. However, we encountered an intraprocedural death in one patient with massive main pulmonary artery clot who was hypotensive and moderately hypoxemic prior to initiation of the catheter-directed treatment. Upon activation of the over-the-wire Trerotola device in the main pulmonary, the patient developed electrical-mechanical dissociation on our procedure table and could not be resuscitated. The experience with this device remains very limited and its safety in native pulmonary arteries is unproven.

Thrombus Fragmentation Catheters and Balloons

The theoretical advantage of the fragmentation technique is that the central pulmonary artery volume is roughly 50% of the volume of the branch pulmonary arterial segments. Therefore, by achieving immediate redistribution of the occlusive thrombus from the central main pulmonary artery to the more peripheral pulmonary artery branches, the afterload on the right ventricle is immediately reduced. In addition, following clot fragmentation, a greater surface area of the thrombus is exposed to allow greater activation of clot-bound plasminogen to plasmin by the infused lytic agents, if thrombolysis is used in combination with the fragmentation technique.

Balloon Catheters

Balloon angioplasty (6–16 mm in diameter) for fragmentation of large central pulmonary emboli has been used in association with local thrombolytic infusion with encouraging results. Recovery rates of 87.5%, as measured by pulmonary artery pressures, blood O_2 values, and clinical outcomes, have been reported with use of this technique.[25]

Angiographic and Pigtail Catheters

Various angiographic or pigtail catheter devices have been used to fragment centrally located emboli by direct mechanical action. The majority of the reported patients were also treated with local or systemic thrombolysis[26,27] (Table 21.1); therefore, it is unclear whether thrombus fragmentation with a catheter without thrombolysis is effective.

The rotatable pigtail catheter is a custom-made 5F pigtail catheter. It is 110 cm in length and has 10 side holes for contrast injection (Figure 12.5). The catheter is introduced via a flexible 5.5F sheath. The catheter is designed to be used over an 0.035-in movable-core J wire. An electrical motor is connected to a luer lock adapter on the proximal hub end of the catheter and can generate rotational speeds up to 500 rpm. The pigtail catheter is designed to rotate within the sheath with a guidewire exiting through the distal side hole. The sheath prevents precessing of the catheter shaft, thereby minimizing damage along the venous access route. The wire serves as a rigid central axis for pigtail rotation. During activation of the electrical motor, the catheter can be advanced and pulled back over the wire. The catheter can also be used for follow-up angiograms after clot fragmentation.[8] In 20 patients with massive PE, catheter intervention with the rotatable pigtail catheter showed a 33% recanalization rate by fragmentation, but the catheter was more effective with adjuvant thrombolytic therapy. The mortality rate in this series was 20%.[28] A recent study reported on the use of a modified rotatable pigtail catheter with or without thrombolytics and showed shorter hospital stay and higher survival rate when utilizing catheter fragmentation and aspiration without thrombolytics than when thrombolytics are added.[29]

In summary, clot fragmentation techniques have been employed with success,

but usually in combination with catheter-directed thrombolysis or suction embolectomy via large guiding catheters (10F). Distal migration of large clot fragments does remain a concern with clot fragmentation techniques without adjuvant thrombolysis, as it may lead to acute worsening in the hemodynamic status of the patient depending upon how the clot redistributes.

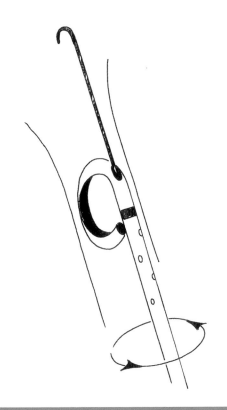

FIGURE 12.5.   The drawing depicts the rotation of the pigtail catheter about the axis of a stationary guidewire. Emboli are fragmented by the mechanical action of the rotating catheter loop. During rotation, the pigtail catheter can be advanced or withdrawn over the guidewire. Side holes are present within the catheter to allow contrast injection following the fragmentation procedure. The authors would like to acknowledge Leanne Lessley for her expert help in image illustration.

Suction Embolectomy with Guide Catheters/Sheaths

Manual suction embolectomy had been used alone or as an adjunct to other techniques. An 8F–16F guiding catheter/sheath is advanced into the thrombus in the main right or left pulmonary artery (PA). A 10- to 30-mL syringe with a luer lock connector is then used to apply suction while the catheter is moved slowly to and fro over several centimeters within the PA. During advancement, it is important to be aware of any resistance, which may indicate subintimal passage. When blood readily enters the syringe, the material has cleared the catheter. The syringe is then removed and its contents are expressed over a gauze-draped basin. It is necessary to readvance the catheter into the PAs for each successive aspiration. This technique has been described with or without local thrombolytics.[30,31] In a recent study, clinical success was 100% in 15 patients utilizing an 8Fr guiding catheter. In another study, the survival rate utilizing this technique was 72%. The study also showed that this technique is more efficacious with acute PE when the procedure is performed < 48 hours from the onset of symptoms.[32]

Hydrodynamic Thrombectomy Devices

Although none of the currently available hydrodynamic or rheolytic catheter devices were designed for the treatment of large arteries, they have been successfully used in an off-label fashion for the treatment of patients with massive PE. The Hydrolyzer (Cordis; Warren, NJ) is a 7F, 80-cm over-the-wire catheter, with a large side hole near the distal tip. The larger catheter lumen is used for aspiration of the fragmented clots, and the smaller lumen serves as the injec-tion channel with metallic tubing looped 180° to enable retrograde injection of fluid at high velocities. High-velocity injection through the small lumen of the metallic tubing creates lower pressure dynamics in the larger lumen. A Bernoulli effect is created, resulting in a vortex, causing fragmentation of the clots by the pressure gradient.[8] The fragmented clots can then be aspirated via the larger lumen. The Hydrolyzer has been reported to be effective in removing an acute clot from vessels up to 9 mm in diameter. The device is no longer available in the United States.

The AngioJet Xpeedior (MEDRAD, Inc.) is a 6F over-the-wire mechanical thrombectomy device and is probably the most efficacious catheter among the currently available hydrodynamic devices (see Figure 8.1 on page 91). Power saline jets at speeds up to 300 miles per hour are injected in a retrograde fashion to create a low-pressure zone around the catheter tip, causing a Bernoulli effect and a recirculating vortex. The injected saline is removed in a euvolemic fashion via a suction port on the catheter. The thrombus is withdrawn toward the catheter into the vortex and fragmented into small particles that are, in theory, removed along with the injected fluid through the suction port of the device. Since the AngioJet Xpeedior was not designed to treat vessels larger than 12 mm in diameter, it is also of limited effectiveness in the treatment of central PE located in larger arteries. However, the resultant disruption of the clot with the device and enhancement in pulmonary perfusion often is sufficient to improve hemodynamics and clinical outcomes in these patients.[7,33-36] In one study, 14 patients were treated with this device. Adjunctive local thrombolysis was performed in 5 patients. Clinical success was obtained in 86% of patients. Procedural mortality occurred in one patient who presented in cardiogenic shock and nonfatal hemoptysis occurred in one patient.[35] In another study, 51 patients were treated with the AngioJet device, 21% of whom also received local thrombolytic therapy. The in-hospital mortality rate was 15%.[36]

The use of this device close to the heart is commonly associated with bradyarrhythmias, including transient asystole, which can cause significant symptoms and hinder its use in some patients. The incidence of the bradyarrhythmias appears to increase with the proximity of the device to the heart and the duration of device activation. The incidence of bradyarrhythmias with the use of this device is 20% to 79% in patients undergoing coronary artery thrombectomy.[37] In one series, 2 of 17 patients (12%) who underwent pulmonary thrombectomy with the AngioJet had bradyarrhythmias.[34] In another series 8% of patients required tranvenous pacing for significant bradycardia.[36] The cause of AngioJet-induced bradyarrhythmia remains unknown. Some authors suggest that the arrhythmias could be related to activation of stretch receptors by the high-pressure jets. The effect of adenosine released from lysed cells on the atrioventricular node has also been suggested as a possible mechanism. Most typically, the bradyarrhythmias will stop within 10 seconds of deactivating the device. In addition, activation of the device for short bursts (ie, less than 10 seconds) with 15- to 20-second pauses between device activation minimizes the occurrence of the bradyarrhythmias. A few procedural-related deaths with use of the AngioJet for acute PE have been described in the literature, which leads many operators to recommend against using this device in the pulmonary circulation. It is worth mentioning, however, that we have used the AngioJet device in combination with local thrombolytics for pulmonary embolectomy in 16 patients and have had no procedural-related mortalities. Bradyarrhythmias were common, but transient (Figure 12.6). We emphasize that careful monitoring of the cardiac rhythm and hemodynamic parameters is paramount during the use of this device. As mentioned earlier, mechanical ventilation is encouraged as the activation of this device in the

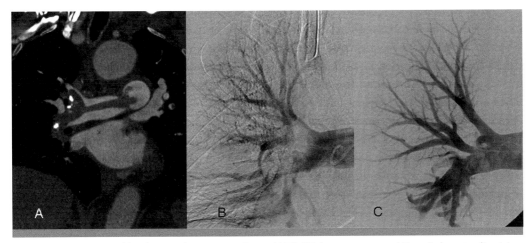

FIGURE 12.6.   72-year-old with acute chest pain. **A.** Coronal MPR CT demonstrates a saddle embolus extending into right main PA. Echocardiogram showed moderate right atrium dilatation and right ventricular dysfunction. **B.** Right pulmonary angiogram demonstrates right PA embolus. Mean PAP on initial study was 34 mm Hg. **C.** Post AngioJet and 12 hours of thrombolysis angiogram demonstrates significant decrease in clot burden. Mean PAP was 15 mm Hg.

pulmonary circulation is commonly associated with the patient complaining of a sense of difficulty breathing and, on occasion, becoming apneic. Again, a judicious protocol of a short duration of device activation, followed by a discrete pause, seems to minimize the occurrence of bradyarrhythmias.

Other complications related to this device include hemoglobinuria and renal insufficiency. Therefore, we will often employ a sodium bicarbonate drip to alkalinize the urine and facilitate excretion of the free hemoglobin when we use the AngioJet device.

Aspirex PE Catheter

The 11F Aspirex catheter thrombectomy device (Straub Medical; Wangs, Switzerland) was specifically designed and developed for percutaneous interventional treatment of acute PE in arteries ranging from 6 to 14 mm in caliber. The central part of the catheter system is a high-speed rotational coil (40,000 revolutions per minute) within the catheter body that creates negative pressure through an L-shaped aspiration port at the catheter tip. The rotating coil macerates aspirated thrombus, and removes thrombus fragments via an augerlike action (Figure 12.7). The distal part of the catheter has

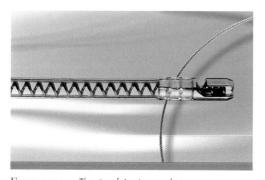

Figure 12.7. The tip of Aspirex catheter thrombectomy device. Used with permission from Straub Medical, Wangs, Switzerland.

enhanced flexibility, which facilitates its passage through the right side of the heart into the pulmonary arteries. A recent study on the use of this device in 11 patients reported a clinical success rate of 88%.[38] A cohort study is currently being performed in Europe to investigate the effectiveness and safety of the Aspirex device in patients with acute, massive PE and a contraindication for thrombolysis.[7]

Complications of Catheter-Directed Interventions

Complications of catheter-directed interventions for acute PE include perforation or dissection of cardiovascular structures, pericardial tamponade, pulmonary hemorrhage, distal thrombus embolization, and death.[7,39] Other potential complications include chest pain, hemoptysis, blood loss, arrhythmias, contrast-induced nephropathy, anaphylactic reaction to iodine contrast, hemolysis, and vascular access complications such as hematoma, access site thrombosis, arterial puncture, pseudoaneurysm, or arteriovenous fistula. To minimize the risk of vascular perforation or dissection, mechanical thrombectomy should be performed only in the main and lobar pulmonary arteries, not in the segmental pulmonary arteries. The procedure should be performed with a guiding sheath positioned in the main pulmonary to minimize trauma to the heart and the induction of arrhythmias. The procedure should be terminated as soon as hemodynamic improvement is achieved, regardless of the angiographic result.[7,8]

Fewer hemorrhagic complications should be seen with catheter-directed thrombolysis than with bolus intravenous infusion, but no randomized control data have demonstrated this difference. However, the rate of major bleeding was reported at 6% with catheter-directed infusion of rtPA compared with 27% and 12%, respectively, for peripherally infused urokinase in phases I and II of the UPET study.[8]

IVC Filter Placement

In patients with a contraindication to anticoagulation, an IVC filter is placed before initiation of catheter-directed therapy. In patients with compromised hemodynamics, even if they can be anticoagulated, an optional IVC filter is often placed prior to initiation of catheter-directed interventions for massive PE. We then work through the filter to perform our catheter-directed therapy if the access is from the femoral vein. Once we have completed treatment of the PE, if the patient can be fully anticoagulated and has no further need for the IVC filter, the filter is removed. If the clinical status of the patient is tenuous, the IVC filter remains in place until all consultants agree that there is no further need for the filter.

Conclusion

Once the diagnosis of acute PE has been established, therapy should be initiated as soon as possible to minimize the morbidity and mortality associated with the embolic event and to enhance the chances for pulmonary artery recanalization. Patients who do not have any underlying cardiopulmonary disease and are not compromised by their acute embolic event can usually be treated with a 3- to 6-month course of anticoagulation. Patients who have a moderate volume of clot (>1 lobe) and are hemodynamically compromised (tachycardia, systemic hypotension, right ventricle dysfunction by echocardiogram or other imaging modality, and/or marked pulmonary hypertension), or

persistently hypoxemic despite appropriate anticoagulation and supplemental oxygen administration, should be considered for more aggressive intervention.

Thrombolytic therapy appears to be useful in rapidly restoring more normal hemodynamics and may prove to be useful in reducing the sequela of chronic pulmonary hypertension. With a greater understanding of the risks associated with fibrinolysis, bleeding complications can be reduced. The use of the intravenous route is favored when there is diffuse, bilateral acute PE, the patient is young, and the patient has absolutely no contraindication to thrombolysis. In situations in which there is markedly asymmetric clot burden or the patient is at some risk for bleeding, or the patient is very hemodynamically compromised and there is asymmetric clot burden, catheter-directed techniques rather than IV therapy are recommended. Direct intrathrombus infusion of lower doses of the thrombolytic agent may also reduce bleeding complications without decreasing the beneficial fibrinolytic affect.

Although percutaneous embolectomy and fragmentation techniques are intriguing, most of the devices are not widely available. Despite the lack of availability of these percutaneous devices, several studies have shown that simple catheter techniques aiming at mechanical fragmentation of the clot using angioplasty balloons and pigtail catheters, coupled with either suction embolectomy and/or local thrombolytic administration, have resulted in dramatic improvements in patients with massive, acute PE.[27,40] However, older, more organized thrombus may be refractory to thrombolysis and mechanical fragmentation and require surgical intervention. Use of optional IVC filters will likely help in the acute period, since the patient is likely still at risk for recurrence of additional emboli.

Acknowledgments

The authors would like to acknowledge Ms. Leanne Lessley for her expert help in image illustration.

References

1. Dalen JE, Alpert JS. Natural history of pulmonary embolism. Prog Cardiovas Dis. 1975;17:259-70.

2. Hermann RE, Davis JH, Holden WD. Pulmonary embolism: a clinical and pathologic study with emphasis on the effect of prophylactic therapy with anticoagulants. Am J Surg. 1961;102:19-28.

3. Barritt DW, Jordan SE. Anticoagulant drugs in the treatment of pulmonary embolism: a controlled trial. Lancet. 1960;1:1309-12.

4. Benotti JR, Dalen JE. The natural history of pulmonary embolism. Clin Chest Med. 1984;5:403-10.

5. Kucher N, Rossi E, De Rosa M, Goldhaber SZ. Prognostic role of echocardiography among patients with acute pulmonary embolism and a systolic arterial pressure of 90 mm Hg or higher. Arch Intern Med. 2005;165:1777-81.

6. Schoepf UJ, Kucher N, Kipfmueller F, Quiroz R, Costello P, Goldhaber SZ. Right ventricular enlargement on chest computed tomography: a predictor of early death in acute pulmonary embolism. Circulation. 2004;110:3276-80.

7. Kucher N. Catheter embolectomy for acute pulmonary embolism. Chest. 2007;132:657-63.

8. Uflacker R. Interventional therapy for pulmonary embolism. J Vasc Interv Radiol. 2001;12:147-64.

9. National Institutes of Health Consensus Panel. Thrombolytic therapy and thrombosis: a National Institutes of Health consensus development conference. Ann Intern Med. 1980;93:141-4.

10. Goldhaber SZ. Thrombolysis for pulmonary embolism. Prog Cardiovas Dis. 1991;34:113-34.

11. Anderson DR, Levine MN. Thrombolytic therapy for the treatment of acute pulmonary embolism. Can Med Assoc J. 1992;146:1317-24.

12. Konstantinides S, Geibel A, Heusel G, Heinrich F, Kasper W. Management Strategies and Prognosis of Pulmonary Embolism-3 Trial Investigators. Heparin plus alteplase compared with heparin alone in patients with submassive pulmonary embolism. N Engl J Med. 2002;347:1143-50.

13. Terrin M, Goldhaber SZ, Thompson B. The TIPE Investigators. Selection of patients with acute pulmonary embolism for thrombolytic therapy: the thrombolysis in pulmonary embolism (TIPE) patient survey. Chest. 1989;95:279S-81S.

14. Molina JE, Hunter DW, Yedlicka JW, Cerra FB. Thrombolytic therapy for post operative pulmonary embolism. Am J Surg. 1992;163:375-81.

15. González-Juanatey JR, Valdés L, Amaro A, Iglesias C, Alvarez D, García Acuña JM, et al. Treatment of massive pulmonary thromboembolism with low intrapulmonary dosages of urokinase: short-term angiographic and hemodynamic evolution. Chest. 1992;102:341-6.

16. Verstraete M, Miller GAH, Bounameaux H, Charbonnier B, Colle JP, Lecorf G, et al. Intravenous and intrapulmonary recombinant tissue-type plasminogen activator in the treatment of acute massive pulmonary embolism. Circulation. 1988;77:353-60.

17. Kandarpa K. Technical determinants of success in catheter-directed thrombolysis for peripheral arterial occlusions. J Vasc Interv Radiol. 1995;6:55S-61S.

18. Chamsuddin A, Nazzal L, Kang B, Best I, Peters G, Panah S, et al. Catheter-directed thrombolysis with the EndoWave system in

the treatment of acute massive pulmonary embolism: a retrospective multicenter case series. J Vasc Interv Radiol. 2008;19(3):372-6.

19. Meyer G, Tamisier D, Sors H, Stern M, Vouhé P, Makowski S, et al. Pulmonary embolectomy: a 20-year experience at one center. Ann Thorac Surg. 1991;51:232-6.

20. Leacche M, Unic D, Goldhaber SZ, Rawn JD, Aranki SF, Couper GS, et al. Modern surgical treatment of massive pulmonary embolism: results in 47 consecutive patients after rapid diagnosis and aggressive surgical approach. J Thorac Cardiovasc Surg. 2005;129(5):1018-23.

21. Greenfield LJ, Proctor MC, Williams DM, Wakefield TW. Long-term experience with transvenous catheter pulmonary embolectomy. J Vasc Surg. 1993;18:450-8.

22. Uflacker R, Strange C, Vujic B. Massive pulmonary embolism: preliminary results of treatment with the Amplatz thrombectomy device. J Vasc Interv Radiol. 1996;7:519-28.

23. Müller-Hülsbeck S, Brossmann J, Jahnke T, Grimm J, Reuter M, Bewig B, et al. Mechanical thrombectomy of major and massive pulmonary embolism with use of the Amplatz thrombectomy device. Invest Radiol. 2001;36:317-22.

24. Rocek M, Peregrin J, Velimsky T. Mechanical thrombectomy of massive pulmonary embolism using an Arrow Trerotola percutaneous thrombolytic device. Eur Radiol. 1998;8:1683-5.

25. Fava M, Loyola S, Flores P, Huete I. Mechanical fragmentation and pharmacologic thrombolysis in massive pulmonary embolism. J Vasc Interv Radiol. 1997;8:261-6.

26. Schmitz-Rode T, Janssens U, Hanrath P, Günther RW. Fragmentation of massive pulmonary embolism using a pigtail rotation catheter: possible complication. Eur Radiol. 2001;11:2047-9.

27. De Gregorio MA, Gimeno MJ, Mainar A, Herrera M, Tobio R, Alfonso R, et al. Mechanical and enzymatic thrombolysis for

massive pulmonary embolism. J Vasc Interv Radiol. 2002;13:163-9.

28. Schmitz-Rode T, Janssens U, Schild HH, Basche S, Hanrath P, Günther RW. Fragmentation of massive pulmonary embolism using a pigtail rotation catheter. Chest. 1998;114:1427-36.

29. Yoshida M, Inoue I, Kawagoe T, Ishihara M, Shimatani Y, Kurisu S, et al. Novel percutaneous catheter thrombectomy in acute massive pulmonary embolism: rotational bidirectional thrombectomy (ROBOT). Catheter Cardiovasc Interv. 2006;68:112-7.

30. Lang EV, Barnhart WH, Walton DL, Raab SS. Percutaneous pulmonary thrombectomy. J Vasc Interv Radiol. 1997;8:427-32.

31. Tajima H, Murata S, Kumazaki T, Nakazawa K, Kawamata H, Fukunaga T, et al. Manual aspiration thrombectomy with a standard PTCA guiding catheter for treatment of acute massive pulmonary thromboembolism. Radiat Med. 2004;22:168-72.

32. Timsit JF, Reynaud P, Meyer G, Sors H. Pulmonary embolectomy by catheter device in massive pulmonary embolism. Chest. 1991;100:655-8.

33. Siablis D, Karnabatidis D, Katsanos K, Kagadis GC, Zabakis P, Hahalis G. AngioJet rheolytic thrombectomy versus local intrapulmonary thrombolysis in massive pulmonary embolism: a retrospective data analysis. J Endovasc Ther. 2005;12: 206-14.

34. Zeni PT, Blank BG, Peeler DW. Use of rheolytic thrombectomy in treatment of acute massive pulmonary embolism. J Vasc Interv Radiol. 2003;14:1511-5.

35. Chauhan MS, Kawamura A. Percutaneous rheolytic thrombectomy for large pulmonary embolism: a promising treatment option. Catheter Cardiovasc Interv. 2007;70: 123-30.

36. Chechi T, Vecchio S, Spaziani G, Giuliani G, Giannotti F, Arcangeli C, et al. Rheolytic

thrombectomy in patients with massive and submassive acute pulmonary embolism. Catheter Cardiovasc Interv. 2009;73:506-13.

37. Dwarka D, Schwartz SA, Smyth SH, O'Brien MJ. Bradyarrhythmias during use of the AngioJet system. J Vasc Interv Radiol. 2006;17:1693-5.

38. Eid-Lidt G, Gaspar J, Sandoval J. Combined clot fragmentation and aspiration in patients with acute pulmonary embolism. Chest. 2008;134:45-60.

39. Skaf E, Beemath A, Siddiqui T, Janjua M, Patel NR, Stein PD. Catheter-tip embolectomy in the management of acute massive pulmonary embolism. Am J Cardiol. 2007;99:415-20.

40. Kuo WT, van den Bosch MA, Hofmann LV, Louie JD, Kothary N, Sze DY. Catheter-directed embolectomy, fragmentation, and thrombolysis for the treatment of massive pulmonary embolism after failure of systemic thrombolysis. Chest. 2008;134;250-4.

Thoracic Outlet Syndrome

Venous thoracic outlet remains a niche practice in contemporary vascular surgery, and management in this area generates some controversy. While all agree that an upper extremity DVT requires anticoagulation in accordance with the current American College of Chest Physicians (ACCP) criteria, the choice of patient who requires decompression is practice dependent. Drs. Thompson and Johansen have kindly provided a balanced and contemporary overview of the subject and demonstrate the consensus and the differences in the patterns of care, from resolution of the immediate problem with thrombolysis to pharmacological or surgical intervention. There is no level I evidence to support either the use of thrombolysis or decompression similar to that used for the treatment of the lower extremity DVT. One point that should be emphasized is that due to the anatomy, endovascular interventions (angioplasty or stent placement) without decompression have no role in the management of primary axillosubclavian DVT.

Primary Axillosubclavian Venous Thrombosis
Observational Care

Kaj H. Johansen

Thrombosis of the deep veins of the upper extremities may occur for diverse reasons. Most commonly, axillosubclavian venous thrombosis (ASVT) is *secondary* to a pacemaker wire or a chronic indwelling catheter inserted for hemodialysis access or for the long-term administration of antibiotics, chemotherapeutic agents, or blood products.[1-3]

Also presenting, like those with secondary ASVT, with a swollen, discolored, sometimes painful arm, are individuals who have suffered a spontaneous, or *primary*, ASVT. Alternatively known as Paget-Schroetter syndrome, the condition is also termed "effort" thrombosis as a consequence of the observation that a number of such individuals, usu-

ally young and active, develop this problem after extensive or untoward physical exertion with the affected arm.

In the lower extremities, deep venous thrombosis (DVT) commonly is followed by the development of chronic swelling, pain, prominent veins, and skin changes, all manifestations of the postphlebitic or postthrombotic syndrome (PTS). The condition can also follow untreated upper extremity DVT. To varying degrees, PTS can be vexing, disfiguring, or even disabling whether it occurs in the lower or the upper extremities.

Because patients with primary ASVT have been thought to be at substantial risk for chronic postthrombotic symptoms, they are advised to undergo thoracic outlet decompression. If the axillosubclavian vein is partially or completely occluded, various venous reconstructive procedures are recommended so that such patients can enjoy a durable return of upper extremity function.

Venous Thromboembolic Disease. Contemporary Endovascular Management series. © 2011 Mark G. Davies MD and Alan B. Lumsden MD, eds. Cardiotext Publishing, ISBN 978-1-935395-22-5.

Anatomy and Pathophysiology of Primary ASVT

Upper extremity deep venous thrombosis not related to a prior indwelling catheter or electrode wire is generally thought to arise consequent to extrinsic compression of the subclavian vein as it traverses the costoclavicular space. It has been surmised that chronic trauma to the subclavian vein at this site results in a neointimal hyperplastic stenosis within the vein that, over time, narrows to the point that partial or complete thrombosis of the vein occurs, resulting in the characteristic venous congestive symptoms and signs that characterize the clinical presentation of primary ASVT. Substantial venous collaterals then develop around the shoulder and the clavicle, some of them becoming visible in the subcutaneous tissues of the upper arm, shoulder, and chest wall. Thrombus generally extends throughout the subclavian vein and may extend in a retrograde fashion out into the axillary and even upper brachial and basilic veins: the cephalic vein commonly remains patent and may be a major outflow collateral for the congested upper extremity venous system.

Over time, as with deep vein clots elsewhere, the axillosubclavian thrombus may reduce in size, partially recanalize, or even lyse completely. Another explanation for a reduction in size of the clot burden in the axillosubclavian vein is pulmonary embolization.[4]

Initial arm swelling in ASVT may be severe, and upon rare occasion, phlegmasia cerulea dolens has been reported.[5] Because of the aforementioned venous collateralization and clot resolution, as well as the fact that such patients generally present early after presentation and catheter-directed venous thrombolysis is commonly instituted, arm swelling rapidly returns to normal in a large majority of patients with primary ASVT.

General Principles

Only when the natural history of a disease state is well understood can the advantages and disadvantages of various therapies be evaluated. For example, for many decades peptic ulcer disease was thought to be the consequence of a metabolic disorder leading to gastric acid hypersecretion. It was assumed that if the condition was left untreated, recurrent foregut ulceration, perforation, bleeding, and obstruction were certain and would be treatable only by major operations that either altered the neurophysiology of gastric acid secretion or rearranged the anatomy of the esophagus, stomach, and duodenum. Entire academic careers rose and fell on whether a vagotomy should be truncal or selective, and a generation of medical students and residents strained to differentiate among the different postgastrectomy syndromes.

But because of the epochal discovery[6] that peptic ulcers are almost always the result of a bacterial colonization of the stomach, are easily treated by an oral medication, and are thereafter almost never associated with recurrent symptoms, the underlying condition has all but disappeared from contemporary surgical consciousness. Complicated peptic ulcer disease, treated properly, is only uncommonly diagnosed in contemporary medical practice and is widely understood to be a benign and self-limited condition.

What do we truly know about the natural history of deep venous disease of the upper extremities?

The Natural History of ASVT: Older Data

Beginning in the 1960s, numerous papers regarding the natural history of primary ASVT were published.[7-9] These series were of substantial size and had extended and relatively complete follow-up. They demonstrated that, once patients presented with upper extremity DVT, their course, in 40% to 70% of cases, was quite morbid, with recurrent episodes of arm swelling, pain and discoloration, and other manifestations of the postthrombotic syndrome. Many of these patients were thought to be disabled.

Given the data, appropriate means to mitigate or even relieve patients' chronic PTS symptoms were contemplated, developed, and assessed. Because ASVT has been thought by many to be a consequence of extrinsic compression of the subclavian vein in the costoclavicular space between the clavicle and the first rib, initial efforts were directed toward thoracic outlet decompression, generally by first rib resection or claviculectomy.[9,10] Patients whose axillosubclavian veins had remained patent or only moderately stenotic appeared to do well.

However, in ASVT patients whose axillosubclavian vein had been left occluded or highly stenotic, simple thoracic outlet decompression was not adequate. In fact, the effort to remove the first rib potentially interrupted periclavicular venous collaterals and potentially worsening patients' postthrombotic symptoms. So efforts to reconstruct the blocked vein by thrombectomy, venous patch angioplasty, or bypass grafting began to be performed. Several relatively recent series suggest these very large operations (which continue to include first rib resection besides axillosubclavian venous reconstruction and, sometimes, peripheral AV fistula formation) show good to excellent results—relatively durable venous patency and resolution of postthrombotic symptoms—in 80% to 90% of cases.[11-15] While complications of these major operations may be severe,[16,17] they are relatively uncommon in series reported from high-volume centers.[11-15]

Natural History of ASVT: Recent Data

Beginning in the late 1990s, a series of reports began to appear suggesting that patients with primary ASVT who had been treated at the time of their initial presentation by venous thrombolysis (often associated with an effort at venous angioplasty) and oral anticoagulation appeared to have a remarkably benign course, notwithstanding their having undergone no surgical intervention at all. These series often arose from audits of vascular laboratory experiences following patients who had presented with primary ASVT[18] or from vascular medicine or thrombosis specialists.[19-22] But several surgical series described patients in whom initial thrombolysis and anticoagulation had been performed but an operation had been reserved for patients with recurrent or persistent, unremitting symptoms; a majority of these patients appeared to have done well without operation as well.[23-25]

It could be readily concluded from these more recent studies that patients with primary ASVT treated by thrombolysis and anticoagulation at the time of their initial presentation ultimately do well, without development of recurrent thrombosis or postthrombotic symptoms, in 80% to 90% of cases.

Comment

The proper choice among differing treatments for a particular condition should revolve around relative safety, efficacy, durability, and when possible, cost-effectiveness. The choice of therapy also depends upon an up-to-date understanding of the natural history of the condition.

But physicians' understanding of the natural history of a particular condition should also be informed by new evidence. This is particularly true when a condition's subsequent course has been substantially altered by early treatment. As noted previously, the landscape for surgical management of peptic ulcer disease has been transformed by the contemporary demonstration that the condition is predominantly an infectious disease[6] that can be mostly prevented by the administration of oral antimicrobial agents and antacids.[26]

Historical analyses of patients who had suffered from primary deep venous thrombosis of the upper extremity veins demonstrated that, if untreated, a large majority of patients had persistent arm swelling, pain, discoloration, and other manifestations of the postthrombotic syndrome.[7-9] It was entirely reasonable that a surgical approach to diminishing the risk of recurrent thrombosis (by thoracic outlet decompression) and, later, persistently obstructed venous flow (by venous reconstruction or bypass) were developed and perfected. In recent series, a large majority of patients so treated have appeared to enjoy durable relief of their prior arm problems and have returned to normal activities.[11-15]

However, prior historical series evaluated the outcomes of primary ASVT patients who had received no initial treatment: no thrombolysis and sometimes not even consistent anticoagulation.[7-10] More recently, the immediate anticoagulation in these patients—not only to prevent thrombus progression but also to eliminate the risk of pulmonary embolization[4]—has become the standard of practice. Since the early 1980s, catheter-directed thrombolysis of the upper extremity veins has become routine.[27] Indeed, when thrombolysis is partially or completely successful, the use of other endovascular techniques is commonplace. Some of these treatments, such as balloon angioplasty of venous stenosis, may be effective,[28] whereas others (venous stenting) are not.[29]

Follow-up of ASVT patients subjected to contemporary initial management suggests a much more benign course than historical controls. Evidence from multiple series of such patients undergoing contemporary initial treatment of their primary ASVT[19-25] suggests that the majority do *not* develop recurrent stenoses or significant ongoing evidence for postthrombotic symptoms. Indeed, while the optimal circumstance would obviously be complete restoration of axillosubclavian venous patency by either endogenous or exogenous thrombolysis, the evidence is that a substantial number of individuals with persistent venous stenoses or even occlusions collateralize around this relatively focal obstruction in such robust fashion that they are asymptomatic at rest and even after upper extremity exertion.[23-25]

Thus, approximately the same percentage of individuals followed by observation alone have an excellent, or at least as good as, outcome as individuals who undergo first rib resection and axillosubclavian venous reconstruction. With the presumption that these patient populations are similar, the routine recommendation for thoracic outlet decompression/upper extremity vein reconstruction operation for patients who have suffered primary ASVT would seem to overreach.

Indeed, the major debate has been not whether to carry out such surgical reconstruction for primary ASVT or not, but whether to wait for a period for postthrombosis inflammation to clear rather than operating immediately.[30]

It has been proposed that an aggressive operative reconstructive approach to primary ASVT may be particularly appropriate for certain individuals who might be expected to be sensitive to even minimal amounts of arm swelling—younger individuals or elite athletes,[31] for example. This assertion may be correct. However, it is impossible to prove that a subset of primary ASVT patients exist for whom aggressive operative reconstruction should be the norm because of the absence of a control group of such individuals who have *not* been reconstructed in this fashion.

Indeed, the dilemma in what to advise patients who have suffered primary ASVT, after they have undergone thrombolysis and 3 months of anticoagulation, is that no level I, or even level II, evidence is available to permit a truly informed decision by the patient. Instead, if a primary ASVT patient presents to a major academic medical center in Baltimore, St. Louis, or Denver, the patient is likely to undergo thoracic outlet decompression and, if necessary, major upper extremity venous reconstructive surgery. The same patient appearing at a similar institution in Palo Alto, Seattle, or Vancouver will likely simply be urged to exercise vigorously and will be offered an operation only if, during long-term follow-up, persistent or recurrent postthrombotic symptoms persist or recur—an extremely uncommon event.

At the very least, the necessity for *immediately* decompressing and reconstructing primary ASVT patients' axillosubclavian veins should be reexamined. There are no compelling data that demonstrate improved outcome following axillosubclavian vein decompression and reconstruction with an immediate operation vs. a period of observation. Noting recent data,[19-25] a skeptical observer might wonder whether, if observation continued long enough, a substantial number of such patients would be asymptomatic and might not need an operation at all. One study comparing outcomes of operations for venous and neurogenic thoracic outlet syndrome by means of a validated functional tool [32] noted that primary ASVT patients were minimally symptomatic preoperatively and were not improved by operation.[33]

Optimally, given the fact that this is a relatively stereotypic patient population that presents soon after the onset of upper extremity symptoms, a prospective randomized trial of immediate operation vs. observation should be launched. An excellent venue for this could be the nascent Consortium on Outcomes Research and Education for Thoracic Outlet Syndrome (CORE-TOS), chaired by Robert Thompson, MD, of St. Louis, and Julie Freischlag, MD, of Baltimore. A multicenter enrollment of primary ASVT patients, all of them undergoing initial anticoagulation and thrombolysis and then randomized either to operation or observation, should soon yield credible results regarding whether there is an advantage to operative intervention for such patients. Such a randomized control trial is under discussion.

References

1. Linenburger ML. Catheter-related thrombosis: risks, diagnosis and management. J Natl Compr Cancer Netw. 2006;4:889-901.
2. Mandolfo S, Piazza W, Galli F. Central venous catheter and the hemodialysis patient: a difficult symbiosis. J Vasc Access. 2002;3:64-73.
3. Rozmus G, Danbert JP, Huang DT, Rosero

S, Hall B, Francis C. Venous thrombosis and stenosis after implantation of pacemakers and defibrillators. J Interv Card Electrophysiol. 2005;13:9-19.

4. Monreal M, Lafoz E, Ruiz J, Valls R, Alastrue A. Upper-extremity deep venous thrombosis and pulmonary embolism. Chest. 1991;99:280-3.

5. Kammen BF, Soulen MC. Phlegmasia cerulean dolens of the upper extremity. J Vasc Interv Radiol. 1995;6:283-6.

6. Marshall BJ, Warren JR. Unidentified curved bacilli in the stomach of patients with gastritis and peptic ulceration. Lancet. 1984;1: 1311-5.

7. Tilney NL, Griffiths HJG, Edwards EA. Natural history of major venous thrombosis of the upper extremity. Arch Surg. 1970;101: 792-6.

8. Gloviczki P, Kazmier FS, Hollier LH. Axillary-subclavian venous occlusion: the morbidity of a non-lethal disease. J Vasc Surg. 1986;4:333-7.

9. Kunkel JM, Machleder HI. Treatment of Paget-Schroetter syndrome. Arch Surg. 1989;124:1153-8.

10. Green RM, Waldman D, Ouriel K, Riggs P, Deweese JA. Claviculectomy for subclavian venous repair: long-term functional results. J Vasc Surg. 2000;32:315-21.

11. Urschel HC, Razzuk MA. Improved management of the Paget-Schroetter syndrome secondary to thoracic outlet compression. Ann Thorac Surg. 1991;52: 1217-21.

12. Machleder HI. Evaluation of a new treatment strategy for Paget-Schroetter syndrome: spontaneous thrombosis of the axillary-subclavian vein. J Vasc Surg. 1993;17:305-17.

13. Thompson RW, Schneider PA, Nelken NA, Skioldebrand CG, Stoney RJ. Circumferential venolysis and paraclavicular thoracic outlet decompression for "effort thrombosis" of the subclavian vein. J Vasc Surg. 1992;16:723-32.

14. Adelman MA, Stone DH, Riles TS, Lamparello PJ, Giangola G, Rosen RJ. A multidisciplinary approach to the treatment of Paget-Schroetter syndrome. Ann Vasc Surg. 1997;11:149-54.

15. Molina JE. Need for emergency treatment in subclavian vein effort thrombosis. J Am Coll Surg. 1995;181:414-20.

16. Melliere D, Becquemin JP, Etienne G, Lecheviller B. Severe injuries resulting from operations for thoracic outlet syndrome: can they be avoided? J Cardiovasc Surg (Torino). 1991;32:599-603.

17. Chang DC, Lidor AO, Matsen SL, Freischlag JA. Reported in-hospital complications following rib resections for neurogenic thoracic outlet syndrome. Ann Vasc Surg. 2007;21:564-70.

18. Hingorani A, Ascher E, Lorenson E, DePippo P, Salles-Cunha S, Scheinman M, et al. Upper extremity deep venous thrombosis and its impact on morbidity and mortality rates in a hospital-based population. J Vasc Surg. 1997;26:853-60.

19. Heron E, Lozinguez O, Emmerich J, Laurian C, Fiessinger JN. Long-term sequelae of spontaneous axillary-subclavian venous thrombosis. Ann Intern Med. 1999;131:510-3.

20. Lechner D, Wiener C, Weltermann A, Eischer L, Eichinger S, Kyrle PA. Comparison between idiopathic deep vein thrombosis of the upper and lower extremity regarding risk factors and recurrence. J Thromb Haemost. 2008;6: 1269-74.

21. Martinelli I, Battaglioli T, Bucciarelli P, Passamonti SM, Mannucci PM. Risk factors and recurrence rate of primary deep vein thrombosis of the upper extremities. Circulation. 2004;110:566-70.

22. Elman EE, Kahn SR. The post-thrombotic syndrome after upper extremity deep venous thrombosis in adults: a systematic review. Thromb Res. 2006;117:609-14.

23. Lee WA, Hill BB, Harris EJ Jr, Semba CP, Olcott C IV. Surgical intervention is not required for all patients with subclavian vein thrombosis. J Vasc Surg. 2000;32:57-67.

24. Lokanathan R, Salvian AJ, Chen JC, Morris C, Taylor DC, Hsiang YN. Outcome after thrombolysis and selective thoracic outlet decompression for primary axillary vein thrombosis. J Vasc Surg. 2001;33:783-8.

25. Johansen K. Does axillosubclavian ("effort") thrombosis oblige first-rib resection? Arch. Surg., in press.

26. Chan FKL, Leung WK. Peptic ulcer disease. Lancet. 2002;360:933-41.

27. Taylor LM, McAllister WR, Dennis DL, Porter JM. Thrombolytic therapy followed by first rib resection for spontaneous ("effort") subclavian vein thrombosis. Am J Surg. 1985;149:644-7.

28. Glanz S, Gordon DH, Lipkowitz GS, Butt KM, Hong J, Sclafani SJ. Axillary and subclavian vein stenosis: percutaneous angioplasty. Radiology. 1988;168:371-3.

29. Bjarnason H, Hunter DW, Crain MR, Ferral H, Miltz-Miller SE, Wegryn SA. Collapse of a Palmaz stent in the subclavian vein. AJR Am J Roentgenol. 1993;160:1123-4.

30. Capparelli DJ, Freischlag J. A unified approach to axillosubclavian venous thrombosis in a single hospital admission. Semin Vasc Surg. 2005;18:153-7.

31. Melby SJ, Vedantham S, Narra VR, Paletta GA Jr, Khoo-Summers L, Driskill M, et al. Comprehensive surgical management of the competitive athlete with effort thrombosis of the subclavian vein (Paget-Schroetter syndrome). J Vasc Surg. 2008;47:809-20.

32. Beaton DE, Wright JG, Katz JG. The Upper Extremity Collaborative Group. Development of the QuickDASH: comparison of three item-reduction approaches. J Bone Joint Surg. 2005;87A:1038-46.

33. Cordobes-Gual J, Lozano-Vilardell P, Torreguitart-Mirada N, Lara-Hernandez R, Riera-Vazquez R, Julia-Montoya J. Prospective study of the functional recovery after surgery for thoracic outlet syndrome. Eur J Vasc Endovasc Surg. 2008;35: 79-83.

Axillary-Subclavian Venous Effort Thrombosis
Surgical Care

Valerie B. Emery and Robert W. Thompson

Primary axillary-subclavian venous effort thrombosis, also known as the Paget-Schroetter syndrome, is a relatively rare condition that affects young, active, otherwise healthy individuals.[1] Effort thrombosis is caused by compression and repetitive injury of the subclavian vein between the first rib and overlying clavicle, and it is therefore considered a form of thoracic outlet syndrome (TOS). Axillary-subclavian venous effort thrombosis is distinct from other forms of deep venous thrombosis (DVT) with respect to pathophysiology, clinical presentation, functional consequences, and treatment. In this chapter we review the management of axillary-subclavian venous effort thrombosis, with an emphasis on current approaches to surgical treatment.

Venous Thromboembolic Disease. Contemporary Endovascular Management series. © 2011 Mark G. Davies MD and Alan B. Lumsden MD, eds. Cardiotext Publishing, ISBN 978-1-935395-22-5.

Pathophysiology

Patients with venous TOS typically present with the axillary-subclavian venous effort thrombosis syndrome, characterized by the abrupt, spontaneous swelling of the entire arm, often with cyanotic (bluish) discoloration, heaviness, and pain.[2] Rather than being caused by an underlying coagulation disorder, the pathogenesis of effort thrombosis involves extrinsic compression of the subclavian vein between the clavicle and first rib, particularly during activities involving arm elevation or exertion (Figure 14.1). With repetition over many months, this focal type of venous injury leads to progressive fibrous stenosis of the vein at the level of the first rib, involving scar tissue formation and contraction around the outside of the vein, as well as fibrosis and wall thickening within the wall of the vein itself. This initial phase of venous TOS is usually asymptomatic, due to the simultaneous expansion of dense collat-

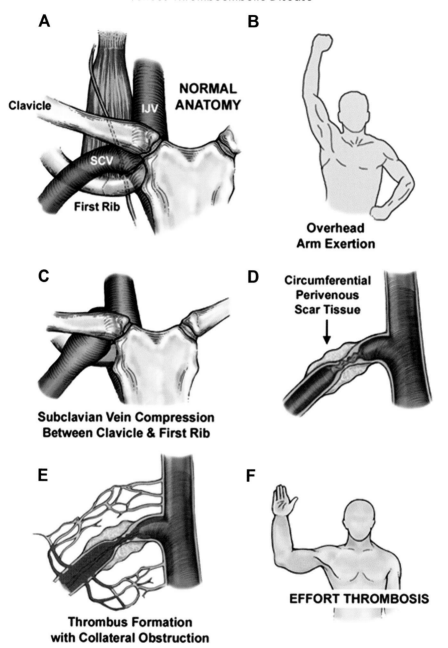

FIGURE 14.1 Pathogenesis of axillary-subclavian venous thrombosis. **A.** Normal anatomy of the thoracic outlet illustrating relationship of the internal jugular vein (IJV) and subclavian vein (SCV) to the clavicle and first rib. **B.** Vigorous activities requiring overhead positions of the arm are associated with the development of axillary-subclavian venous effort thrombosis. **C.** Subclavian vein compression between the clavicle and first rib results in focal vein wall injury. **D.** Chronic repetitive compression injury of the subclavian vein leads to formation of circumferential perivenous scar tissue, which can severely constrict the lumen. **E.** Thrombus formation within the lumen of the constricted subclavian vein causes complete obstruction of the subclavian vein, with extension of thrombus to the axillary vein causing obstruction of collateral veins. **F.** Symptomatic presentation of axillary-subclavian venous effort thrombosis. Adapted and redrawn from Melby et al., Comprehensive surgical management of the competitive athlete with effort thrombosis of the subclavian vein (Paget-Schroetter syndrome). J Vasc Surg 2008; 47:809-820, Supplement A Figure III.

eral veins. Thrombotic occlusion eventually occurs due to stagnant and turbulent blood flow in the narrowed segment of the subclavian vein. Peripheral extension of thrombus into the axillary vein can then result in further obstruction of critical collateral veins, resulting in the acute clinical presentation. Pulmonary embolism from the subclavian vein may also occur (currently estimated to occur in approximately 10% of patients with effort thrombosis), but this is infrequent compared to deep venous thrombosis in the lower extremities.

Diagnosis

Clinical Presentation

In the absence of an indwelling central venous catheter, any young, healthy, active individual presenting with the sudden onset of arm swelling and cyanotic discoloration should be suspected of having axillary-subclavian venous effort thrombosis. This condition most frequently occurs in individuals between 15 and 35 years of age, with an equal distribution between males and females. Most patients are physically active, with many engaged in work-related or recreational activities that involve vigorous use of the upper extremities in repetitive overhead positions and/or heavy lifting. The magnitude of arm swelling is usually quite substantial, with the diameter of the affected extremity increased as much as twice that of the opposite side. Most patients also describe fatigue, tightness, heaviness, and pain in the arm, especially with use or overhead positioning. Many patients will exhibit visible distention of subcutaneous veins in the upper arm, around the shoulder, or in the upper anterior chest wall. In the vast majority of situations, the clinical diagnosis of ax-

illary-subclavian venous effort thrombosis is apparent from the stereotypical history and physical examination findings.

Some patients with venous TOS may present with a more protracted history of arm swelling, fatigue, heaviness, and pain that occurs only on an intermittent basis, especially following vigorous use of the arm. Such patients may have nonthrombotic positional obstruction of the subclavian vein at the level of the first rib, which has not yet evolved to produce axillary-subclavian venous thrombosis. Another subset of patients may present with a chronic history of upper extremity venous insufficiency that has caused persistent or progressive limitations in activity over a period of many months to several years. These individuals are often found to have had previous axillary-subclavian venous thrombosis that was unrecognized and/or untreated. Finally, up to 20% of patients with venous TOS describe symptoms of pain, numbness, and/or tingling in the hand and fingers that suggest the concomitant presence of neurogenic TOS. This may occur as a result of a localized inflammatory response to subclavian venous thrombosis that has extended to the surrounding tissues of the scalene triangle, producing perineural fibrosis similar to that seen in patients with neurogenic TOS.

Vascular Laboratory Tests

Upper extremity duplex imaging is most often used as the initial diagnostic study to detect axillary-subclavian venous thrombosis, as it is noninvasive, inexpensive, and readily available. Duplex studies are of value if they are positive for axillary-subclavian vein obstruction, helping to confirm the clinical diagnosis. However, duplex imaging of the subclavian vein is complicated by the superimposed clavicle and the depth of the vein in the neck, and is highly technician-dependent. Expanded collateral veins may also be mistaken for the subclavian vein, and indirect hemodynamic measures of venous flow may not accurately reflect the status of the proximal subclavian vein. Duplex imaging studies have a false-negative rate as high as 30% for effort thrombosis and are thereby not sufficiently accurate to exclude the diagnosis of venous TOS if negative.

Radiologic Imaging

In current practice, either contrast-enhanced computed tomography (CT) or magnetic resonance (MR) angiography are being used with greater frequency as the initial noninvasive diagnostic studies for axillary-subclavian venous effort thrombosis. Both of these studies are highly accurate in detecting axillary-subclavian vein occlusion and/or focal stenosis at the level of the first rib (Figure 14.2A-B). They can also demonstrate the presence or absence of enlarged collateral veins, may provide information on the age of any thrombus present, and can be performed with the arms in elevated positions as well as at rest to elucidate evidence of positional subclavian vein obstruction. Additional information can also be obtained by comparisons with the contralateral upper extremity. Since CT or MR venography provide more anatomic information than venous duplex imaging, these studies can be used to accurately exclude the diagnosis of venous TOS when negative.

The most direct and definitive means to confirm the diagnosis of axillary-subclavian venous effort thrombosis and venous TOS is through catheter-directed contrast venography. Direct venography provides complete anatomic information regarding the site and extent of thrombosis, and it allows definitive evaluation of the collateral venous pathways.

Direct venography is also required to undertake catheter-based venous thrombolysis, the preferred initial step in treatment of almost all patients presenting with effort thrombosis. Taking all of these factors into consideration, we believe the most practical, efficient, and cost-effective approach to evaluating the patient with suspected effort thrombosis is to go directly to catheter-based venography, rather than utilize duplex studies or other noninvasive imaging tests.

Blood Coagulation Tests

Although considered to be a "mechanical" anatomical problem unrelated to an increased propensity toward thrombosis, it has been reported that up to 70% of patients with venous TOS may have associated abnormalities in coagulation tests.[3] Since such abnormalities may influence subsequent patient management, a panel of coagulation studies should be obtained either during the initial diagnostic evaluation or in follow-up, including tests for protein C and protein S activities, antithrombin III levels, plasma homocysteine, the presence of anticardiolipin antibodies and lupus anticoagulant, and mutations in the genes encoding prothrombin (G20210A), factor V (Leiden, G1692A), plasminogen activator inhibitor-1 (PAI-1, 4G/5G), and methyltetrahydrofolate reductase (MTHFR, C677T). These tests are usually negative and thereby add little to the initial diagnosis or management of effort thrombosis.

Goals of Treatment and Initial Management

There are 4 principal goals of treatment for axillary-subclavian venous effort thrombo-

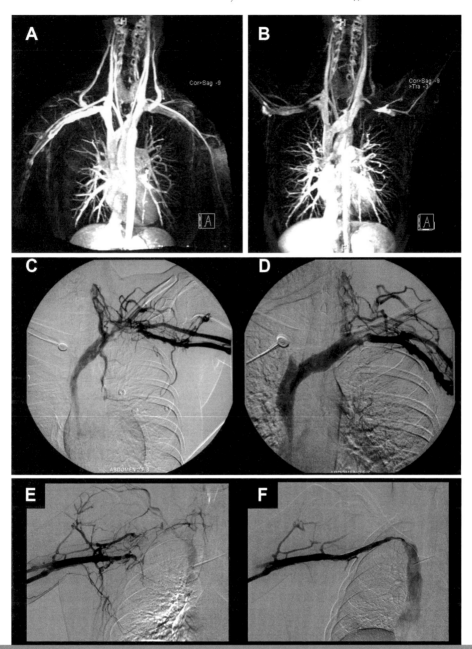

FIGURE 14.2   Imaging studies in venous TOS. **A** and **B**: Positional magnetic resonance venography. With the arms at rest (**A**), there is a patent right subclavian vein and an occluded left subclavian vein. With the arms elevated overhead (**B**), there is moderate stenosis of the right subclavian vein and persistent occlusion of the left subclavian vein. **C** and **D**: Thrombolytic therapy for left-sided axillary-subclavian venous effort thrombosis. Initial venogram (**C**) demonstrates a segmental occlusion of the subclavian vein with dense collaterals. Following thrombolytic therapy (**D**), most of the axillary and subclavian vein has been cleared of thrombus, with a residual focal high-grade stenosis at the level of the first rib. **E** and **F**: Thrombolytic therapy for right-sided axillary-subclavian venous effort thrombosis. Initial venogram (**E**) demonstrates a long occlusion of the entire axillary and subclavian veins, with relatively limited development of collaterals. Following thrombolytic therapy (**F**), most of the axillary and subclavian vein has been cleared of thrombus, with a moderate residual stenosis at the level of the first rib.

sis: (1) provide prompt relief of acute symptoms of upper extremity venous congestion and prevention of pulmonary embolism; (2) reduce the likelihood of recurrent venous thrombosis following initial management; (3) avoid the development of upper extremity postthrombotic syndrome; and (4) return to normal upper extremity activity without medications. The first of these goals is best met by prompt anticoagulation and thrombolytic therapy.

Anticoagulation

In the absence of any contraindications, once the diagnosis of axillary-subclavian venous effort thrombosis is suspected, almost all patients should be anticoagulated with intravenous or subcutaneous heparin. This can be done while additional diagnostic studies are being performed and/or prior to patient transfer from one hospital to another, and is important to help prevent the extension of thrombus within the axillary and subclavian veins. Treatment with an antiplatelet agent, such as aspirin or clopidogrel (Plavix), is often included.

Thrombolytic Therapy

Current approaches to venous TOS emphasize early diagnosis by contrast venography and prompt use of catheter-based thrombolytic therapy to reduce the amount of thrombus within the axillary and subclavian veins (Figure 14.2C-F).[4] Venous thrombolysis has traditionally been performed by continuous infusion of the thrombolytic drug directly into a multihole catheter that has been placed within the axillary-subclavian vein at the time of the initial venogram. Infusion is continued with repeat venograms performed at follow-up intervals for a period of 24 to 48 hours, until a maximum effect is achieved,

requiring monitoring in an acute-care setting (eg, intermediate-care or intensive-care unit) for several days. In recent years, it has become more typical to perform thrombolysis with catheter-based pharmacomechanical thrombectomy, in which a mechanical device on the tip of the catheter is used to rapidly break up the clot, along with localized infusion of a much smaller amount of thrombolytic agent.[5] The great advantage of this approach is that it can usually be completed in a single stage, often within several hours, thereby avoiding a long stay in a monitored hospital setting.

Balloon Angioplasty

The goal of thrombolysis is to clear any fresh or recent clot from the axillary-subclavian and collateral veins. This usually results in a marked improvement in the venographic appearance of the vein and a prompt reduction in symptoms of venous obstruction. Following thrombolysis a focal occlusion or high-grade stenosis of the proximal subclavian vein is usually identified at the level of the first rib; this is not composed of thrombus, but represents the underlying scar tissue caused by subclavian vein compression, injury, and tissue repair. In some cases, balloon angioplasty may be used at the same time in an attempt to reduce the degree of stenosis in the subclavian vein. However, because the vein is usually obstructed by scar tissue in the wall of the vein as well as external compression between the clavicle and first rib, balloon angioplasty is often unsuccessful, and even when improvement is obtained it is usually short-lived. There is also abundant evidence demonstrating that vascular stents should not be placed in the subclavian vein, at least prior to surgical decompression, due to an inevitably high rate of failure.[6] We therefore rarely recommend the use of balloon angioplasty for subclavian vein stenosis following thrombolysis. Following thrombolysis, the patient should remain on systemic anticoagulation.

Nonsurgical Management

Conservative treatment of axillary-subclavian venous effort thrombosis has traditionally consisted of chronic anticoagulation, intermittent arm elevation, long-term restrictions in arm activity, and the use of compression sleeves, with the hope that increased collateral development will eventually compensate for axillary-subclavian vein occlusion. Many studies in the medical literature have shown that this approach rarely results in symptom-free use of the arm and is associated with a significant incidence of chronic venous congestion, particularly with active use of the arm, requiring considerable limitations in young, active patients (Table 14.1).[7-11] Unlike lower extremity DVT, the proper duration of anticoagulation treatment for subclavian venous effort thrombosis is not known. Because this condition is caused by compression of the vein rather than a disorder of blood clotting, many recommend lifelong anticoagulation unless there has been a defined alteration in the underlying anatomy. It is notable that there is still a significant risk of recurrent thrombosis following thrombolysis and anticoagulation alone, with published estimates ranging from 50% to 70%. As summarized by Aziz et al., "Medical therapy, consisting either of anticoagulation or thrombolytic therapy, results in an unsatisfactory clinical outcome because it does not correct the underlying mechanical abnormality."[12]

Indications and Protocols for Surgical Treatment

Surgical treatment provides definitive management for axillary-subclavian venous effort thrombosis and venous TOS, and should be considered in almost all patients with this condition. Operative treatment is centered on 2 goals: (1) decompression of the subclavian vein and collateral venous pathways through the thoracic outlet by removal of the first rib and associated scalene and subclavius muscles, and (2) restoration and maintenance of normal blood flow through the subclavian vein, by removing constricting scar tissue from around the vein, by adjunctive balloon angioplasty, or by direct venous reconstruction when necessary.

TABLE 14.1 **Reported Outcomes of Conservative Management for Axillary-Subclavian Venous Effort Thrombosis**

Author	Year	# Patients	Outcomes
Adams et al.[7]	1965	NA	Disabling symptoms >70%
Tilney et al.[8]	1970	48	Disabling symptoms in 74%
Donayre et al.[9]	1986	41	Disabling symptoms >50%
Gloviczki et al.[10]	1986	95	Late sequelae in 30%
Lindblad et al.[11]	1988	73	Moderate disability 25%

The vast majority of patients with recent axillary-subclavian venous effort thrombosis are excellent candidates for surgical treatment, particularly within the first several weeks of undergoing successful thrombolytic therapy. However, patients with longstanding untreated subclavian vein occlusion, or those that exhibit a long segment of residual venous occlusion extending into the axillary vein despite thrombolysis, are often considered to be unsuitable candidates for surgical treatment. This judgment depends in large part upon the surgical experience available and the surgical approaches to venous TOS preferentially used in a particular center.

Thrombolysis → Anticoagulation 3 Months → Staged Surgery vs. Anticoagulation

Over the past 3 decades since the advent of thrombolytic therapy, protocols for the management of axillary-subclavian venous effort thrombosis have evolved considerably. The first comprehensive approach to this problem was described by Machleder and colleagues at the University of California-Los Angeles, involving a 3-month period of anticoagulation followed by transaxillary first rib resection.[13-15] As reported in a series of publications, approximately 70% of patients following the Machleder protocol required surgery for persistent symptoms after 3 months of anticoagulation, with up to 30% having had recurrent thrombosis. Clinical outcomes were largely influenced by the status of the subclavian vein following decompression: at final assessment, 90% to 95% of those with a patent subclavian vein were free of symptoms, as compared to 64% of those with an occluded subclavian vein.

Thrombolysis → Anticoagulation 1 Month → Staged Surgery vs. Anticoagulation

Reports from other centers indicate that the interval for reevaluation of patients on anticoagulation can be effectively reduced to 1 month following thrombolysis.[16,17] In an initial report of 22 patients following this staged approach, Lee et al. found that 13 (59%) required surgery and 9 (41%) did not, with uniformly successful outcomes in each treatment group.[16] However, in a follow-up report of a larger series (64 patients), 29 (45%) had surgery within 3 months of thrombolysis and 35 (55%) continued with nonoperative management. It is notable that 8 (23%) of these conservatively managed patients also had recurrent thrombosis requiring later surgical treatment (overall 58% requiring surgery).[17]

Thrombolysis → Anticoagulation → Early Surgery → Interval Angioplasty

With the recognition that the vast majority of patients with axillary-subclavian venous effort thrombosis will require surgical treatment within 1 to 3 months of initial thrombolytic therapy, others have sought to reduce the overall duration of treatment by proceeding with surgery within days to weeks after thrombolysis. As it has also become clearer that long-term results for patients undergoing surgery are better for those with a patent subclavian vein, attempts to further improve outcomes have coupled transaxillary first rib resection with postoperative balloon angioplasty at various intervals after operation.[18-20] Although excellent results have been reported with these strategies, the actual outcomes of delayed balloon angioplasty for venous TOS remain unclear and there may remain a substantial proportion of patients who have residual subclavian vein obstruction refractory to intervention, for which long-term anticoagulation may be recommended.

Thrombolysis → Early Surgery with Subclavian Vein Reconstruction

The most recent step in the evolution of treatment protocols for axillary-subclavian venous effort thrombosis has involved wider use of anterior approaches to thoracic outlet decompression and direct reconstruction of the subclavian vein at the time of operation.[21-28] Molina and colleagues reported results with immediate surgery using subclavicular decompression and subclavian vein patch angioplasty in 114 patients.[26] Of 97 (85%) patients treated within 2 weeks of symptoms, the outcomes were uniformly successful. However, of 17 (15%) patients treated more than 2 weeks after the onset of symptoms, all had developed progressive subclavian vein fibrosis, with 12 (70%) having postoperative restenosis and 5 (30%) being considered inoperable. In extending this strategy to offer definitive surgical treatment to a broader group of patients, our group has long advocated use of paraclavicular thoracic outlet decompression that involves incisions above and below the clavicle.[21,24,28] This approach permits more complete first rib resection and more thorough venous decompression than can be obtained through alternative approaches, as well as optimal exposure to accomplish direct subclavian vein reconstruction when necessary. This approach also allows completion of these steps to be accomplished during a single operative procedure and hospital stay, with excellent functional outcomes in a large and ongoing clinical series of patients with venous TOS.

Selection of Surgical Approach

Transaxillary first rib resection remains one of the most frequently employed approaches to the treatment of venous TOS. This typically involves partial resection of the first rib and division of its scalene muscle attachments. Because it is not feasible to fully expose or control the subclavian vein from the transaxillary approach, direct evaluation and/or reconstruction of the subclavian vein is not performed. Rather, transaxillary first rib resection is usually coupled with the subsequent use of intraoperative or postoperative venography and performance of balloon angioplasty and/or stent placement to deal with any residual stenosis in the subclavian vein.[29] Current estimates indicate that 40% to 50% of patients will demonstrate a residual subclavian vein stenosis requiring balloon angioplasty, even several weeks after first rib resection. Because these lesions are typically composed of dense scar tissue within and around the wall of the vein, balloon angioplasty may be relatively ineffective in this setting. Although placement of subclavian vein stents may be considered in this situation, the long-term effectiveness of stents in this position is limited. Long-term anticoagulation may therefore need to be considered in an effort to reduce the potential for recurrent venous thrombosis. For these reasons we prefer more direct and thorough approaches to the management of patients with venous TOS.

The paraclavicular approach combines the advantages of the supraclavicular exposure used for neurogenic and arterial forms of TOS with an infraclavicular incision that permits complete resection of the medial first rib, as well as wide exposure of the subclavian vein to permit vascular reconstruction. With this approach we offer operative decompression to virtually all patients with symptomatic venous TOS or recent effort thrombosis, regardless of the interval between initial diagnosis and referral, previous treatment, or adverse findings on contrast venography. Operative procedures based on paraclavicular exposure thereby provide the most versatile, comprehensive, and safe approach to the treatment of venous TOS.[27,28]

Paraclavicular Thoracic Outlet Decompression

Thoracic outlet decompression for venous TOS begins with supraclavicular exposure (Figure 14.3A). The patient is positioned supine with the head of the bed elevated 30 degrees, and the neck, chest, and affected upper extremity are prepped into the field to permit movement of the arm during the operation and access to the forearm and wrist. A transverse supraclavicular incision is made, subplatysmal flaps are developed to expose the scalene fat pad, and the omohyoid muscle is divided. The scalene fat pad is detached and progressively elevated in a medial to lateral direction, exposing the surface of the anterior scalene muscle and the phrenic nerve. Small blood vessels and lymphatics are secured between ligatures and, if necessary, the thoracic duct is ligated and divided. Lateral mobilization of the scalene fat pad continues until there is ample exposure of the anterior scalene muscle and phrenic nerve, the brachial plexus nerve roots, and the middle scalene muscle. The long thoracic nerve is observed emerging from the middle scalene muscle and crossing the posterolateral aspect of the first rib. The scalene fat pad is held in position with several retraction sutures.

The anterior scalene muscle is circumferentially dissected at the level of its insertion upon the first rib and sharply divided under direct vision (Figure 14.2B). The remaining muscle is lifted superiorly and detached from the underlying tissues, carrying the dissection superiorly to the level of its origin on the C6 transverse process, and the muscle is divided and removed. Each of the 5 nerve roots comprising the brachial plexus (C5, C6, C7, C8, and T1) are identified, mobilized, and protected from injury, and any aberrant fibrous bands, ligaments, or fascial attachments that may contribute to neurovascular compression are resected.

With the brachial plexus nerve roots gently retracted in an anteromedial direction, the attachment of the middle scalene muscle is carefully divided from the top of the first rib (Figure 14.2C). The intercostal muscles along the posterolateral aspect of the first rib are divided, and the tip of a right-angle clamp is passed underneath the posterior neck of the first rib. The posterior aspect of the first rib is divided with a modified Stille-Giertz rib cutter, and a Kerrison bone rongeur is used to smooth the posterior end of the bone to a level medial to the course of the T1 nerve root (Figure 14.3D-E). The proximal end of the first rib is elevated and a fingertip is passed underneath the rib to bluntly separate additional extrapleural fascia and intercostal muscle attachments. The anterior portion of the first rib is not yet divided at this stage.

To accomplish complete resection of the anteromedial portion of the first rib, a second transverse skin incision is made one fingerbreadth below the medial clavicle (Figure 14.3F). A plane of separation is created between the upper and middle portions of the pectoralis major muscle, and the cartilaginous portion of the first rib is identified. This is facilitated by applying downward

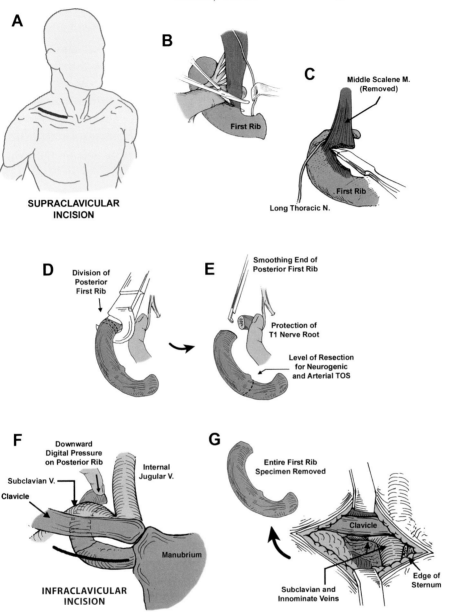

FIGURE 14.3 Paraclavicular thoracic outlet decompression. **A.** Paraclavicular decompression begins with a supraclavicular incision. **B.** The anterior scalene muscle is divided from the first rib and removed. **C.** The middle scalene muscle is divided from the first rib and removed. **D** and **E.** The posterior aspect of the first rib is divided (**D**) with protection of the C8 and T1 brachial plexus nerve roots under direct vision, and the remaining edge of the rib is trimmed to a level proximal to the nerve roots (**E**). The anterior first rib is not yet divided at this stage of the procedure, as it is in operations for neurogenic or arterial TOS. **F.** An infraclavicular incision is made overlying the anteromedial aspect of the first rib and the rib is exposed, facilitated by pressure on the posterior end of the rib to separate the costoclavicular space. **G.** The anteromedial aspect of the first rib is divided at the edge of the sternum and the entire first rib is removed, allowing complete dissection of the axillary-subclavian vein throughout the thoracic outlet, to its junction with the internal jugular and innominate veins. Adapted and redrawn from Thompson RW, Venous Thoracic Outlet Syndrome: Paraclavicular Approach. Operative Techniques in General Surgery 2008; 10:113-121 (Figures 1-7).

pressure to the divided posterior segment of the first rib with a finger placed within the supraclavicular incision, placing the attachments between the medial first rib and clavicle under tension and allowing the medial portion of the first rib to be dissected from its soft tissue attachments through the infraclavicular incision.

The subclavius muscle tendon, the costoclavicular ligament, and the muscles of the first intercostal space are divided under direct vision and the cartilaginous portion of the first rib is divided adjacent to the sternum, with the first rib removed from the operative field as a single specimen (Figure 14.3G). The axillary-subclavian vein is identified underneath the clavicle and carefully separated from the subclavius muscle, with ligation and division of any collateral vein branches that enter the subclavian vein, and the subclavius muscle is resected. Further exposure of the subclavian vein is undertaken through the supraclavicular exposure and continued medially toward the junction of the subclavian and internal jugular veins to form the innominate vein. The internal jugular vein is fully exposed several centimeters superior to its junction with the subclavian vein, and the innominate vein is exposed for several centimeters into the upper mediastinum. The course of the phrenic nerve into the upper mediastinum is also noted, and the nerve is protected where it passes underneath the subclavian vein.

Any pathological changes in the central portion of the subclavian vein are assessed visually and by digital palpation. As the subclavian vein is typically found to harbor a focal area with fibrous wall thickening resulting from chronic repetitive injury, any residual scar tissue surrounding the vein is completely excised ("circumferential external venolysis") (Figure 14.4A). This often results in reexpansion of the previously

constricted segment of the vein, and if the vein is soft and easily compressible to palpation, and shows evidence of rapid filling and emptying with respiratory variation, it is likely that no further venous reconstruction is necessary (in our experience, this is the case in approximately 50% of patients with venous TOS, even in those with long-segment stenosis prior to operation). When external venolysis does not alleviate subclavian vein obstruction, or when intraoperative venography demonstrates a residual stenosis despite the apparent success of external venolysis, additional venous reconstruction is performed. Following systemic anticoagulation (Dextran and heparin), clamp control is obtained of the distal subclavian and internal jugular veins and a pediatric Satinsky clamp is passed around the upper portion of the innominate vein. A longitudinal venotomy is created along the superior aspect of the subclavian vein and the lumen is thoroughly inspected. If the luminal surface is smooth and free of thrombus and/or irregularity, a vein patch angioplasty is performed using greater saphenous vein or a segment of cryopreserved femoral vein (Figure 14.4B). It is considered important to construct the patch to span the entire length of the affected subclavian vein, with an extension into the lateral aspect of the internal jugular vein or the anteromedial aspect of the innominate vein.

When dense fibrosis remains within the wall of the subclavian vein despite external venolysis, the affected segment of the subclavian vein is replaced by interposition bypass (Figure 14.4C). The intervening segment of the native subclavian vein is excised (Figure 14.4D), and an interposition graft is constructed using a widely beveled end-to-end anastomosis to the unaffected distal axillary-subclavian vein. The proximal anastomosis is constructed in a wide end-to-side anastomosis, using an extension of the graft

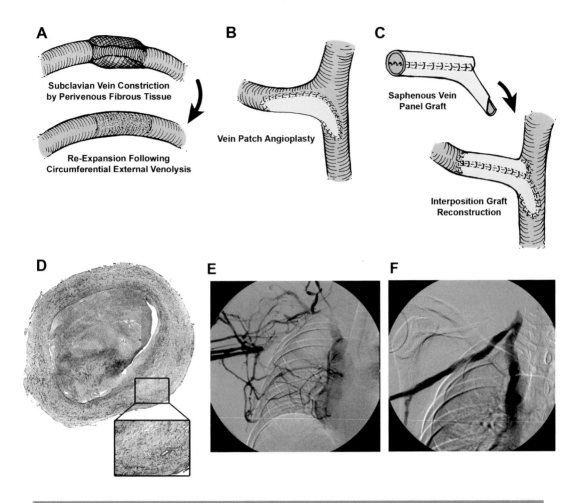

FIGURE 14.4   Subclavian vein reconstruction in venous TOS. **A.** Circumferential external venolysis to remove constricting fibrous scar tissue from around the subclavian vein, which may allow the vein to re-expand to a normal diameter. **B.** When subclavian vein reconstruction is necessary and the lumen of the vein is found to be smooth and free of chronic thrombus, vein patch angioplasty is sufficient for reconstruction. **C.** When subclavian vein reconstruction is necessary but the luminal surface is unsuitable for patch angioplasty, replacement of the subclavian vein is accomplished with an interposition bypass using a saphenous vein panel graft. **D.** Microscopic cross-sectional appearance of the chronically occluded subclavian vein in effort thrombosis. The lumen is occluded with chronic organized thrombus and inflammatory cell infiltrates, and the vein wall is markedly thickened with fibrosis, loss of the normal elastic architecture, and previous intramural hemorrhage (Verhoeff van Giesen stain). **E** and **F.** Venography in right-sided axillary-subclavian venous effort thrombosis. The initial venogram **(E)** demonstrates long occlusion of the axillary and subclavian veins with widespread collaterals. Venogram performed 12 weeks after surgical treatment **(F)**, which had involved creation of an axillary-innominate subclavian vein interposition bypass reconstruction. Adapted and redrawn from Melby et al., Comprehensive surgical management of the competitive athlete with effort thrombosis of the subclavian vein (Paget-Schroetter syndrome). J Vasc Surg 2008; 47:809-820, Supplement A Figure III; and Thompson RW, Venous Thoracic Outlet Syndrome: Paraclavicular Approach. Operative Techniques in General Surgery 2008; 10:113-121 (Figures 1-7).

onto the lateral aspect of the internal jugular vein or the anteromedial aspect of the innominate vein. Because the caliber of the saphenous vein is usually too small to match the subclavian vein, use of the saphenous vein requires creation of a panel graft with twice the diameter of the native saphenous vein. Alternatively, subclavian vein interposition bypass can be performed using a suitable segment of cryopreserved femoral vein.

Finally, intraoperative venography is used to confirm satisfactory subclavian vein reconstruction, typically performed through the cephalic vein in the distal forearm. Our operative approach also includes frequent construction of a temporary radiocephalic arteriovenous (AV) fistula between the end of the distal cephalic vein and the side of the radial artery, used as an adjunct to increase upper extremity venous blood flow during the first several months after operation. This is subsequently ligated under local anesthesia at 12 weeks after surgical treatment, at which time a follow-up contrast venogram is also performed (Figure 14.4E-F).

Postoperative care includes ample use of pain medications, muscle relaxants, and anti-inflammatory agents. The potential complications of surgery are similar to those considered in other operations for thoracic outlet syndromes, as well as those related to venous reconstruction, as follows:

- Subclavian artery injury/intraoperative hemorrhage
- Subclavian vein injury/intraoperative hemorrhage
- Brachial plexus nerve injury or postoperative paresis
- Phrenic nerve injury or postoperative paresis
- Long thoracic nerve injury or postoperative paresis

- Pneumothorax or pleural effusion
- Postoperative lymph leak
- Residual subclavian vein obstruction or early postoperative rethrombosis
- Postoperative bleeding/wound hematoma/excessive anticoagulation
- Late postoperative axillary or subclavian vein obstruction or rethrombosis

The expected hospital stay is 5 days, with the closed-suction drain removed approximately 7 days after operation. Inpatient physical therapy is started the day after operation to maintain range of motion, with postoperative rehabilitation then overseen by a physical therapist with expertise in the management of TOS, and no restrictions placed on upper extremity activity beyond 12 weeks after operation. Therapeutic anticoagulation (heparin/warfarin plus clopidogrel) is initiated several days after operation and then discontinued at 12 weeks. Recovery is typically complete within 3 months of operation, and a full return to previous levels of function can usually be expected.

References

1. Hughes ESR. Venous obstruction in the upper extremity (Paget-Schroetter's syndrome). Int Abstr. Surg. 1949;88:89-127.
2. Sanders RJ. Thoracic Outlet Syndrome: A Common Sequelae of Neck Injuries. Philadelphia: J. B. Lippincott Company; 1991.
3. Cassada DC, Lipscomb AL, Stevens SL, Freeman MB, Grandas OH, Goldman MH. The importance of thrombophilia in the treatment of Paget-Schroetter syndrome. Ann Vasc Surg. 2006;20:596-601.
4. Rutherford RB. Primary subclavian-axillary vein thrombosis: the relative roles of thrombolysis, percutaneous angioplasty, stents,

and surgery. Semin Vasc Surg. 1998;11: 91-5.

5. Schneider DB, Curry TK, Eichler CM, Messina LM, Gordon RL, Kerlan RK. Percutaneous mechanical thrombectomy for the management of venous thoracic outlet syndrome. J Endovasc Ther. 2003;10:336-40.

6. Urschel HC Jr, Patel AN. Paget-Schroetter syndrome therapy: failure of intravenous stents. Ann Thorac Surg. 2003;75:1693-6.

7. Adams JT, McEvoy RK, DeWeese JA. Primary deep venous thrombosis of the upper extremity. Arch Surg. 1965;91:29-42.

8. Tilney NL, Griffiths HJG, Edwards E. Natural history of major venous thrombosis of the upper extremity. Arch Surg. 1970;101:792-5.

9. Donayre CE, White GH, Mehringer SM, Wilson SE. Pathogenesis determines late morbidity of axillosubclavian vein thrombosis. Am J Surg. 1986;152:179-84.

10. Gloviczki P, Kazmier FJ, Hollier LH. Axillary-subclavian venous occlusion: the morbidity of a nonlethal disease. J Vasc Surg. 1986;4:333-7.

11. Lindblad B, Tengborn L, Bergqvist D. Deep vein thrombosis of the axillary-subclavian veins: epidemiologic data, effects of different types of treatment and late sequelae. Eur J Vasc Surg. 1988;2:161-5.

12. Aziz S, Straehley CJ, Whelan TJ Jr. Effort-related axillosubclavian vein thrombosis. A new theory of pathogenesis and a plea for direct surgical intervention. Am J Surg. 1986; 152:57-61.

13. Kunkel JM, Machleder HI. Spontaneous subclavain vein thrombosis: a successful combined approach of local thrombolytic therapy followed by first rib resection. Surgery. 1989;106:114.

14. Kunkel JM, Machleder HI. Treatment of Paget-Schroetter syndrome: a staged, multidisciplinary approach. Arch Surg. 1989;124:1153-7.

15. Machleder HI. Evaluation of a new treatment strategy for Paget-Schroetter syndrome:

16. Lee WA, Hill BB, Harris EJ Jr, Semba CP, Olcott CI. Surgical intervention is not required for all patients with subclavian vein thrombosis. J Vasc Surg. 2000;32:57-67.

17. Lee JT, Karwowski JK, Harris EJ, Haukoos JS, Olcott C IV. Long-term thrombotic recurrence after nonoperative management of Paget-Schroetter syndrome. J Vasc Surg. 2006;43:1236-43.

18. Urschel HC Jr, Razzuk MA. Improved management of the Paget-Schroetter syndrome secondary to thoracic outlet compression. Ann Thorac Surg. 1991;52:1217-21.

19. Angle N, Gelabert HA, Farooq MM, Ahn SS, Caswell DR, Freischlag JA, et al. Safety and efficacy of early surgical decompression of the thoracic outlet for Paget-Schroetter syndrome. Ann Vasc Surg. 2001;15:37-42.

20. Caparrelli DJ, Freischlag J. A unified approach to axillosubclavian venous thrombosis in a single hospital admission. Semin Vasc Surg. 2005;18:153-7.

21. Thompson RW, Schneider PA, Nelken NA, Skioldebrand CG, Stoney RJ. Circumferential venolysis and paraclavicular thoracic outlet decompression for "effort thrombosis" of the subclavian vein. J Vasc Surg. 1992;16:723-32.

22. Molina JE. Surgery for effort thrombosis of the subclavian vein. J Thorac Cardiovasc Surg. 1992;103:341-6.

23. Molina JE. Need for emergency treatment in subclavian vein effort thrombosis. J Am Coll Surg. 1995;181:414-20.

24. Thompson RW, Petrinec D, Toursarkissian B. Surgical treatment of thoracic outlet compression syndromes. II. Supraclavicular exploration and vascular reconstruction. Ann Vasc Surg. 1997;11:442-51.

25. Azakie A, McElhinney DB, Thompson RW, Raven RB, Messina LM, Stoney RJ. Surgical management of subclavian vein "effort"

thrombosis secondary to thoracic outlet compression. J Vasc Surg. 1998;28:777-86.

26. Molina JE, Hunter DW, Dietz CA. Paget-Schroetter syndrome treated with thrombolytics and immediate surgery. J Vasc Surg. 2007;45:328-34.

27. Melby SJ, Vedantham S, Narra VR, Paletta GA, Jr., Khoo-Summers L, Driskill M, Thompson RW. Comprehensive surgical management of the competitive athlete with effort thrombosis of the subclavian vein (Paget-Schroetter syndrome). J Vasc Surg. 2008;47:809-20.

28. Melby SJ, Thompson RW. Supraclavicular (paraclavicular) approach for thoracic outlet syndrome. In: Pearce WH, Matsumura JS, Yao JST, editors. Operative Vascular Surgery in the Endovascular Era. Evanston: Greenwood Academic; 2008. p434-45.

29. Urschel HC, Jr., Razzuk MA. Paget-Schroetter syndrome: what is the best management? Ann Thorac Surg. 2000;69:1663-8.

Central Venous Disease

Central venous diseases (DVT and stenosis) are a frequent area of consultation for vascular specialists as the interest in direct intervention on iliofemoral and innominate disease is growing. We have sufficient level I evidence to support anticoagulation in cases of DVT. Interventions for these categories of acute occlusive disease have become more commonplace due to the rapid resolution of symptoms with thrombolytic therapy. May-Thurner syndrome is well treated with lysis and stent placement. Introduction of intravascular ultrasonogrraphy in the venous system has increased the understanding and incidence of stenotic disease in the system. In a different area of vascular surgery, central venous occlusive disease has developed as the Achilles' heel of dialysis access and is posing a difficult area to treat with either endovascular or open interventions. No intervention is proving successful. Renal vein thrombosis has become recognized as a unique problem in renovascular disease and requires intensive imaging, good clinical judgment, and therapy. We have only limited case series to guide clinical decision-making in these areas. Mesenteric venous thrombosis and Budd-Chiari syndrome are distinct and important gastrointestinal venous diseases.

Iliofemoral
Deep Venous Thrombosis

Mark G. Davies

Iliofemoral deep venous thrombosis (iliofemoral DVT) is a distinct entity with distinct anatomic and functional implications for the patient. Isolated left lower extremity swelling secondary to left iliac vein compression was first described by McMurrich in 1908, and defined anatomically by May and Thurner in 1957 and clinically by Cockett and Thomas in 1965. The left iliac vein is usually located posterior to the right iliac artery and can be compressed between the artery and the fifth lumbar vertebrae. Symptoms include left lower extremity edema, pain, varicosities, venous stasis changes, and deep venous thrombosis. Historically, the evaluation of these patients

included a venous duplex scan to rule out deep venous thrombosis and an abdominal computed tomography (CT) scan to rule out pelvic mass.

Medical Management and Open Surgical Thrombectomy

Medical therapy comprising appropriate identification by imaging, adequate immediate and long-term anticoagulation, and mobilization with compression are now recommended for all patients with DVT, including iliofemoral DVT. Until recently, this was the only standard management of an iliofemoral DVT except in extreme limb salvage situations where open venous thrombectomy was considered appropriate. The

Venous Thromboembolic Disease. Contemporary Endovascular Management series. © 2011 Mark G. Davies MD and Alan B. Lumsden MD, eds. Cardiotext Publishing, ISBN 978-1-935395-22-5.

goal of venous thrombectomy is to remove thrombus from the iliofemoral segments of a lower extremity in patients who are unsuitable for catheter-directed thrombolysis (CDT) and in danger of limb loss.[1] The chapter by Bo Eklöf clearly illustrates the role of surgical venous thrombectomy in the modern management of iliofemoral DVT. Surgical extraction of venous thrombi should be used in the management of patients with extensive iliofemoral disease in which limb loss is imminent, such as in "phlegmasia cerulea dolens." In these patients, there are benefits to avoiding limb loss, preventing pulmonary embolism, and reducing the severity of postthrombotic syndromes. Surgical thrombectomy should not be performed in DVT that does not involve the iliofemoral segment, in nonambulatory patients or in high-risk surgical patients, and is generally reserved for young patients. Early mortality is generally 1% if proper selection criteria are applied. Early iliac vein rethrombosis is 13%. Cumulative patency is 75% at 4 years. In the presence of nonadherent clots, the patency is 92%, while in patients with adherent clots, the patency is 45%.[2] In patients with successful venous thrombectomy, 37% are symptom-free compared to 18% in patients treated conservatively. Those patients with no symptoms had significantly lower ambulatory venous pressures, improved venous emptying, and a better calf pump function. These physiological changes portend to a lower incidence of chronic venous insufficiency in the longer term. In a study that examined the efficacy of stent placement after infrainguinal loco-regional thrombolysis and iliac thrombectomy of acute DVT in patients with May-Thurner syndrome, technical success defined as complete vein patency and normal valve function was documented in all patients. The calculated cumulative primary patency rate for venous iliac stents

was 82%, and the assisted patency rate was 91%, which remained unchanged over a mean follow-up of 22 months. There was mild reflux with few clinical symptoms of postthrombotic syndrome.[3] In the only published randomized trial, Plate et al. showed that, although the operated group (venous thrombectomy) had better outcomes than the group treated with anticoagulation, neither of the 2 groups did very well in the long run.[4]

Endovascular Management

The management of iliofemoral DVT is undergoing an evolution with increased recognition that early intervention may benefit the well-selected patient. The indications for endovascular intervention are phlegmasia cerulea dolens, acute/subacute inferior vena cava (IVC) thrombosis, acute iliofemoral DVT, acute femoropopliteal DVT, and subacute/chronic iliofemoral DVT. This evolution is prompted by accruing evidence of benefit and spurred on by the 2008 ACCP guidelines as discussed by Comerota in chapter 5. As described in previous chapters by Henke, Wakefield, and Bush in this book, the etiology of DVT is multifactorial and must be individualized for each patient. Iliofemoral DVT may be due to extrinsic compression, wall damage secondary to catheters, and transient and permanent hypercoaguable states. Iliac vein compression is the most probable cause of iliofemoral DVT. One-half to two-thirds of patients with left-sided iliofemoral DVT have intraluminal webs or spurs from chronic extrinsic compression of the left iliac vein at the crossing point of the right common iliac artery. Approximately 2% to 5% of those with chronic deep venous insufficiency of the left leg may have iliac vein compression syndrome. Iliac vein compression syndrome occurs when compression of the common iliac vein is severe enough to inhibit the rate of venous outflow. In its more severe manifestation, iliac vein compression syndrome is known to cause acute iliofemoral DVT. Iliac vein compression syndrome is caused by the combination of compression and the vibratory pressure of the right iliac artery on the iliac vein, which is pinched between the artery and the pelvic bone. In oncology patients requiring staging CT scans of the thorax, abdomen, and pelvis, there is a prevalence of 6.8% unsuspected iliofemoral, 1.2% unsuspected common iliac, and 0.3% unsuspected inferior vena cava DVT.[5] In a series of patients treated medically for iliofemoral DVT, 50% of the limbs had a pathological (deep reflux or obstructive change) finding in the popliteal segment after a 20-month follow-up. The rate of recanalization was high. There was no difference between calf and more proximal DVTs. Pain (62%), edema (46%), and pigmentation (35%) were common, and only 27% of the legs with DVT were asymptomatic. One study suggests that the development of the postthrombotic syndrome begins quite early. The frequency of the subjective symptoms is high.[6] The introduction of catheter-directed thrombolysis, rheolytic catheters, and the combination pharmacomechanical thrombectomy (PMT) were initiated with the goals of (1) eliminating iliofemoral venous thrombus, (2) providing unobstructed venous drainage from the affected limb, and (3) preventing recurrent thrombosis; these approaches appear to be associated with better clinical outcome compared with either systemic fibrinolysis and standard anticoagulation (Table 15.1).[7-10] The specifics of the catheters, techniques, and results are illustrated in chapters by Davies, Meissner, and Arko in this book.

Patients suitable for catheter-directed thrombolysis include young, active individuals who have an acute (<10 days) deep venous thrombosis and those with isolated infrainguinal disease. Additionally, any patient who has signs/symptoms of phlegmasia cerulea dolens, regardless of their clinical condition or age, should be considered for thrombolytic therapy. The algorithm for care is shown in Figure 15.1. The incidence of major clinical hemorrhage after fibrinolysis for DVT is between 6% and 30%, a 3-fold increase compared to standard heparin therapy. Infusion of thrombolysis is associated with increased risk of local hematoma formation at the site of catheter insertion and a lower risk of distant bleeding. The National Multicenter Venous Registry recommends that any acute deep venous thrombosis without a prior history of thrombosis will yield the greatest degree of lysis, which is predictive of long-term benefit and a significant decrease in the likelihood of the development of chronic venous insufficiency. Endovascular management of iliofemoral DVT due to May-Thurner syndrome in patients with protein C and/or S deficiency is clinically effective in the short term.[11] The incidence of clinical signs and symptoms of venous insufficiency and duplex-scan findings of valvular reflux was significantly lower in the patients in which lytic therapy succeeded and patency was kept, compared with patients experiencing acute therapeutic failure or rethrombosis (P <.01).[12]

Catheter-directed thrombolytic therapy for the treatment of acute extensive iliofemoral DVT due to May-Thurner syndrome is an effective method for restoring venous patency, preventing valvular insufficiency, and providing relief of the acute symptoms.[13] In a study by Dake et al., initial technical success was achieved in 34 of 39 patients (87%). The overall patency rate at 1 year was 79%.

TABLE 15.1. **Outcomes of Trials of Iliofemoral DVT Interventions**

Author	Study	Type	Patients	Drug	Anatomic	Clinical
Catheter-Directed Therapy						
Semba	1994	Observational	21	UK	85	85
Bjarnason	1997	Prospective Cohort	77	UK	79	79
Verhaeghe	1997	Observational	25	TPA	76	76
Raju	1998	Observational	24	UK	88	-
Mewissen	1999	Prospective Registry	287	UK	83	-
Patel	2000	Observational	10	UK	100	100
O'Sullivan	2000	Observational	39	UK	87	-
Kasirajan	2001	Observational	17	UK/TPA/RPA	82	82
Chang	2001	Observational	10	TPA	100	100
Ouriel	2001	Prospective Registry	11	RPA	91	-
Shortell	2001	Observational	31	UK/tPA	80	-
AbuRahma	2001	Prospective Controlled	51	UK/tPA	89	-
Castaneda	2002	Prospective Cohort	25	rPA	92	-
Vedantham	2002	Observational	20	UK/tPA/rPA	89	82
Razavi	2002	Prospective Cohort	31	TNK	89	-
Elsharawy	2002	Randomized Trial	35	SK	100	-
Sugimoto	2003	Observational	54	UK/tPA	-	85
Grunwald	2004	Observational	74	UK/tPA/rPA	98	-
Vedantham	2004	Observational	18	RPA	100	96
Lin	2006	Observational	46	tPA	64	-
Kim	2006	Observational	23	UK	81	-
Martinez	2008	Observational	21	tPA	60	-
Pharmacomechanical Therapy						
Kasirajan	2001	Observational	17	tPA	80	82
Vedantham	2002	Observational	20	UK/rPA/RPA	62	-
Bush	2004	Observational	22	UK/rPA/RPA	65	100
Jackson	2006	Observational	28	TNK	100	80
Lin	2006	Observational	52	tPA	68	-
Kim	2006	Observational	14	UK	84	-
Arko	2007	Observational	14	TNK	80	90
Martinez	2008	Observational	22	tPA	80	-
Rao	2009	Observational	43	tPA	95	93
Shi	2009	Observational	16	UK	89	-
Li	2010	Observational	36	tPA	80	83
EKOS						
No large studies						

Abbreviations: EKOS = EkoSonic Endovascular System; rPA = reteplase; SK = streptokinase; TNK = tenecteplase; tPA = tissue plasminogen activator; UK = urokinase. Adapted from Vedantham S et al. J Vasc Interv Radiol. 2009 Jul;20(7 suppl):S227-39.

Symptomatically, 85% of patients were completely or partially improved compared with findings before treatment. There were no deaths, pulmonary embolus, cerebral hemorrhage, or major bleeding complications.[14] AbuRahma et al. reported a technical success in 16 of 18 patients (89%) receiving CDT and primary iliofemoral venous patency rates at 1, 3, and 5 years of 24%, 18%, and 18% and 83%, 69%, and 69% for medical therapy and endovascular therapy, respectively. Long-term symptom resolution was achieved in 30% for medical therapy vs. 78% endovascular therapy.[15] Kwak et al. demonstrated a technical success rate of 96% (26 of 27 stents) and a clinical success rate of 95% (21 of 22 patients). The causes of common iliac vein obstruction were May-Thurner syndrome (n = 16), pelvic mass (n = 2), and unknown (n = 4). Overall, the 1-year and 2-year primary patency rates were both 95%, and the 1-year and 2-year secondary patency rates were both 100%.[16] From a national registry of patients (n = 473) with

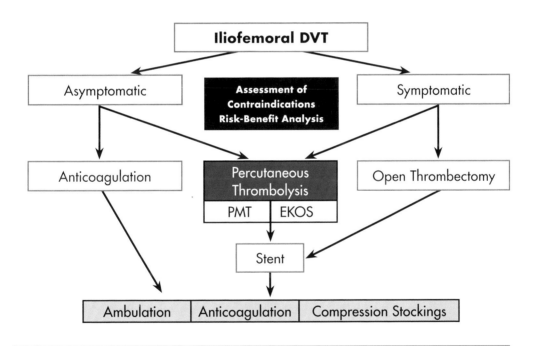

FIGURE 15.1 Algorithm for iliofemoral DVT prevention. Patients diagnosed with an iliofemoral DVT should be stratified into symptomatic and asymptomatic and then assessed for contraindications to thrombolysis. Concomitant with this, a risk-benefit analysis should also be performed. If in the clinician's opinion declotting needs to be done and there are no contraindications for lysis, percutaneous lysis is performed with use of simple lyse and wait, mechanical thrombectomy, pharmacomechancial (PMT), or ultrasound-assisted lysis (EKOS). If the patient is symptomatic with a significant clot burden and contraindications to thrombolysis, open thrombectomy should be performed. Venography and correction of underlying lesions with stent placement is recommended. Standard therapy thereafter is anticoagulation, ambulation, and compression stockings.

symptomatic lower limb DVT, results of 312 urokinase infusions in 303 limbs of 287 patients were analyzed. After thrombolysis, grade III (complete) lysis was achieved in 96 (31%) infusions; grade II (50%–99% lysis) in 162 (52%); and grade I (< 50% lysis) in 54 (17%). For acute thrombosis, grade III lysis occurred in 34% of cases of acute and in 19% of cases of chronic DVT (P < .01). Major bleeding complications occurred in 54 (11%) patients, most often at the puncture site. At 1 year, the primary patency rate was 60%. Lysis grade was predictive of 1-year patency rate (grade III, 79%; grade II, 58%; grade I, 32%; P < .001).[17] There was no difference found in physical functioning and well-being between the groups before the development of deep venous thrombosis. Following treatment, patients receiving catheter-directed thrombolysis reported better overall physical functioning, less stigma, less health distress, and fewer postthrombotic symptoms compared to those patients treated with anticoagulation alone.[18] A 10-year study by Kölbel et al. demonstrated a technical success of 100% and a clinical success of 96%. While cumulative patency was 89%, clinically 68% of limbs were asymptomatic, 18% of limbs were moderately improved, and the remainder were unchanged or moderately worse.[19] In another study to assess venous reflux and the obstruction pattern after catheter-directed and systemic thrombolysis of deep iliofemoral venous thrombosis, valvular competence was preserved in 44% of patients treated with catheter-directed thrombolysis compared with 13% of those treated with systemic thrombolysis (P = 0.049). Reflux in any deep vein was present in 44% of patients treated by catheter-directed lysis compared with 81% of patients receiving systemic thrombolysis (P = 0.03).[20] Bjarnason et al. have reported a 2-year patency of 78% and Ly et al. found

that all of those who initially had complete lysis remained patent at 20 months, whereas those with only partial lysis had a lower patency rate.[21,22]

Use of rheolytic mechanical thrombectomy catheters has been shown to be effective in the treatment of ilifemoral deep venous thrombosis. Additional infusion of thrombolytic agents via the device creates a novel treatment strategy of pharmacomechanical thrombectomy, which further enhances thrombectomy efficacy (Figure 15.2). In a preliminary experience, pharmacomechanical catheter-directed iliofemoral DVT thrombectomy with early stent placement was safe and effective.[23] The Amplatz device is reported as having removal of thrombus at 75% to 83% in lower extremity acute DVT within 6 months and a patency of 77%.[24,25] The Arrow-Trerotola device, when used clinically in addition to thrombolytic therapy and angioplasty with stents, has been reported to have technical and clinical success in 100% of patients with a 16-month clinical success of 92%. Concerns about valve and intimal damage, although justified, have not been reported.[26] In a study without adjunctive preprocedural thrombolytic therapy, Kasirajan et al[27] reported that half of the patients treated with the AngioJet device had ≥50% of their thrombus removed. Patency was restored in 77% of those patients with ≥50% thrombus removal. Improved results have been observed in a similar study in which the AngioJet was used without preprocedural thrombolytics. Sixty-five percent of patients had complete thrombus removal while partial thrombus removal was observed in the remaining 35%.[28] The Trellis catheter can provide segmental and controlled pharmacomechanical thrombectomy. It is associated with a greater technical success rate, a lower rate of bleeding, and a lower cost than that reported for CDT.[29,30] The emission of

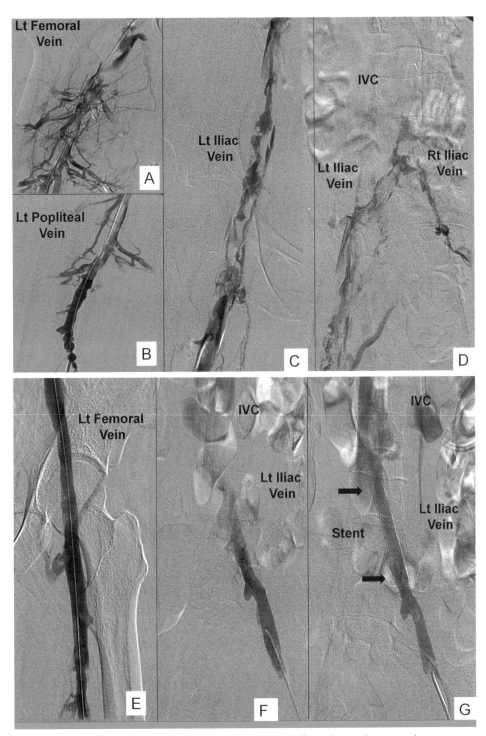

FIGURE 15.2   32-year-old patient presenting with symptomatic iliofemoral DVT. She is 6 weeks postpartum. She underwent transpopliteal venogram in the prone position. The venograms show iliofemoral DVT (**A-D**). The final result after PMT and 24 hours of EKOS-supplemented tPA infusion, which reveals a stenosis consistent with May-Thurner syndrome (**E and F**). Final image shows a patent vein and an intact, fully deployed stent indicated by the arrows (**G**).

ultrasound waves from an infusion catheter delivering lytic agent is an interesting new adjunct to catheter-directed thrombolysis. A recent study evaluated the success of lysis and clinical outcomes in patients treated with ultrasound (US)-accelerated thrombolysis for DVT using an EKOS device. Complete lysis (≥90%) was seen in 70% cases and overall lysis (complete plus partial) was seen in 91%. No lysis occurred in 5 cases (9%), 4 of which were chronic. It appears that the addition of ultrasound reduces total infusion time and provides a greater incidence of complete lysis.[31] In another retrospective study, patients undergoing CDT showed complete or partial thrombus removal in 32 (70%) and 14 (30%) cases, respectively. When compared to CDT in this study, PMT provides similar treatment success with reduced ICU and total hospital length of stay and hospital costs.[32] Subclinical thrombus embolization during CDT/PMT is a common phenomenon in patients with iliofemoral DVT.[33] A study by Protack et al. demonstrated that when using a mixed modality (CDT/PMT) approach, 83%, 83%, and 75% of patients were free of recurrent DVT at 1, 2, and 3 years, respectively. Furthermore, it appears that CDT/PMT without universal prophylactic IVC filter placement is safe and effective in treating acute iliofemoral DVT. Selective rather than routine IVC filter placement is a safe and appropriate approach.[34]

Several reports suggest that long-term results of CDT are not satisfactory because of the high recurrence rate of DVT, with stent length more than 6 cm being a poor prognostic factor[35] and only a marginal reduction in the incidence and severity of postthrombotic limb syndromes.[36] Furthermore, extent of thrombolysis is a statistically significant factor affecting the freedom of rethrombosis and chronic change.[37] In a retrospective study of iliofemoral and femoral DVT treated with thrombolysis and best medical therapy, a significantly greater proportion of iliofemoral patients (73%) than femoral patients (31%) remained asymptomatic at the end of their follow-up ($P <0.025$); 82% of iliofemoral limbs showed partial or complete lysis 4 weeks after diagnosis of clot. No significant difference in reflux development was observed between the 2 groups. Although the extent of reflux development was similar in both groups, iliofemoral patients still showed fewer clinical symptoms after follow-up.[38]

In a small randomized trial of local thrombolysis and anticoagulation vs. anticoagulation alone in patients with iliofemoral DVT, the patency rate at 6 months was better in cases treated with thrombolysis (13/18 [72%] vs. 2/17 [12%], $P < 0.001$). Venous reflux was higher in patients treated with anticoagulant (7 patients [41%] vs. 2 [11%], $P = 0.04$).[39] In an open multicenter, randomized, controlled trial, 103 patients (64 men, mean age 52 years) were allocated to CDT (n = 50) or standard treatment alone (n = 53). After CDT, grade III (complete) lysis was achieved in 24 and grade II (50%–90%) lysis in 20 patients. After 6 months, iliofemoral patency was found in 32 patients (64.0%) in the CDT group vs. 19 (35.8%) controls, corresponding to an absolute risk reduction (RR) of 28.2% (95% CI: 9.7%–46.7%; $P = 0.004$). Venous obstruction was found in 10 patients (20.0%) in the CDT group vs. 26 (49.1%) controls; absolute RR 29.1% (95% CI: 20.0%–38.0%; $P = 0.004$). Femoral venous insufficiency did not differ between the two groups.[40]

Conclusion

CDT reduced clot burden and DVT recurrence, and it may prevent the formation of postthrombotic syndrome. Indications for its use include younger individuals with a long life expectancy and few comorbidities, limb-threatening thromboses, and proximal iliofemoral DVTs. There is a marked lack of randomized controlled trials examining CDT-related mortality and long-term outcomes compared to anticoagulation alone. Published studies on endovascular DVT treatments have been limited by nonstandardized reporting, lack of long-term follow-up, and use of surrogate outcomes measures. The Society of Interventional Radiology has published reporting and quality improvement guideline documents that should be followed in any future trials. [41,42] The effectiveness of combined pharmacomechanical thrombectomy, although promising, needs to be investigated further, as does the role of caval filters in preventing DVT-associated pulmonary emboli.[43]

References

1. Comerota AJ, Gale SS. Technique of contemporary iliofemoral and infrainguinal venous thrombectomy. J Vasc Surg. 2006;43(1):185-91.

2. Elliott G. Thrombolytic therapy for venous thromboembolism. Curr Opin Hematol. 1999;6(5):304-8.

3. Husmann MJ, Heller G, Kalka C, Savolainen H, Do DD, Schmidli J, Baumgartner I. Stenting of common iliac vein obstructions combined with regional thrombolysis and thrombectomy in acute deep vein thrombosis. Eur J Vasc Endovasc Surg. 2007;34(1):87-91.

4. Plate G, Akesson H, Einarsson E, Ohlin P, Eklof B. Long-term results of venous thrombectomy combined with temporary arteriovenous fistula. Eur J Vasc Surg. 1990;4:483-9.

5. Cronin CG, Lohan DG, Keane M, Roche C, Murphy JM. Prevalence and significance of asymptomatic venous thromboembolic disease found on oncologic staging CT. Am J Roentgenol. 2007;189(1):162-70.

6. Saarinen J, Kallio T, Lehto M, Hiltunen S, Sisto T. The occurrence of the postthrombotic changes after an acute deep venous thrombosis. A prospective two-year follow-up study. J Cardiovasc Surg (Torino). 2000;41(3):441-6.

7. Comerota AJ, Aldridge SC, Cohen G, Ball DS, Pliskin M, White JV. A strategy of aggressive regional therapy for acute iliofemoral venous thrombosis with contemporary venous thrombectomy or catheter-directed thrombolysis. J Vasc Surg. 1994;20(2):244-54.

8. Comerota AJ, Gravett MH. Iliofemoral venous thrombosis. J Vasc Surg. 2007;46(5):1065-76.

9. Comerota AJ, Paolini D. Treatment of acute iliofemoral deep venous thrombosis: a strategy of thrombus removal. Eur J Vasc Endovasc Surg. 2007;33(3):351-60; discussion 361-2.

10. Semba CP, Dake MD. Catheter-directed thrombolysis for iliofemoral venous thrombosis. Semin Vasc Surg. 1996;9(1):26-33.

11. Cho YP, Ahn JH, Choi SJ, Han MS, Jang HJ, Kim YH, et al. Endovascular management of iliofemoral deep venous thrombosis due to iliac vein compression syndrome in patients with protein C and/or S deficiency. J Korean Med Sci. 2004;19(5):729-34.

12. Casella IB, Presti C, Aun R, Benabou JE, Puech-Leão P. Late results of catheter-directed recombinant tissue plasminogen activator fibrinolytic therapy of iliofemoral deep venous thrombosis. Clinics (Sao Paulo). 2007;62(1):31-40.

13. Patel NH, Stookey KR, Ketcham DB, Cragg AH. Endovascular management of acute extensive iliofemoral deep venous thrombosis caused by May-Thurner syndrome. J Vasc Interv Radiol. 2000;11(10):1297-302.

14. O'Sullivan GJ, Semba CP, Bittner CA, Kee ST, Razavi MK, Sze DY, et al. Endovascular management of iliac vein compression (May-

Thurner) syndrome. J Vasc Interv Radiol. 2000;11(7):823-36.

15. AbuRahma AF, Perkins SE, Wulu JT, Ng HK. Iliofemoral deep vein thrombosis: conventional therapy versus lysis and percutaneous transluminal angioplasty and stenting. Ann Surg. 2001;233(6): 752-60.

16. Kwak HS, Han YM, Lee YS, Jin GY, Chung GH. Stents in common iliac vein obstruction with acute ipsilateral deep venous thrombosis: early and late results. J Vasc Interv Radiol. 2005;16(6):815-22.

17. Mewissen MW, Seabrook GR, Meissner MH, Cynamon J, Labropoulos N, Haughton SH. Catheter-directed thrombolysis for lower extremity deep venous thrombosis: report of a national multicenter registry. Radiology. 1999 Apr;211(1):39-49.

18. Comerota AJ. Quality-of-life improvement using thrombolytic therapy for iliofemoral deep venous thrombosis. Rev Cardiovasc Med. 2002;3 suppl 2:S61-7.

19. Kölbel T, Lindh M, Holst J, Uher P, Eriksson KF, Sonesson B, et al. Extensive acute deep vein thrombosis of the iliocaval segment: midterm results of thrombolysis and stent placement. J Vasc Interv Radiol. 2007;18(2):243-50.

20. Laiho MK, Oinonen A, Sugano N, Harjola VP, Lehtola AL, Roth WD, et al. Preservation of venous valve function after catheter-directed and systemic thrombolysis for deep venous thrombosis. Eur J Vasc Endovasc Surg. 2004;28(4):391-6.

21. Bjarnason H, Kruse JR, Asinger DA, Nazarian GK, Dietz CA, Caldwell MD, et al. Iliofemoral deep venous thrombosis: safety and efficacy outcome during 5 years of catheter-directed thrombolytic therapy. J Vasc Interv Radiol. 1997;8:405-18.

22. Ly B, Njaastad AM, Sandbæk G, Solstrand R, Rosales A, Slagsvold CE. Kateterbasert trombolytisk behandling af bekkenvenetrombose. Tidsskr Nor Lægeforen. 2004;124:478-80.

23. Vedantham S, Vesely TM, Sicard GA, Brown D, Rubin B, Sanchez LA, et al. Pharmaco-mechanical thrombolysis and early stent placement for iliofemoral deep vein thrombosis. J Vasc Interv Radiol. 2004;15(6):565-74.

24. Gandini R, Maspes F, Sodani G, Masala S, Assegnati G, Simonetti G. Percutaneous ilio-caval thrombectomy with the Amplatz device: preliminary results. Eur Radiol. 1999;9(5): 951-8.

25. Delomez M, Beregi JP, Willoteaux S, Bauchart JJ, Janne DB, Asseman P, et al. Mechanical thrombectomy in patients with deep venous thrombosis. Cardiovasc Intervent Radiol. 2001;24(1):42-8.

26. Lee KH, Han H, Lee KJ, Yoon CS, Kim SH, Won JY, et al. Mechanical thrombectomy of acute iliofemoral deep vein thrombosis with use of an Arrow-Trerotola percutaneous thrombectomy device. J Vasc Interv Radiol. 2006;17(3):487-95.

27. Kasirajan K, Gray B, Ouriel K. Percutaneous AngioJet thrombectomy in the management of extensive deep venous thrombosis. J Vasc Interv Radiol. 2001;12(2):179-85.

28. Bush RL, Lin PH, Bates JT, Mureebe L, Zhou W, Lumsden AB. Pharmacomechanical thrombectomy for treatment of symptomatic lower extremity deep venous thrombosis: safety and feasibility study. J Vasc Surg. 2004;40(5):965-70.

29. Hilleman DE, Razavi MK. Clinical and economic evaluation of the Trellis-8 infusion catheter for deep vein thrombosis. J Vasc Interv Radiol. 2008;19(3):377-83.

30. O'Sullivan GJ, Lohan DG, Gough N, Cronin CG, Kee ST. Pharmacomechanical thrombectomy of acute deep vein thrombosis with the Trellis-8 isolated thrombolysis catheter. J Vasc Interv Radiol. 2007;18(6): 715-24.

31. Parikh S, Motarjeme A, McNamara T, Raabe R, Hagspiel K, Benenati JF, et al. Ultrasound-accelerated thrombolysis for the treatment of deep vein thrombosis: initial clinical experience. J Vasc Interv Radiol. 2008;19(4):521-8.

32. Lin PH, Zhou W, Dardik A, Mussa F, Kougias P, Hedayati N, et al. Catheter-direct thrombolysis versus pharmacomechanical thrombectomy for treatment of symptomatic lower extremity deep venous thrombosis. Am J Surg. 2006;192(6):782-8.

33. Kölbel T, Alhadad A, Acosta S, Lindh M, Ivancev K, Gottsäter A. Thrombus embolization into IVC filters during catheter-directed thrombolysis for proximal deep venous thrombosis. J Endovasc Ther. 2008;15(5):605-13.

34. Protack CD, Bakken AM, Patel N, Saad WE, Waldman DL, Davies MG. Long-term outcomes of catheter directed thrombolysis for lower extremity deep venous thrombosis without prophylactic inferior vena cava filter placement. J Vasc Surg. 2007;45(5):992-7; discussion 997.

35. Park YJ, Choi JY, Min SK, Lee T, Jung IM, Chung JK, et al. Restoration of patency in iliofemoral deep vein thrombosis with catheter-directed thrombolysis does not always prevent post-thrombotic damage. Eur J Vasc Endovasc Surg. 2008;36(6): 725-30.

36. Comerota A, Aldridge S. Thrombolytic therapy for deep vein thrombosis: a clinical review. Can J Surg. 1993;36:359-64.

37. Park YJ, Choi JY, Min SK, Lee T, Jung IM, Chung JK, et al. Restoration of patency in iliofemoral deep vein thrombosis with catheter-directed thrombolysis does not always prevent post-thrombotic damage. Eur J Vasc Endovasc Surg. 2008 Dec;36(6): 725-30.

38. Singh H, Masuda EM. Comparing short-term outcomes of femoral-popliteal and iliofemoral deep venous thrombosis: early lysis and development of reflux. Ann Vasc Surg. 2005;19(1):74-9.

39. Elsharawy M, Elzayat E. Early results of thrombolysis vs anticoagulation in iliofemoral venous thrombosis. A randomised clinical trial. Eur J Vasc Endovasc Surg. 2002;24(3):209-14.

40. Enden T, Kløw NE, Sandvik L, Slagsvold CE, Ghanima W, Hafsahl G, et al; CaVenT Study Group. Catheter-directed thrombolysis vs. anticoagulant therapy alone in deep vein thrombosis: results of an open randomized, controlled trial reporting on short-term patency. J Thromb Haemost. 2009;7(8): 1268-75.

41. Vedantham S, Grassi CJ, Ferral H, Patel NH, Thorpe PE, Antonacci VP, et al; Technology Assessment Committee of the Society of Interventional Radiology. Reporting standards for endovascular treatment of lower extremity deep vein thrombosis. J Vasc Interv Radiol. 2009;20(7 suppl):S391-408.

42. Vedantham S, Thorpe PE, Cardella JF, Grassi CJ, Patel NH, Ferral H, et al; CIRSE and SIR Standards of Practice Committees. Quality improvement guidelines for the treatment of lower extremity deep vein thrombosis with use of endovascular thrombus removal. J Vasc Interv Radiol. 2009;20(7 suppl):S227-39.

43. Gogalniceanu P, Johnston CJ, Khalid U, Holt PJ, Hincliffe R, Loftus IM, et al. Indications for thrombolysis in deep venous thrombosis. Eur J Vasc Endovasc Surg. 2009;38(2):192-8.

Management of Central Venous Stenosis

Michael J. Reardon and Mark G. Davies

With increasing use of both short-term and long-term central venous access systems and with the growing dialysis access population, central venous stenosis and/or occlusion are becoming a more frequent event in clinical vascular practice. There is also renewed interest in Budd-Chiari syndrome, Paget-Schroetter syndrome, and May-Thurner syndrome. The global incidence of subclavian vein stenoses is 15.6%, jugular vein stenoses is 2.7%, and femoral vein stenoses is 0% to 3.8%. Asymptomatic subclavian vein stenoses, detected by venograms, represent only 23% to 33% of all subclavian vein stenoses. Most reports show a higher incidence of asymptomatic vs. symptomatic lesions: for subclavian vein ste-noses, it is 41% vs. 3.3%; for asymptomatic jugular vein stenoses, it is 9% vs. 1.6%.[1] In about 20% of the cases, however, the cause is benign.

Etiology of extrathoracic central venous obstruction is most often anatomic (May-Thurner and Paget-Schroetter), iatrogenic or traumatic (thrombosis or fibrosis related to indwelling dialysis catheters, pacemakers, defibrillators, or central venous lines), while intrathoracic central venous obstruction is commonly an extension of bronchopulmonary neoplasm or mediastinal disease.[2] Onset of symptoms is often slow and insidious, with tolerance in the early stages being explained by the development of an effective collateral circulation. Symptoms usually regress after medical treatment, sometimes requiring thrombolysis; however, in 10% of patients, major functional impairment may require bypass surgery or transluminal angioplasty.[3] The surgical treatment of central

Venous Thromboembolic Disease. Contemporary Endovascular Management series. © 2011 Mark G. Davies MD and Alan B. Lumsden MD, eds. Cardiotext Publishing, ISBN 978-1-935395-22-5.

venous stenosis has been reserved for significantly symptomatic patients who have an obstruction or stenosis that is not amenable to an endovascular approach, who have failed endovascular intervention, or who have venous resection as part of a planned en bloc tumor resection.[4]

Intrathoracic Malignant Disease

In the presence of known malignant disease of the thorax, percutaneous management of complete superior vena cava (SVC) occlusion with thrombolysis and/or clot aspiration followed by stent insertion is safe and effective, giving sustained symptomatic relief.[5] Primary patency in malignant and benign cases at 1 year was 64% and 76%, respectively. Overall symptom-free survival ranged from 1 to 34 months.[6] Resection for malignant tumor involvement was long considered an absolute contraindication to resection. Increasingly, resection and graft replacement have been used in selected cases in which en bloc resection could be achieved.[7,8] Infiltration of the SVC due to advanced non small cell lung cancer (NSCLC) or thymoma can be treated by prosthetic replacement or tangential resection. It should not be considered as palliative treatment because of the perioperative risks. SVC tangential resection involves fewer surgical problems. However, since this procedure is used mostly for N2 NSCLC subjects, patients have a low mean survival in spite of adjuvant therapy.[9] Surgical reconstruction of the superior vena cava with an ePTFE (expanded polytetrafluoroethylene) prosthesis provided immediate and long-term relief of symptoms of superior vena cava obstruction with a low surgical morbidity, even in patients with unresectable

malignancy.[10] When replacing the superior vena cava combined with resection of mediastinal malignancies, reconstruction of a left brachiocephalic vein alone results in a significant rate of occlusion and development of superior vena cava syndrome. Single right brachiocephalic vein reconstruction or bilateral brachiocephalic vein reconstruction in this setting, and separate reconstruction of the veins, is preferable to use of a Y graft.[11] Replacement grafts can include PTFE,[1] spiral vein graft,[12] or pericardium, although no data exist to support the superiority of one over the other. Our preference for superior vena cava reconstruction has been a self-constructed pericardial tube graft (Figure 16.1). Vessel involvement by soft tissue sarcoma can classified as type I, artery and vein; type II, artery only; type III, vein only; and type IV, neither artery nor vein. In patients with retroperitoneal soft tissue sarcoma, the most common vascular involvement pattern was vein only (type III, 64%). The inferior vena cava (6 ePTFE tube grafts, 3 ePTFE patches, 2 venoplasties), iliac vein (1 ePTFE bypass, 1 Dacron bypass, 1 venous patch), and superior mesenteric vein (1 anastomosis, 1 Dacron bypass) were restored in 80% of the patients (n = 16). Morbidity was 36% and mortality was 4%. At a median follow-up of 19.3 months, the venous patency rate was 93.8% (primary and secondary).[13]

Intrathoracic Benign Disease

The need for intervention for benign etiologies is increasing as the use of indwelling catheters for dialysis and cardiac therapy such as pacemakers and implantable defibrillators increases. Endovascular treatment of benign iliocaval occlusive disease is a safe

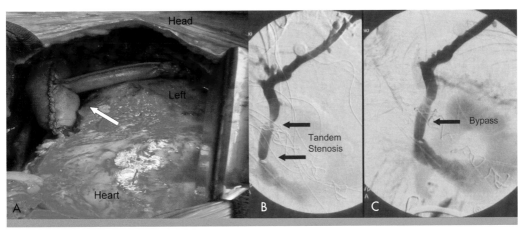

FIGURE 16.1   Central venous bypass. **A.** Superior vena cava reconstruction with a self-constructed pericardial tube graft (arrow). **B.** Innominate vein tandem stenosis on venography resistant to angioplasty or stent placement. **C.** Venogram of a superior vena cava reconstruction with a self-constructed pericardial tube graft.

and efficient minimally invasive technique with good midterm patency rates. Moreover, it improves cases with obstruction only, as well as cases with associated reflux and obstruction. Primary stenting should always be performed by using self-expanding stents deployed under general anesthesia to avoid lumbar pain. In case of failure, the endovascular procedure does not preclude further surgical reconstruction.[14] Endovascular repair is emerging as a first-line treatment for patients with superior vena cava syndrome of benign etiology. Open surgical repair of benign SVC syndrome is effective, with durable long-term relief from symptoms. Endovascular repair is less invasive but is equally effective in the midterm, albeit at the cost of multiple secondary interventions. It is an appropriate primary treatment for benign SVC syndrome. Open surgical repair remains an excellent choice for patients who are not suited for endovascular repair or in whom the endovascular repair fails.[15] Pacemaker wires can result in stenosis of the superior vena cava and other central veins. SVC stenting is safe and effective in patients who develop the SVC obstruction after cardiac pacemaker

insertion. No pacemaker function dysfunction was encountered in several case series.[16] Reconstruction is usually limited to patients who are significantly symptomatic and have failed endovascular attempts at correction. Reconstruction can be done via mediasternotomy or upper hemisternotomy. Proximal access is generally not difficult, and replacement of the SVC using the right atrium as the outflow site is easily accomplished. For isolated brachiocephalic obstruction, reconstruction has generally been done with ringed PTFE. The major technical issue is vein exposure and control in the arm and thoracic outlet.

Infradiaphragmatic Disease

Occlusive disease of the inferior vena cava (IVC) can arise from old thrombotic events, fibrosis, and extrinsic compression. Endovenous stent therapy has emerged as an effective, minimally invasive discipline for restoring patency in chronic iliofemoral/

caval vein obstruction or the May-Thurner syndrome. Technical success of 90% or greater can be achieved with this approach, and a 3-year assisted primary patency exceeds 80%. Venous reconstructions for iliofemoral or IVC obstruction offers 3-year patency rates of 62%.[14] The Palma procedure with autologous saphenous vein has the best long-term patency, whereas long-term success with ePTFE is more moderate.[17] Tumor lesions of the inferior vena cava can originate from the vein or can develop by malignant tumor infiltration from the surrounding tissue. The resection rate is 83%, with surgical reconstruction of the IVC achievable in all cases. The perioperative morbidity for such a strategy is 33%, with a hospital mortality

of 8.3%. The variable prognosis of the various IVC tumor lesions depends on tumor entity, stage, resection status, and individual risk factors.[18] Palliative relief can be achieved with covered stents to obtain short-term decompression, while other therapies (radiation or chemotherapy) are considered or the natural course of the disease occurs (Figure 16.2).

Budd-Chiari Syndrome

Primary Budd-Chiari syndrome (BCS) is characterized by a blocked hepatic venous outflow tract at various levels from small hepatic veins to inferior vena cava, resulting

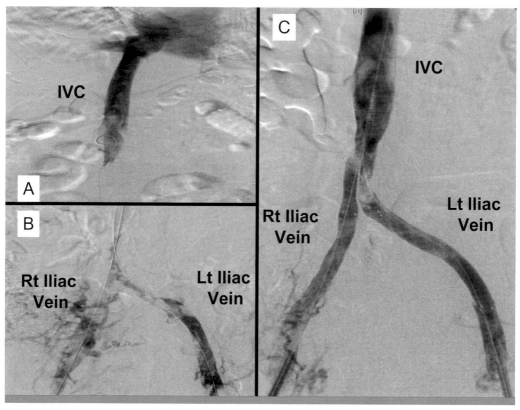

FIGURE 16.2. Stent grafting of the IVC. **A** and **B** demonstrate occlusion of the IVC and the common iliac veins. **C** represents the patency of the IVC and common iliac veins after lytic therapy.

from thrombosis or its fibrous sequellae.[19] This is a rare disease that affects mainly young adults. Multiple risk factors have been identified and are often combined in the same patient. Myeloproliferative diseases of atypical presentation account for nearly 50% of patients; their diagnosis can be made by showing the V617F mutation in Janus tyrosine kinase-2 gene of peripheral blood granulocytes and, should this mutation be absent, by showing clusters of dystrophic megakaryocytes at bone marrow biopsy. Diagnosis can be difficult because of the wide spectrum of presentation of the disease and the varying severity of liver damage. The traditional classification of Budd-Chiari syndrome—as fulminant, acute, or chronic—is not prognostically useful. This makes assessing the benefit of therapy difficult, especially because there is no evidence from randomized studies. Portal-vein thrombosis occurs in 20% to 30% of cases, and acute presentation reflects an acute or chronic syndrome in 60% of Budd-Chiari syndrome cases.[20] Presentation and manifestations are extremely varied, so that the diagnosis must be considered in any patient with acute or chronic liver disease. Doppler ultrasonography, computed tomography (CT), or magnetic resonance imaging (MRI) of hepatic veins and inferior vena cava can demonstrate lesions in the hepatic veins and/or inferior vena cava.

The disease is considered to be spontaneously lethal within 3 years of first symptoms. Budd-Chiari syndrome can be diagnosed and treated on a single occasion in the setting of the radiology department, with hepatic venography, transjugular liver biopsy, retrograde CO_2 portography, and inferior vena cava pressure measurements performed simultaneously with therapies such as dilation or stenting of webs in the inferior vena cava or hepatic veins, and placement of transjugular intrahepatic portosystemic shunts (TIPS).

Disruption of a portal vein thrombus can also be done during the same session. Surgical shunts have been superseded by the use of transjugular intrahepatic portosystemic shunts. Liver transplantation is reserved for fulminant and progressive chronic forms of BCS. Anticoagulation therapy must be used routinely before and after specific therapy regardless of whether a thrombophilic disorder is diagnosed. First-line strategy is anticoagulation, correction of risk factors, diuretics, and prophylaxis for portal hypertension. Second-line strategy consists of angioplasty for short-length venous stenoses[21] followed by TIPS. The final strategy is liver transplantation. Treatment progression is dictated by the response to previous therapy. This tiered strategy has achieved 5-year survival rates approaching 90%. Medium-term prognosis depends on the severity of liver disease. Patients with Budd-Chiari syndrome and portal venous system thrombosis constitute a unique group with limited therapeutic options and poor prognosis (median survival = 1 month).[22] Long-term outcome might be jeopardized by transformation of underlying conditions and hepatocellular carcinoma.

Renal Vein Thrombosis (RVT)

Renal vein occlusion in adults is usually a result of the vein thrombosis, which is frequently associated with the nephrotic syndrome. The anatomy of renal vascularization is of primary importance in understanding its pathophysiological responses and the clinical and diagnostic presentation of patients with this condition.[23] The reaction of the kidney to its vein occlusion is determined by the balance between the acuteness of the disease, extent of the development of collateral circulation, involvement of one or both kidneys, and the origin of the underlying disease. Renal vein occlusion is generally a complication of some other condition but may also be a primary disease. Renal vein thrombosis is relatively rare. CT angiography is considered the investigation of choice; alternatives include MR angiography or renal venography in highly selected patients.

As the condition is relatively uncommon, consensus on the best form of therapy for this condition has been slow to evolve. The trend in management has shifted to nonsurgical therapies, particularly systemic anticoagulation, except in a highly selected group of patients. The principal mode of treatment includes correction of fluid and electrolyte imbalance, dialysis, antihypertensive drugs, anticoagulation, and in certain cases, thrombolysis. Percutaneous catheter-directed thrombectomy with or without thrombolysis for acute RVT is associated with a rapid improvement in renal function and low incidence of morbidity. It is feasible for native and allograft renal veins and should be considered in patients with acute RVT, particularly in the setting of deteriorating renal function.[24]

May-Thurner Syndrome

The obstruction of the left common iliac vein by the pressure of the anteriorly positioned right common iliac artery, with intimal changes, was first described by May and Thurner in 1956.[25] Nonthrombotic iliac vein lesions, such as webs and spurs described by May and Thurner, are commonly found in the asymptomatic general population. However, the clinical syndrome, variously known as May-Thurner syndrome, Cockett syndrome, or iliac vein compression syndrome, is thought to be a relatively rare contributor of chronic venous disease. Iliac vein compression syndrome (May-Thurner syndrome) is the most probable cause of iliofemoral deep venous thrombosis (DVT). One-half to two-thirds of patients with left-sided iliofemoral DVT have intraluminal webs or spurs from chronic extrinsic compression of the left iliac vein at the crossing point of the right common iliac artery. Approximately 2% to 5% of those with chronic deep venous insufficiency of the left leg may have May-Thurner syndrome. May-Thurner syndrome occurs when compression of the common iliac vein is severe enough to inhibit the rate of venous outflow. In its more severe manifestation, May-Thurner syndrome is known to cause acute iliofemoral DVT.

May-Thurner syndrome is caused by the combination of compression and the vibratory pressure of the right iliac artery on the iliac vein that is pinched between the artery and the pelvic bone. With the advent of catheter-directed thrombolytic therapy for patients presenting with iliofemoral DVT, the underlying cause has been unveiled, and May-Thurner syndrome is gaining recognition. Patients presenting with symptoms of chronic venous insufficiency often fail conservative treatment, and because of their crippling symptoms, they may have a high rate of work absence or are on permanent disability. If May-Thurner syndrome can be identified as the cause and corrected, patients' quality of life would improve. With the advent of endovascular stenting, the underlying cause can be easily corrected, and long-term patency is acceptable[26,27] (Figure 16.3).

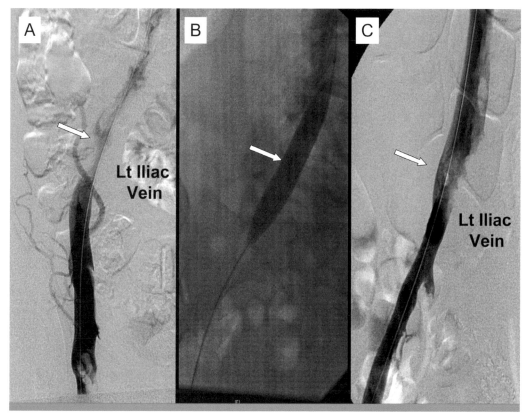

FIGURE 16.3. May-Thurner syndrome. **A.** Stenosis of the common iliac vein with collaterals. **B.** An angioplasty balloon inflated in the area. **C.** Final result: a patent common iliac vein without collaterals.

Paget-Schroetter Syndrome

Paget-Schroetter syndrome refers to spontaneous thrombosis of the axillary and subclavian venous segments in young, healthy individuals. It is a rare but potentially disabling affliction. The diagnosis should be suspected in any young patient presenting with unilateral arm swelling. Typically, the dominant arm is affected, and frequent, repetitive arm use is a common component of the patient's history. While venous duplex may make or infer the diagnosis, cross-sectional imaging or contrast venography is used to confirm the diagnosis because of

the central location of the venous abnormality (Figures 16.4 and 16.5). The underlying pathophysiology of this disorder is felt to be repetitive venous trauma owing to arm motion in the narrow anatomic space between the clavicle and first rib. The treatment of Paget-Schroetter syndrome remains controversial. Prompt anticoagulation is generally accepted as the minimal treatment offered. In the symptomatic individual, a more aggressive endovascular treatment is currently undertaken, with thrombolysis undertaken in the acute situation.[28] Many centers proceed with relief of the anatomic compression of the subclavian vein by first rib resection in all patients, whereas others perform this procedure selectively in cases of persistent

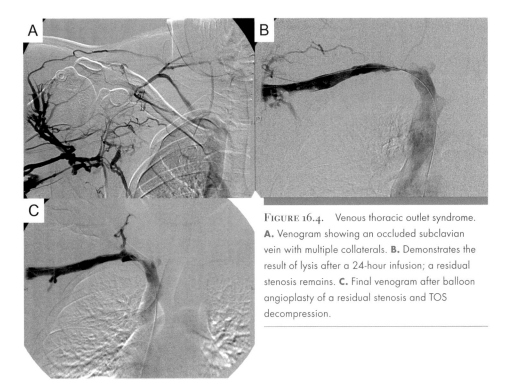

FIGURE 16.4.   Venous thoracic outlet syndrome.
A. Venogram showing an occluded subclavian
vein with multiple collaterals. **B.** Demonstrates the
result of lysis after a 24-hour infusion; a residual
stenosis remains. **C.** Final venogram after balloon
angioplasty of a residual stenosis and TOS
decompression.

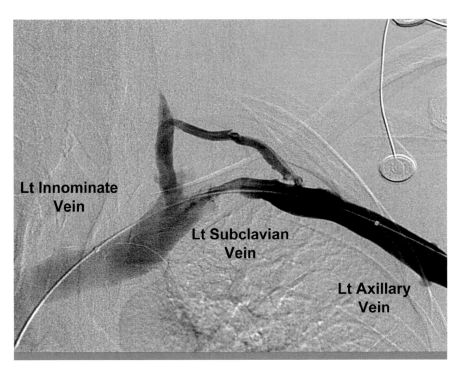

FIGURE 16.5.   Venous thoracic outlet syndrome. Example of a patent subclavian vein with extrinsic
compression and collateral formation representing TOS.

venous stenosis or ongoing symptoms.[29,30] Angioplasty with or without stenting is discouraged without concomitant anatomic decompression but does have an adjunctive role in patients undergoing first rib resection and can avoid the need for jugular turndown or patch angioplasty.

Dialysis Access-Related Central Venous Stenosis

Central venous obstruction is a common problem in patients with chronic renal failure who undergo maintenance hemodialysis. Incidences of central vein stenosis reported within hemodialysis patients have ranged from 11% to 40%.[31-35] Significant stenosis or occlusion of the subclavian vein is known to occur in 20% to 50% of patients who have had central venous catheters inserted into the subclavian vein or the internal jugular vein.[36] Stents provide a temporary benefit in most patients with central or peripheral upper extremity stenosis and obstruction. Incidence of central vein stenosis reported within hemodialysis patients have ranged from 11% to 40%.[31-33,37,38] Regular follow-up and reinterventions are required to maintain patency and achieve long-term clinical success. Stents used for central venous lesions have higher clinical success rates than stents used for peripheral venous lesions. However, endovascular therapy for central venous stenosis in the dialysis access patient, whether via angioplasty or stenting, is safe, with low rates of technical failure. Multiple additional interventions are the rule with both treatment modalities. Although neither offers truly durable outcomes, stent placement does not improve upon the patency rates provided by balloon angioplasty and does not add to the longevity of ipsilateral hemo-

dialysis access sites.[39] Thus, patients with a reasonable life expectancy or who are unable to return for subsequent procedures should be considered for alternative therapy.[40] The right atrial bypass grafting has been used to restore central venous patency in the carefully selected patient, in whom all other access sites are exhausted and in whom percutaneous dilation and/or stenting has failed.[41]

Conclusion

Central venous disease remains a small but significant area of venous disease. The data in the literature are composed of small series and case reports. In most cases, treatment has not been validated by level I evidence. There remains significant potential for clinical research and reporting. The practicing vascular specialist should be cognizant of each of the entities and be prepared to offer the spectrum of medical, radiological, and surgical therapy.

References

1. Huu TC. Central venous stenosis: review of the literature from 1980 to 2000. Nephrologie. 2001;22(8):479-85.

2. Schifferdecker B, Shaw JA, Piemonte TC, Eisenhauer AC. Nonmalignant superior vena cava syndrome: pathophysiology and management. Catheter Cardio Inte. 2005;65:416-23.

3. Marlier S, Bonal J, Cellarier G, Bouchiat C, Talard P, Dussarat GV. Superior vena cava syndromes of benign etiology. Presse Med. 1996;25(26):1203-7.

4. Picquet J, Blin V, Dussaussoy C, Jousset Y, Papon X, Enon B. Surgical reconstruction of the superior vena cava system: indications and results. Surgery. 2009;135:93-9.

5. Crowe MT, Davies CH, Gaines PA. Percutaneous management of superior vena cava occlusions. Cardiovasc Inter Rad. 1995;18(6):367-72.

6. Barshes NR, Annambhotla S, El Sayed HF, Huynh TT, Kougias P, Dardik A, et al. Percutaneous stenting of superior vena cava syndrome: treatment outcome in patients with benign and malignant etiology. Vascular. 2007;15(5):314-21.

7. Suzuki K, Asamura H, Watanbe S, Tsuchiya R. Combined resection of superior vena cava for lung carcinoma: prognostic significance of patterns of superior vena cava invasion. Ann Thoracic Surg. 2004;78:1184-9.

8. Thomas P, Magnan PE, Moulin G, Giudicelli R, Fuentes P. Extended operation for the lung cancer invading the superior vena cava. Eur J Cardiothorac Surg. 1994;8:177-82.

9. Politi L, Crisci C, Montinaro F, Andreani M, Podzemny V, Borzellino G. Prosthetic replacement and tangential resection of the superior vena cava in chest tumors. J Cardiovasc Surg (Torino). 2007;48(3):363-8.

10. Magnan PE, Thomas P, Giudicelli R, Fuentes P, Branchereau A. Surgical reconstruction of the superior vena cava. Cardiovasc Surg. 1994;2(5):598-604.

11. Shintani Y, Ohta M, Minami M, Shiono H, Hirabayashi H, Inoue M, et al. Long-term graft patency after replacement of the brachiocephalic veins combined with resection of mediastinal tumors. J Thorac Cardiovasc Surg. 2005;129(4):809-12.

12. Erbella J, Hess PJ, Huber TS. Superior vena cava bypass with superficial femoral vein for benign superior vena cava syndrome. Ann Vasc Surg. 2006;20:834-8.

13. Schwarzbach MH, Hormann Y, Hinz U, Leowardi C, Böckler D, Mechtersheimer G, et al. Clinical results of surgery for retroperitoneal sarcoma with major blood vessel involvement. J Vasc Surg. 2006;44(1):46-55.

14. Hartung O, Otero A, Boufi M, Decaridi G, Barthelemy P, Juhan C, et al. Mid-term results of endovascular treatment for symptomatic chronic nonmalignant iliocaval venous occlusive disease. J Vasc Surg. 2005;42(6):1138-44.

15. Rizvi AZ, Kalra M, Bjarnason H, Bower TC, Schleck C, Gloviczki P. Benign superior vena cava syndrome: stenting is now the first line of treatment. J Vasc Surg. 2008;47(2):372-80.

16. Teo N, Sabharwal T, Rowland E, Curry P, Adam A. Treatment of superior vena cava obstruction secondary to pacemaker wires with balloon venoplasty and insertion of metallic stents. Eur Heart J. 2002;23(18): 1465-70.

17. Jost CJ, Gloviczki P, Cherry KJJ, McKusick MA, Harmsen WS, Jenkins GD, et al. Surgical reconstruction of iliofemoral veins and the inferior vena cava for nonmalignant occlusive disease. J Vasc Surg. 2001;33(2):320-8.

18. Eder F, Halloul Z, Meyer F, Huth C, Lippert H. Surgery of inferior vena cava associated malignant tumor lesions. Vasa. 2008;37(1):68-80.

19. Valla DC. Primary Budd-Chiari syndrome. J Hepatol. 2009;50(1):195-203.

20. Senzolo M, Cholongitas EC, Patch D, Burroughs AK. Update on the classification, assessment of prognosis and therapy of Budd-Chiari syndrome. Nat Clin Pract Gastr. 2005;2(4):182-90.

21. Lee BB, Villavicencio L, Kim YW, Do YS, Koh KC, Lim HK, et al. Primary Budd-Chiari syndrome: outcome of endovascular management for suprahepatic venous obstruction. J Vasc Surg. 2006;43(1):101-8.

22. Mahmoud AE, Helmy A, Billingham L, Elias E. Poor prognosis and limited therapeutic options in patients with Budd-Chiari syndrome and portal venous system thrombosis. Eur J Gastr Hepat. 1997;9(5):485-9.

23. Asghar M, Ahmed K, Shah SS, Siddique MK, Dasgupta P, Khan MS. Renal vein thrombosis. Eur J Vasc Endovasc Surg. 2007;34(2):217-23.

24. Kim HS, Fine DM, Atta MG. Catheter-directed thrombectomy and thrombolysis for acute renal vein thrombosis. J Vasc Interv Radiol. 2006;17(5):815-22.

25. May R, Thurner J. Em Gefsssporn in der v.iliaca corn. sin. als wahrscheinliche Ursacheder uberwiegend liknsseitigen Beckenvenenthrombose. Z Kreisl-Forsch. 1956;45:912.

26. Mussa FF, Peden EK, Zhou W, Lin PH, Lumsden AB, Bush RL. Iliac vein stenting for chronic venous insufficiency. Tex Heart Inst J. 2007;34(1):60-6.

27. Lin PH, Zhou W, Dardik A, Mussa FF, Kougias P, Hedayati N, et al. Catheter-direct thrombolysis versus pharmacomechanical thrombectomy for treatment of symptomatic lower extremity deep venous thrombosis. Am J Surg. 2006;192(6):782-8.

28. Landry GJ, Liem TK. Endovascular management of Paget-Schroetter syndrome. Vascular. 2007;15(5):290-6.

29. Molina JE, Hunter DW, Dietz CA. Protocols for Paget-Schroetter syndrome and late treatment of chronic subclavian vein obstruction. Ann Thorac Surg. 2009;67(2):416-22.

30. Molina JE, Hunter DW, Dietz CA. Paget-Schroetter syndrome treated with thrombolytics and immediate surgery. J Vasc Surg. 2007;45(2):328-34.

31. Schumacher KA, Wallner B, Weidenmaier W, Friedrich JM. Venous occlusions distant to the shunt as malfunction factors during hemodialysis. Fortschr Röntgenstr. 1989;150:198-201.

32. Haage P, Vorwerk D, Piroth W, Schuermann K, Guenther RW. Treatment of hemodialysis-related central venous stenosis or occlusion: results of primary wallstent placement and follow-up in 50 patients. Radiology. 1999;212:175-80.

33. Schwab SJ, Quarles LD, Middleton JP, Cohan RH, Saeed M, Dennis VW. Hemodialysis-associated subclavian vein stenosis. Kidney Int. 1988;33:1156-9.

34. Surratt RS, Picus D, Hicks ME, Darcy MD, Kleinhoffer M, Jendrisak M. The importance of preoperative evaluation of the subclavian vein in dialysis access planning. Am J Roentgenol. 1991;156:623-5.

35. Lumsden AB, MacDonald MJ, Isiklar H, Martin LG, Kikeri D, Harker LA, et al. Central venous stenosis in the hemodialysis patient: incidence and efficacy of endovascular treatment. Cardiovasc Surg. 1997;5:504-9.

36. Chandler NM, Mistry BM, Garvin PJ. Surgical bypass for subclavian vein occlusion in hemodialysis patients. J Am Coll Surg. 2002;194(4):416-21.

37. Lumsden AB, MacDonald MJ, Isiklar H, Martin LG, Kikeri D, Harker LA, et al. Central venous stenosis in the hemodialysis patient: incidence and efficacy of endovascular treatment. Cardiovasc Surg. 1997;5:504-9.

38. Surratt RS, Picus D, Hicks ME, Darcy MD, Kleinhoffer M, Jendrisak M. The importance of preoperative evaluation of the subclavian vein in dialysis access planning. Am J Roentgenol. 1991;156:623-5.

39. Bakken AM, Protack CD, Saad WEA, Lee D, Waldman DL, Davies MG. Longterm outcomes of primary angioplasty versus primary stenting in the management of central venous stenoses in the hemodialysis patient. J Vasc Surg. 2007;45:776-83.

40. Oderich GS, Treiman GS, Schneider P, Bhirangi K. Stent placement for treatment of central and peripheral venous obstruction: a long-term multi-institutional experience. J Vasc Surg. 2000;32(4):760-9.

41. El-Sabrout RA, Duncan JM. Right atrial bypass grafting for central venous obstruction associated with dialysis access: another treatment option. J Vasc Surg. 1999;29(3):472-8.

Mesenteric Venous Thrombosis

Hosam F. El Sayed

Mesenteric venous thrombosis (MVT) is a distinct clinical entity that is responsible for 5% to 15% of all cases of mesenteric ischemia.[1] The low incidence of the disease, the nonspecific symptoms, the insidious onset, and the low awareness among clinicians may be responsible for the relatively high mortality rate of 32% to 44% reported in recent series.[2] The disease was first described by Elliot in 1895[3] and was later recognized in 1926 by Cokkinis.[4] However, Warren and Eberhard in 1935 were the first to recognize it as a cause of intestinal infarction distinct from mesenteric arterial occlusion.[5]

The disease represents 2 per 100,000 hospital admissions and comprises approxi-mately 0.01% of all emergency surgical ser-vice admissions. Studies have shown that the incidence of the disease has not changed over the past 3 decades; however, there was a higher proportion of elderly population in recent years.[6] There is no sex predilection for the disease and the median age at presenta-tion is 65 years old, with the highest inci-dence in patients between 70 and 79 years of age.[6] In a recent report by Rhee et al.,[7] MVT comprised only 6.2% of all patients treated for mesenteric ischemia.

The diagnosis has often been delayed, and most cases were identified either at lapa-rotomy or at autopsy.[1] The recent improve-ments in imaging techniques have led to both earlier diagnosis and a better idea of the etiology of mesenteric venous thrombosis, which has in turn led to significant changes in the treatment and perhaps reduction of the morbidity and mortality associated with this clinical syndrome.

Venous Thromboembolic Disease. Contemporary Endovascular Management series. © 2011 Mark G. Davies MD and Alan B. Lumsden MD, eds. Cardiotext Publishing, ISBN 978-1-935395-22-5.

Etiology

Mesenteric venous thrombosis can be classified as either primary or secondary. When an etiologic factor is found, the patient is classified as having secondary mesenteric venous thrombosis, and when no obvious cause is found, it is said to be a primary case. With continued improvements in the recognition of various etiologic factors for mesenteric venous thrombosis, the proportion of primary cases continues to decline. Currently, the etiologic factor for mesenteric venous thrombosis is found in about three-quarters of patients.[1] Many studies have also shown that a significant portion of patients with secondary MVT have multiple risk factors.[1,6,8]

The conditions associated with MVT fall into 3 main categories (Table 17.1)[6]: direct injury, local venous congestion or stasis, and hypercoagulable states or thrombophilia. These are essentially the same factors that were explained by Rudolph Virchow when he described his triad in 1856. His work was central to the evolution of the concept of thrombo-hemorrhagic balance. This theory states that there is a fine balance between fibrin degradation and fibrin production, and dominance of the latter leads to a hypercoagulable state.[9]

Factors that cause direct endothelial injury include major abdominal trauma, especially blunt traumas, and after major abdominal surgeries, especially splenectomy. This is much more common in the case of large splenomegaly and splenectomy for hematologic malignancies possibly secondary to thrombocytosis. MVT affects almost 5% of patients with these disorders undergoing splenectomy.[10] Local inflammatory intra-abdominal conditions are also associated with increased risk of mesenteric venous thrombosis.[11] This includes cases of pancreatitis, inflammatory bowel disease, and intra-abdominal infections.

Local venous congestion or stasis in the portal venous system is another significant risk factor for MVT. This is most commonly represented in cases with portal hypertension, especially in cases of liver cirrhosis. It is also manifested in cases with severe congestive heart failure, causing a form of posthepatic portal hypertension. Patients with morbid obesity (BMI >40) are also prone to develop MVT.[6]

TABLE 17.1 **Conditions Associated with MVT**

Direct Injury

Abdominal trauma

Postsurgical trauma (eg, post-splenectomy)

Pancreatitis

Inflammatory bowel disease

Local Venous Congestion or Stasis

Portal hypertension/liver cirrhosis

Severe congestive heart failure (EF < 20%)

Morbid obesity (BMI > 40)

Hypercoagulable States (Thrombophilia)

Inherited

Activated protein C resistance

Protein C deficiency

Protein S deficiency

Antithrombin III deficiency

Prothrombin gene mutation

Acquired

Malignancy (pancreatic cancer, metastatic abdominal cancer)

Hematologic disorders:

    Polycytemia rubra vera

    Essential thrombocytosis

    Leukemia

Hormonal therapy (oral contraceptive pills)

Lupus anticoagulants

Heparin-induced thrombocytopenia

However, the most common cause of secondary MVT remains thrombophilia or hypercoagulable conditions. In fact, more than half of all cases of MVT have an identifiable hypercoagulable condition.[6,12] Hypercoagulable conditions can be either inherited when the subject is born with a genetic defect or acquired. The acquired types of hypercoagulable conditions refer to those systemic diseases that have been known and proven to be associated with thrombosis. However, the true frequency of these disorders in patients with MVT is difficult to estimate since most studies in the literature included patients with all forms of deep venous thrombosis. One study suggested that an acquired or inherited hypercoagulable state was more likely in patients with isolated MVT compared with those with concomitant involvement of the portal or splenic veins.[13] A list of the hypercoagulable conditions associated with MVT can be found in Table 17.1.

Inherited Hypercoagulable Conditions

The available data suggest that the most common inherited hypercoagulable condition associated with MVT is the activated protein C resistance, secondary to factor V Leiden mutation. In one epidemiologic study of cases with documented MVT, factor V Leiden mutation was present in 45% of those cases.[6] Activated protein C resistance can also occur due to other forms of mutations in another 10% of cases.[14]

Another cause of inherited hypercoagulable conditions is the deficiency of the natural anticoagulant proteins that maintain the balance between the coagulant and anticoagulant activity of the blood. Deficiencies of protein C, protein S, and antithrombin III (AT III), collectively, are present in about 10% of cases with MVT.[6,14]

Mutation of the prothrombin gene has also been associated with increased risk of thrombotic events. This mutation leads to higher plasma prothrombin levels and is 4 times as common in patients with a history of venous thrombosis compared to their controls.[15] In one small study, this mutation was found in 40% of cases with idiopathic portal vein thrombosis.[16]

Acquired Hypercoagulable Conditions

Multiple risk factors are associated with acquired hypercoagulable states. The most common of these conditions are malignancy, hormonal therapy, and antiphospholipid antibodies.

Malignancy has been a known risk factor for hypercoagulable state and venous thrombosis. This is particularly more common in older patients and in those malignancies associated with advanced disease at the time of diagnosis (eg, pancreas).[17] Certain cancers are particularly more associated with MVT. Myeloproliferative disorders, especially polycythemia vera and essential thrombocythemia, are strongly associated with MVT.[1] In a small series of patients with MVT, 10% had associated polycythemia vera.[18] Pancreatic cancer and metastatic abdominal cancers are also strongly associated with MVT. In one series, abdominal cancer was present in 24% of all cases of documented MVT, with pancreatic cancer present in half of those cases.[6]

Hormonal therapy is also highly associated with venous thrombosis in general and MVT in particular. Historically, oral contraceptive use accounted for 9% to 18% of the episodes of MVT in young women.[12,19] In a more recent study, oral contraceptives or estrogen hormonal replacement therapy was present in 12% of women diagnosed with MVT.[6] Antiphospholipid antibodies are directed against plasma proteins bound to anionic phospholipids and are associated with venous thrombosis. The antiphospholipid antibodies, including the cardiolipin antibodies and the lupus anticoagulants, are present in another 5% to 10% of cases.[6,8]

Pathophysiology

The celiac, superior mesenteric, and inferior mesenteric arteries are the visceral branches of the aorta supplying the gut. The branches from these arteries terminate as the arteriae rectae in the distal parts of the correspond-

ing mesenteries, supplying the wall of the gut. The venous drainage follows a similar pattern, with the venae rectae forming the venous arcades, which drain the gut into the inferior mesenteric and superior mesenteric veins. The inferior mesenteric vein joins the splenic vein before the confluence with the superior mesenteric vein behind the neck of the pancreas to form the portal vein that supplies the liver parenchyma (Figure 17.1).

There are multiple extrinsic and intrinsic mechanisms that control the blood flow to the bowel wall. This is mainly controlled via changes in the resistance of the mesenteric arterioles, which accounts for the marked

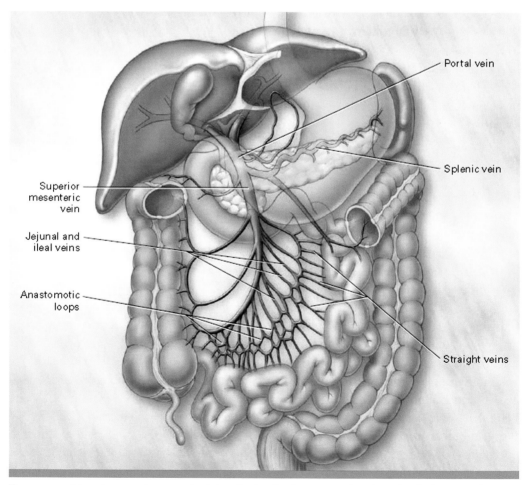

FIGURE 17.1   Normal mesenteric venous circulation. Reprinted with permission from Agur AM, Dailey, AF, Boileau Grant JC. Grants Atlas of Anatomy. 11th ed. Philadelphia, PA: Lippincott Williams & Wilkins; 2004.

variation in the splanchnic blood flow, between 10% and 35% of the cardiac output, depending on variable conditions such as fasting and postprandial states and systemic hypotension. The bowel can withstand an acute 75% reduction of the mesenteric blood flow for up to 12 hours without significant damage occurring.[20] When ischemic injury of the intestine develops, progressive vasoconstriction develops in the affected vascular bed, thereby reducing collateral flow. Vasoconstriction can persist even after blood flow has been restored, leading to continued bowel ischemia and providing the rationale for therapeutic infusion of the vasodilator papaverine for treatment of acute mesenteric ischemia.[20,21]

The location of the initial thrombosis within the mesenteric venous circulation varies with the etiology. Thrombosis due to intra-abdominal causes such as cirrhosis, neoplasm, or operative injury starts at the large vessels (eg, superior mesenteric vein or portal vein) and progresses peripherally to involve the smaller venous arcades and arcuate channels. However, thrombosis due to an underlying hypercoagulable state begins in the small vessels and progresses to involve the larger vessels.[1,13] Intestinal infarction rarely occurs unless the branches of the peripheral arcades and the microcirculation are thrombosed, even when the junction of the portal vein and the superior mesenteric vein is occluded. In a recent large series of patients diagnosed with MVT, bowel infarction occurred in 33% of them that required bowel resection.[22] Inferior mesenteric vein thrombosis leading to infarction has been reported in fewer than 6% of cases with mesenteric venous thrombosis.[21]

When acute MVT happens, the venous drainage of the affected segment of the bowel is compromised. The intramural blood volume increases as the arterial blood keeps flowing into the bowel wall in patients with venous compromise. This leads to increased intravascular hydrostatic pressure, which dilates the blood vessels and widens the fenestrations between the vascular endothelial cells. This results in extravasation of plasma and red blood cells into the bowel wall or lumen. Tension in the submucosal extravascular compartment or prolonged stasis-induced thrombosis of the microvasculature may result in interruption of the arterial blood flow.[23] Grossly, the bowel wall is swollen and looks cyanotic, with intramural hemorrhage. These changes also affect the nearby mesentery. The transition from the affected bowel segment to the normal bowel is usually gradual, unlike that seen with arterial occlusion, which makes it more difficult to accurately evaluate viable from nonviable bowel during surgery. The arterial pulsations are present up to the bowel wall, but arterial vasoconstriction frequently intervenes, which accentuates the compromised intramural blood flow in the congested bowel. Later on, transmural infarction of the bowel sets in, and at that point it may be impossible to differentiate venous from arterial occlusion as a cause of the bowel infarction. Transmural bowel infarction happens in 16% of patients suffering from acute MVT.[24] Serosanguineous peritoneal fluid accompanies early hemorrhagic infarction. When a large segment of the bowel is affected, it leads to extensive third space fluid loss with systemic hypovolemia.[13,20,21]

Two factors contribute to the bowel injury when affected by acute MVT, the first being transmural ischemia secondary to cessation of the blood flow. The second factor is reperfusion injury if restoration of flow is achieved. Most of the damage is due to reperfusion injury after a brief period of ischemia, while the detrimental effects of hypoxia predominate with longer periods of ischemia.[25]

MVT can lead to presinusoidal portal hypertension in the long run and is classified as chronic mesenteric venous thrombosis. This usually happens when patients have no symptoms at the time of the initial thrombosis but secondary pathologic changes develop over the time. This usually manifests as gastrointestinal bleeding from esophageal and/or intestinal varices. Most of these patients have associated thrombosis of the major veins such as the portal or splenic vein. It was reported that portal hypertension develops in 25% of patients who suffered from acute MVT.[24]

Clinical Presentation

MVT can present with acute onset within hours, subacute within days to even weeks, or chronic that is usually asymptomatic until late complications occur. Patients with the acute presentation are at the highest risk for developing bowel infarction and peritonitis. On the other hand, the subacute form is more indolent, where abdominal pain is prominent but neither infarction nor variceal bleeding is likely. In less common situations, the subacute form will evolve over the period of days or weeks into intestinal infarction and peritonitis, blurring the distinction between the acute and the subacute presentation.[1] In the chronic form of the disease, patients are essentially asymptomatic, and their presentation can be upper or lower gastrointestinal bleeding secondary to esophageal or intestinal varices. Those patients can also develop hypersplenism with pancytopenia or secondary thrombocytopenia.[21,26]

The hallmark of mesenteric ischemia, whether it is due to arterial or to venous thrombosis, is abdominal pain that is out of proportion to the physical findings. With the exception of the abdominal pain, which

is present in almost all patients with acute and subacute MVT, no other symptoms are pathognomonic of MVT. The pain is usually central abdominal and colicky in nature. The duration of pain varies, but 75% of cases had the symptoms for more than 48 hours, a very important distinction from mesenteric arterial causes where the presentation is much earlier.[7] Mathews and White[27] found that approximately 50% of their patients had pain from 5 to 30 days before seeking medical attention, and 27% reported abdominal pain for more than 1 month. It was also reported that patients who presented with symptoms more than 5 days had a better prognosis than patients presenting earlier, possibly due to a more benign disease form that allowed them to delay seeking medical attention for so long.[21]

Anorexia, nausea, vomiting, and diarrhea are also common in acute MVT, occurring in more than 50% of cases. Clinical gastrointestinal bleeding in the form of bloody diarrhea or melena is present in 15% of cases. Hematemesis is also present in an additional 13% of cases. Actually, the presence of hematemesis, as well as bleeding per rectus, should alert the physician to the possibility of mesenteric ischemic catastrophe.[21] However, occult blood in stool is found in nearly 50% of cases.[12]

Initial physical findings in acute MVT vary greatly, reflecting both different stages and degrees of bowel injury. Most of the patients will have some degree of abdominal tenderness and decreased bowel sounds with abdominal distention. However, a minority of patients will develop peritoneal signs in the form of rebound tenderness and abdominal rigidity, which signifies the presence of intestinal infarction with peritonitis. In a large series of patients with MVT, this occurred in 33% of cases.[22] Hemodynamic instability can also occur if a large segment

of the bowel is affected due to fluid seques-
tration within the bowel lumen or the abdominal cavity. It also appears later in the
disease as a manifestation of septic shock
secondary to the bowel infarction and septic
peritonitis. It was consistently shown that the
presence of hemodynamic instability with a
systolic blood pressure of less than 90 mm
Hg denotes a poor prognosis.[28] About half
of the patients have a personal or family history of deep venous thrombosis, pulmonary
embolism, or a heritable hypercoagulable
state, and this is an important point to in-
quire about as it can guide the diagnosis and
therapy of the case.[7]

Laboratory studies in all forms of intestinal ischemia have low sensitivity and specificity. While abnormal laboratory values may
be helpful in bolstering suspicion for acute
mesenteric ischemia, normal laboratory values do not exclude it and do not justify delay-
ing management when clinical suspicion is
present. There is no specific laboratory test
that is pathognomonic of MVT. The presence of increased serum lactate levels and
metabolic acidosis may serve to identify patients with established bowel infarction, but
this is a late finding.[1] Elevated serum amy-
lase levels have been observed in half the patients with intestinal ischemia. An elevated
phosphate level has also been observed in
80% of cases. Creatine kinase (CK)-BB iso-
enzyme elevations have been found to correlate with bowel infarction while total CK
levels were not found to be useful. Lactate
dehydrogenase (LDH) elevation was present
in 75% of cases with bowel infarction but did
not differentiate between ischemia and infarction.[29-31] In fact, the simple leukocytosis
with a white cell count above 12,000/cu mm
with an increase in the proportion of poly-
morphonuclear cells is the most clinically
helpful lab test and is present in two-thirds
of cases. Currently, laboratory tests can only

suggest the diagnosis of intestinal ischemia.[21]
A useful clinical guideline is that any patient
with acute abdominal pain and metabolic
acidosis is suspected of having acute mesenteric ischemia until proven otherwise.

Workup

In the absence of any reliable and specific
symptoms, signs, and laboratory studies,
the preoperative diagnosis of acute MVT is
difficult. Also, the severe variability in the
duration and severity of the manifestations
significantly adds to the difficulty. The aim
of the workup is to reach the correct diagnosis of MVT before bowel infarction develops, in which case the prognosis becomes
significantly worse. In the past, the correct
diagnosis of MVT was reached in more than
90% of cases at laparotomy for patients with
peritoneal signs secondary to bowel infarction, signifying that the diagnosis was severely delayed. In recent years, there has been
enormous improvement of diagnostic radiographic modalities that helped in achieving
this goal. Nowadays, most of the patients are
diagnosed prior to surgery, with significant
improvement in morbidity and mortality.

Projectional Radiography

Plain films of the abdomen are nonspecific
and can be normal in 25% of patients. Positive findings include intestinal dilatation,
small bowel pseudo-obstruction pattern,
or paralytic ileus. More specific but far less
common findings include thumbprinting,
in which multiple round, smooth, soft tissue
densities project into the intestinal lumen as
a result of mucosal and submucosal edema
and hemorrhage. Specific but usually late
signs include the presence of air in the wall
of the bowel (peumatosis intestinalis) (Fig-

ure 17.2), portal venous gas or free intra-peritoneal air, which usually signify bowel infarction.[32] It is to be remembered that the use of intraluminal dye studies of the bowel are contraindicated because they interfere with the visualization using angiogram and add little information to the plain film.[21]

Doppler Flow Ultrasonography

Doppler flow ultrasonography of the mesenteric veins can be used to demonstrate thrombi, especially in the large veins like the superior mesenteric vein and portal vein. The findings include lucent filling defects, thickened mesentery, and bowel wall and intraperitoneal free fluid. However, like all acute mesenteric ischemia disorders, because of body habitus, the overlying bowel gas that interferes with proper visualization and patient cooperation, ultrasonography is not typically used in the initial evaluation of acutely ill patients with suspected acute MVT.[33]

Multidetector Computed Tomography

Multidetector computed tomography (MDCT) has become the preferred imaging modality for the evaluation of suspected MVT cases. It can be performed quickly in critically ill patients and is less dependent on operator skill and patient factors than other imaging modalities.[23] In fact, the sensitivity of CT scan in diagnosing MVT was found to be 90% in several studies.[7] CT scan produces volume data that can be manipulated and viewed in different projections evaluating the bowel wall, the mesentery, the surrounding fat, the omenta, and the mesenteric vessels themselves, visualizing both the arteries and veins and any pathologic abnormalities including stenosis, atherosclerotic plaques, and intravascular thrombi.[34] CT scan can exclude other cases of acute abdominal pain. Specifically, in cases of MVT, the CT scan will show failure to opacify the mesenteric veins with intravenous filling defects,

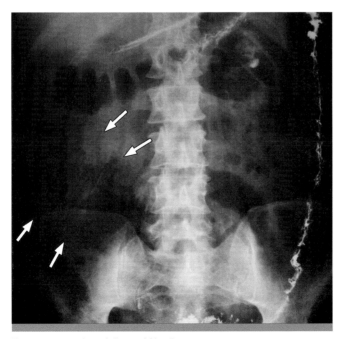

FIGURE 17.2 Plain abdominal film showing extensive pneumatosis intestinalis.

enlarged superior mesenteric vein and persistent enhancement of the bowel wall due to congestion, as well as thickened mesentery (Figure 17.3). In late cases, it will show pneumatosis, portal venous gas, and possibly intraperitoneal free air and fluid.[21]

Magnetic Resonance Imaging/ Magnetic Resonance Angiography

Magnetic resonance imaging (MRI) and magnetic resonance angiography (MRA) can also be used, providing information that is similar to CT scan, with the theoretical advantage of not using ionizing irradiation and using gadolinium-based intravascular contrast rather than iodinated contrast used in CT scans in patient with renal insufficiency, which has been negated by the increased incidence of nephrogenic systemic fibrosis related to the gadolinium-based MR contrast agents.[23] MR, however, is best used in the nonacute setting. The critically ill patient with suspected acute mesenteric ischemia usually has life support apparatus that is incompatible with the MR scanner. Those patients are best scanned with MDCT, which also offers better spatial resolution.[35]

Selective Mesenteric Angiography

Selective mesenteric angiography was the diagnostic modality of choice before the 1990s, when CT scan became available. In fact, a selective mesenteric angiogram is much less sensitive than CT scan in diagnosing MVT, where it was able to diagnose only 55.5% compared to the above 90% sensitivity of CT scan.[22] Nowadays, mesenteric angiogram is performed primarily for transcatheter therapeutic interventions both for arterial and venous mesenteric ischemic disorders. Those interventions include in-

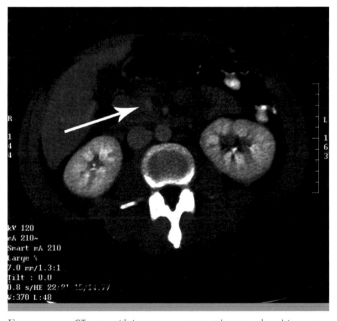

FIGURE 17.3   CT scan with intravenous contrast (venous phase) in a case showing partial occlusion of the superior mesenteric vein by a thrombus (shown by arrow).

fusion of vasodilator agents (papaverine), thrombolytic agents (streptokinase, urokinase, recombinant tissue plasminogen activator), and angioplasty.[36] The angiographic findings of MVT have been determined experimentally and clinically and include[21]:

- Demonstration of a thrombus in the superior mesenteric vein (SMV) on the venous phase of the study with partial or complete occlusion.
- Failure to visualize the SMV or portal vein on delayed views.
- Slow or absent filling of the mesenteric veins.
- Mesenteric arterial spasm with back flushing into the aorta on intra-arterial contrast injection.
- Failure of the arterial arcades to empty.
- Prolonged blush of the wall of the involved bowel segment.
- The angiography can also show slow reconstitution of the mesenteric venous blood flow proximal to the thrombus, which is important in the therapeutic decisions.

The workup of patients with suspected MVT is summarized in the guidelines of management of intestinal ischemia from the American Gastroenterological Association as illustrated in the algorithm in Figure 17.4.[37] Patients presenting with abdominal pain that is severe enough to call to the attention of a physician, whose pain persists for more than 2 or 3 hours, and whose clinical picture does not suggest other abdominal problems (eg, cholecystitis or diverticulitis) should be evaluated and treated for acute mesenteric ischemia. In those patients, suspicion of MVT is signaled by a history of DVT or familial or personal hypercoagulability state, or having

the pain persist for several days before presentation, should have MDCT as their initial evaluation after starting aggressive resuscitation. In cases where MVT was diagnosed, the patient should immediately be started on heparin. If the patient has obvious peritoneal signs, the patient should immediately go the operating room for exploratory laparotomy. A mesenteric angiogram is needed in case of a negative CT scan for MVT or in cases where endovascular interventions are needed. At any time, if the patient starts developing peritoneal signs, the patient has to undergo exploratory laparotomy.

Management

The principles of management of MVT are 3-fold:

- Prevention of further development of venous thrombosis,
- resection of necrotic bowel, and
- prevention of recurrence of venous thrombosis.

Historically, the treatment of acute and sub-acute MVT included anticoagulation with exploratory laparotomy with resection of the necrotic bowel. Laparotomy was an essential part of the management both for diagnostic and therapeutic reasons, as preoperative diagnosis of MVT was not possible. Recently, with the advent of MDCT, the preoperative diagnosis of MVT was possible in most cases. Adding to that the rapid and extensive development of endovascular techniques as minimally invasive therapy options, currently the use of exploratory laparotomy is limited to patients who have persistent peritoneal signs for possible bowel resection. In a one study, that was only needed in 33% of their patients with acute MVT.[22]

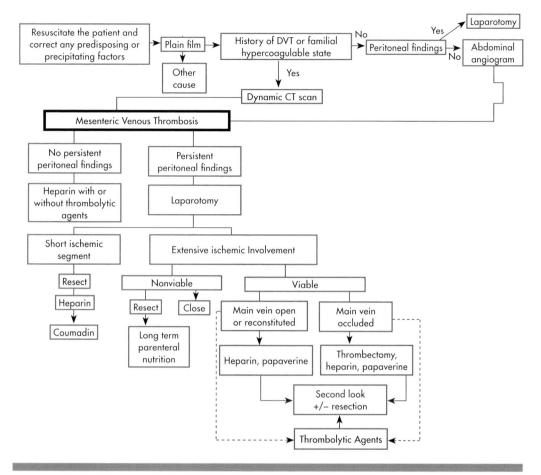

FIGURE 17.4   Diagnosis and treatment of acute mesenteric venous thrombosis. Solid lines indicate accepted management plan; dashed lines indicate alternate management plan. DVT, deep venous thrombosis. (From "American Gastroenterological Association Medical Position Statement: guidelines on intestinal ischemia." Gastroenterology 118(5): 951-3.) With permission from Elsevier.

Currently, the management of acute and subacute MVT includes:

- Anticoagulation
- Exploratory laparotomy
- Endovascular options for recanalizing the thrombosed veins
- Adjunctive supportive measures

Anticoagulation

Heparin is an essential component of therapy in all patients with acute and subacute MVT. The theoretical aim of heparin in such a situation is to prevent progression of the thrombosis and limit the amount of bowel resection, if needed. Contrary to heparin use in acute mesenteric arterial thrombosis and embolism, where the use is delayed for 48 hours postoperatively to avoid postoperative bleeding, in acute and subacute MVT it is started immediately with the diagnosis of the condition, continues intraoperatively, and in the immediate postoperative period. Anticoagulation should be started even in the presence of gastrointestinal bleeding, as the risk of bleeding is outweighed by the benefit of preventing bowel infarction.[1] Anticoagulation has been shown to decrease the rate of recurrence from 25% to 13%. It also reduced mortality from 50% to 13%.[28] Standard anticoagulation with Coumadin is continued for at least 6 months. In cases where there is an underlying hypercoagulable state, the therapy can continue indefinitely.[19,38]

Exploratory Laparotomy

Historically, this was needed in almost all cases because most cases of acute MVT were diagnosed at laparotomy, due to the inability to diagnose the condition preoperatively. Nowadays, with the advent of the advanced radiologic diagnostic modalities including CT, MRA, and mesenteric angiogram, most of the cases are diagnosed preoperatively and many are treated nonoperatively, using the advanced endovascular techniques now available. Exploratory laparotomy is reserved for those cases with persistent peritoneal signs (eg, abdominal tenderness, rebound tenderness, and rigidity). It is also indicated in cases with obvious manifestations of bowel infarction including free intraperitoneal air and portal venous gas.

At laparotomy, the bowel is evaluated for extent of involvement and viability, both clinically and, if necessary, by administration of fluorescein with examination under ultraviolet light. In cases in which there is a localized involvement of the bowel, the segment involved is resected and continuity is restored if the remaining bowel appears absolutely normal. Historically, it was recommended to perform wider resection than the apparently involved bowel because the mesenteric venous thrombosis process extends further in the mesentery; however, recent evidence suggests that there is no need to sacrifice viable bowel. However, if there

is any doubt of involvement of the remaining bowel, continuity may not be restored in the original operation, and the patient is sent back to the intensive care with a second-look laparotomy performed 18 to 24 hours after the initial exploration to check for the remaining bowel condition.[21] An adjunctive measure at that time can be continued infusion of papaverine, a potent vasodilator, in the superior mesenteric artery (SMA) through a catheter inserted via the femoral artery approach. This is because there is a component of mesenteric arterial spasm in the pathologic process of acute MVT and papaverine can help alleviate the vasospasm to improve blood flow, which may avert resection of reversibly ischemic bowel.[28] If no further affection of the bowel is found, the continuity is restored and the abdomen is closed. It is to be stressed that anticoagulation should be continued throughout the process, including intraoperatively.

In some cases, there is extensive involvement of the bowel with obvious bowel necrosis, in which case and at the discretion of the surgeon 1 of 2 options are available, either to perform major resection of the bowel with implementation of lifelong parenteral nutrition due to short loop syndrome, or closing the abdomen as the resection would be incompatible with life. However, if there is extensive involvement of the bowel that is of doubtful viability, in which case the endovascular options are extremely helpful to attempt to recanalize the thrombosed mesenteric veins with saving as much bowel as possible and a second laparotomy to excise the obviously nonviable bowel segments. These techniques can help save some of those patients with extensive disease, which was not possible using the conventional anticoagulation and resection alone.

Historically, there have been some reports of open mesenteric venous thrombectomy using Fogarty balloon thrombectomy catheters, which was performed for cases with extensive bowel involvement with doubtful viability. These were indicated when a long segment of questionable bowel was found and the angiogram or operative findings indicate complete thrombosis of the SMV at its junction with the portal vein, with or without extension into the portal vein. A second-look operation was always performed after the venous thrombectomy. This technique has been reported in only a few patients in the literature, which makes it impossible to define its role in the treatment of acute MVT.[21] Additionally, the endovascular options have largely replaced the need to perform open mesenteric venous thrombectomy.

Endovascular Interventions

Recently, with the extensive development of minimally invasive endovascular interventions, several therapeutic options have evolved in the management of acute and subacute MVT. These interventions are mostly used when nonoperative therapy for acute or subacute MVT is performed to reverse the clinical course and avoid bowel infarction. It is also used in cases when at exploratory laparotomy there is an extensive and diffuse affection of the bowel with large areas of doubtful viability. However, in cases where exploratory laparotomy is used and there is a localized segment of nonviable bowel with no doubtfully viable loops, the therapy remains the standard localized resection and anticoagulation. These interventions can be grouped into 3 options:

- Thrombolysis
- Percutaneous mechanical thrombectomy
- Intra-arterial vasodilator infusion

Thrombolysis

Multiple case reports and small case series have shown thrombolytic therapy to be effective in treating acute MVT. Theoretically, heparin prevents further thrombosis and thrombus propagation; thrombolytic therapy with active clot dissolution may be more effective than traditional treatment of venous thrombosis with anticoagulation and clot stabilization.[39] There are several routes through which the thrombolytic agent is delivered. Systemic intravenous administration of urokinase or tissue plasminogen activator (tPA) has been reported;[40] however, it does not deliver a high concentration of the thrombolytic agent into the mesenteric venous circulation, in addition to the increased bleeding complications with systemic use as well as the need for a higher dose to be effective. The 2 commonly used routes of administration are the transarterial route via a catheter placed in the SMA and direct mesenteric venous administration through a catheter placed in the portal venous system via the transjugular transhepatic approach,[41,42] or via direct percutaneous trans-hepatic approach.[43,44] Whereas the trans-hepatic approaches are successful in clearance of thrombus in the larger mesenteric veins by delivering direct and high concentrations of the thrombolytics and gaining direct access to the mesenteric venous system allowing the performance of percutaneous mechanical thrombectomy, they may not be ideal in addressing thrombus in the smaller secondary and tertiary venous branches. In those cases, the intra-arterial administration of thrombolytics via the SMA is more effective, as it enables the thrombolytic agent to permeate the capillaries and small venules, something that cannot be achieved using the trans-hepatic approach.[39] SMA administration of the thrombolytic also avoids the added risk of bleeding secondary to puncturing the liver parenchyma both through the transjugular approach and especially through the direct percutaneous approach. Very few case reports of thrombolysis via a surgically placed mesenteric venous catheter into one of the small venous tributaries during exploratory laparotomy are found in the literature.[45] Most of the earlier studies of mesenteric venous thrombolysis used urokinase. Nowadays, because urokinase is no longer available on the market, tPA is typically used. The usual dose is an initial bolus of 2 mg followed by infusion of 1 to 2 mg/h for 24 hours. At that time, a catheter check and repeat angiogram to evaluate the response are performed. If there is still residual thrombus left, continued infusion for another 24 hours is performed, after which time the catheter is removed. In the percutaneous trans-hepatic approach, the track has to be sealed with haemostatic glue and coils to avoid intraperitoneal bleeding from the liver track, which can be life-threatening.

The patient should be closely monitored for manifestations of bleeding and fibrinogen levels to avoid overconsumption and excessive thrombolysis. Heparin infusion continues throughout the thrombolytic infusion, however, at a smaller dose (500 units/h), to resume full dose heparinization once thrombolytic infusion has stopped.

Percutaneous Mechanical Thrombectomy

This is another endovascular adjunct procedure for clearing acute MVT. It can be used only when there is trans-hepatic access into the portal venous system. It is also indicated when there is a large clot burden in the main mesenteric veins. Several commercially available percutaneous mechanical thrombectomy devices have been reportedly used for that indication including the AngioJet rheolytic thrombectomy device (MEDRAD, Inc., Warrendale, PA), the Helix Clot Buster

thrombectomy device (ev3, Plymouth, MN), and the Arrow Trerotola device (Arrow International Inc, Reading, PA). Aspiration thrombectomy using a large angulated catheter (at least 8 Fr) has also been described.[42] The aim of these devices is to debulk the mesenteric venous clot, thereby reducing the dose and duration needed for thrombolysis, especially in patients with high risk of bleeding complications. Also, balloon angioplasty has also been described for cases in which there have been venous stenotic lesions or large clot burden not responding to thrombolysis or mechanical thrombectomy because of a large chronic component in the clot. The angioplasty is used to relieve the stenosis with or without use of stents or covered stents. They are also useful to fragment and displace the clot to restore flow within the portal venous system to relieve the congestion in the affected bowel.[42]

Intra-arterial Vasodilator Infusion

Mesenteric arterial vasospasm is commonly present in cases of acute and subacute MVT. It is specifically useful in cases following exploration where there is doubtful bowel left behind for a second-look laparotomy. In this situation, the use of the vasodilators can improve the blood flow to the affected bowel, which in addition to anticoagulation and other endovascular interventions, can help limit the amount of bowel to be resected.[1] Multiple vasodilators can be used for this indication, including tolazoline, nitroglycerin, glucagon, and isoproterenol. However, the most-used vasodilator for this purpose is papaverine. Papaverine is a nonaddictive opium derivative extracted from the poppy plant. It acts by inhibiting the phosphdiesterase enzyme that metabolizes cyclic adenosine monophosphate (cAMP). The net effect is to increase the tissue levels of cAMP, which is a direct vascular smooth muscle relaxant. Ninety percent of papaverine undergoes first-pass metabolism by the liver, which limits its systemic toxicity and side effects.[38] The usual dose is a bolus of 30 to 60 mg, followed by infusion at a rate of 30 to 60 mg/h. The duration of therapy is usually 24 to 48 hours and is guided by clinical and angiographic response. Patients receiving papaverine infusion should be closely monitored in an ICU setting for hypotension. The sudden onset of hypotension in such patients indicates that the catheter has been dislodged from the SMA and that the drug is being infused systemically and requires another trip to the angiography suite for catheter check and replacement.[38]

Supportive Measures

All patients with acute and subacute MVT should be managed in an ICU setting. Adequate resuscitation is mandatory. They must have complete bowel rest with NPO and nasogastric tube suction. Broad-spectrum antibiotic coverage is not indicated in the absence of bowel perforation or peritonitis.[1]

Outcome

The true incidence of MVT is unknown, mainly because it is not diagnosed in many patients because of the vague, mild, and nonspecific manifestations. Because of that, the true outcomes of the condition are essentially unknown, as well. Historically, the mortality rate associated with acute MVT ranged between 20% and 50%.[1] Although high, it was still better than other cases of acute arterial mesenteric ischemia. Survival depends on multiple factors, including age, the presence or absence of coexisting comorbid conditions, and the timing of the diagnosis and surgical intervention. Patients who require surgery and bowel resection are sicker and have longer hospital stays and a more complicated course than those who do not require surgery.[1] However, there has been no correlation between the length of resected bowel and the mortality rate, although it has a detrimental effect on long-term morbidity in the form of short bowel syndrome and its sequelae.[21]

In recent years, the mortality rate has been slightly lower than those from earlier series, now ranging between 13% and 30%.[22] This may be due, in part, to early diagnosis and aggressive management. However, this might also be a selection bias, because we are catching more patients with milder and more benign disease due to the diagnosis of the condition using CT scan instead of the previous reports in which the diagnosis was mostly made at laparotomy, indicating a more severe and advanced disease.[22] Only a few studies have described the long-term outcome in patients who developed MVT. One of the largest series included 60 patients who were followed for a median of 3.5 years. The overall survival at 1 and 5 years was 82% and 78%, respectively. These values were 86% and 82%, respectively, after excluding patients with an underlying malignancy.[46] Long-term survival depends primarily on the cause of the thrombosis. If cancer is the underlying cause, survival is short and determined by the nature of the cancer.[1] The use of endovascular techniques in the management of acute MVT may contribute to the improving mortality rates; however, the use of those techniques remains limited, and their true value remains to be evaluated when more experience is accumulated.

Mesenteric venous thrombosis is a disease with a high rate of recurrence, and recurrences are most common within the first 30 days after presentation.[47] Coumadin therapy significantly reduces the risk of recurrence from 20%–25% to 13%–15%. There is no evidence that long-term Coumadin therapy is beneficial except in cases where there is a persistent hypercoagulable state when lifelong therapy is indicated.[19,38]

The natural history of chronic MVT is not known, but most of the patients appear to be asymptomatic. The percentage of patients with chronic MVT who develop late gastrointestinal bleeding or hypersplenism has not been determined but is probably small. As MVT is recognized more frequently on CT scans done for other disorders, our understanding of the natural history of this disorder should improve.[21]

MVT remains an underdiagnosed and understudied condition that we need to learn more about. Although there has been significant improvement in the diagnosis and management of the disease in recent years, this has not been translated into significant reduction in mortality and morbidity, which tells us that there is still a long way to go to achieve that goal. More is needed to study the natural history of the disease. Also, we need to evaluate the efficacy and refine the new modalities of therapy, especially the minimally invasive endovascular techniques, as well as developing new therapies that can prevent or limit bowel injury, thus reducing the need for open surgery with bowel resection.

References

1.   Kumar S, Sarr MG, Kamath PS. Mesenteric venous thrombosis. N Engl J Med. 2001; 345(23):1683-8.

2.   Schoots IG, Koffeman GI, Legemate DA, Levi M, van Gulik TM. Systematic review of survival after acute mesenteric ischaemia according to disease aetiology. Br J Surg. 2004;91(1):17-27.

3.   Elliot J. The operative relief of gangrene of intestine due to occlusion of the mesenteric vessels. Ann Surg. 1895(21):9-23.

4.   Cokkinis A. Mesenteric Vascular Occlusions. London: Bailliere, Tindall and Cox; 1926. p 1-93.

5.   Warren S, Eberhard TP. Mesenteric venous thrombosis. Surg Gynecol Obstet. 1935;141: 740-2.

6.   Acosta S, Alhadad A, Svensson P, Ekberg O. Epidemiology, risk and prognostic factors in mesenteric venous thrombosis. Br J Surg. 2008;95(10):1245-51.

7.   Rhee RY, Gloviczki P. Mesenteric venous thrombosis. Surg Clin North Am. 1997;77(2):327-38.

8.   Martinelli I, Mannucci PM, De Stefano V, Taioli E, Rossi V, Crosti F, et al. Different risks of thrombosis in four coagulation defects associated with inherited thrombophilia: a study of 150 families. Blood. 1998;92(7):2353-8.

9.   Bagot CN Arya R. Virchow and his triad: a question of attribution. Br J Haematol. 2008;143(2):180-90.

10. Stamou KM, Toutouzas KG, Kekis PB, Nakos S, Gafou A, Manouras A, et al. Prospective study of the incidence and risk factors of postsplenectomy thrombosis of the portal, mesenteric, and splenic veins. Arch Surg. 2006;141(7):663-9.

11. Hatoum OA, Spinelli KS, Abu-Hajir M, Attila T, Franco J, Otterson MF, et al. Mesenteric venous thrombosis in inflammatory bowel disease. J Clin Gastroenterol. 2005;39(1):27-31.

12. Harward TR, Green D, Bergan JJ, Rizzo RJ, Yao JS. Mesenteric venous thrombosis. J Vasc Surg. 1989;9(2):328-33.

13. Kumar S, Kamath PS. Acute superior mesenteric venous thrombosis: one disease or two? Am J Gastroenterol. 2003;98(6): 1299-304.

14. Provan D, O'Shaughnessy DF. Recent advances in haematology. BMJ. 1999;318 (7189):991-4.

15. Margaglione M, Brancaccio V, Giuliani N, D'Andrea G, Cappucci G, Iannaccone L, et al. Increased risk for venous thrombosis in carriers of the prothrombin G→A20210 gene variant. Ann Intern Med. 1998;129(2):89-93.

16. Chamouard P, Pencreach E, Maloisel F, Grunebaum L, Ardizzone JF, Meyer A, et al. Frequent factor II G20210A mutation in idiopathic portal vein thrombosis. Gastroenterology. 1999;116(1):144-8.

17. Elting LS, Escalante CP, Cooksley C, Avritscher EB, Kurtin D, Hamblin L, et al. Outcomes and cost of deep venous thrombosis among patients with cancer. Arch Intern Med. 2004;164(15):1653-61.

18. Alvi AR, Khan S, Niazi SK, Ghulam M, Bibi S. Acute mesenteric venous thrombosis: improved outcome with early diagnosis and prompt anticoagulation therapy. Int J Surg. 2009;7(3):210-3.

19. Abdu RA, Zakhour BJ, Dallis DJ. Mesenteric venous thrombosis—1911 to 1984. Surgery. 1987;101(4):383-8.

20. Rosenblum JD, Boyle CM, Schwartz LB. The mesenteric circulation. Anatomy and physiology. Surg Clin North Am. 1997;77(2):289-306.

21. Boley SJK. Mesenteric ischemic disorders. In: Zinner MJ, ed. Maingot's Abdominal Operations, 10th ed. Upper Saddle River, NJ: Appleton & Lange; 1997.

22. Morasch MD, Ebaugh JL, Chiou AC, Matsumura JS, Pearce WH, Yao JS. Mesenteric venous thrombosis: a changing clinical entity. J Vasc Surg. 2001;34(4):680-4.

23. Gore RM, Thakrar KH, Mehta UK, Berlin J, Yaghmai V, Newmark GM. Imaging in intestinal ischemic disorders. Clin Gastroenterol Hepatol. 2008;6(8): 849-58.

24. Brunaud L, Antunes L, Collinet-Adler S, Marchal F, Ayav A, Bresler L, et al. Acute mesenteric venous thrombosis: case for nonoperative management. J Vasc Surg. 2001;34(4):673-9.

25. Zimmerman BJ, Granger DN. Reperfusion injury. Surg Clin North Am. 1992;72(1):65-83.

26. Warshaw AL, Jin GL, Ottinger LW. Recognition and clinical implications of mesenteric and portal vein obstruction in chronic pancreatitis. Arch Surg 1987;122(4):410-5.

27. Mathews JE, White RR. Primary mesenteric venous occlusive disease. Am J Surg 1971; 122(5):579-83.

28. Boley SJ, Kaleya RN, Brandt LJ. Mesenteric venous thrombosis. Surg Clin North Am. 1992;72(1):183-201.

29. Lange H, Jackel R. Usefulness of plasma lactate concentration in the diagnosis of acute abdominal disease. Eur J Surg. 1994;160(6-7):381-4.

30. Jamieson WG, Marchuk S, Rowsom J, Durand D. The early diagnosis of massive acute intestinal ischaemia. Br J Surg. 1982;69 suppl:S52-3.

31. Fried MW, Murthy UK, Hassig SR, Woo J, Oates RP. Creatine kinase isoenzymes in the diagnosis of intestinal infarction. Dig Dis Sci. 1991;36(11):1589-93.

32. Baker SR, Cho KC. The Abdominal Plain Film with Correlative Imaging. 2nd ed. Stamford (CT): Appleton & Lange; 1999. p 315-29.

33. Dietrich CF, Jedrzejczyk M, Ignee A. Sonographic assessment of splanchnic arteries and the bowel wall. Eur J Radiol. 2007;64(2): 202-12.

34. Horton KM, Fishman EK. Computed tomography evaluation of intestinal ischemia. Semin Roentgenol. 2001;36(2):118-25.

35. Michaely HJ, Dietrich O, Nael K, Weckbach S, Reiser MF, Schoenberg SO. MRA of abdominal vessels: technical advances. Eur Radiol. 2006;16(8):1637-50.

36. Kim ST, Nemcek AA, Vogelzang RL. Angiography and interventional radiology of the hollow viscera. In: Gore RM, Levine MS, eds. Textbook of Gastrointestinal Radiology.

3rd ed. Philadelphia: Saunders; 2008. p117-40.

37. American Gastroenterological Association Medical Position Statement: guidelines on intestinal ischemia. Gastroenterology. 2000;118(5):951-3.

38. Frishman WH, Novak S, Brandt LJ, Spiegel A, Gutwein A, Kohi M, et al. Pharmacologic management of mesenteric occlusive disease. Cardiol Rev. 2008;16(2):59-68.

39. Henao EA, Bohannon WT, Silva MB Jr. Treatment of portal venous thrombosis with selective superior mesenteric artery infusion of recombinant tissue plasminogen activator. J Vasc Surg. 2003;38(6):1411-5.

40. Suzuki S, Nakamura S, Baba S, Sakaguchi S, Ohnuki Y, Yokoi Y, et al. Portal vein thrombosis after splenectomy successfully treated by an enormous dosage of fibrinolytic agent in a short period: report of two cases. Surg Today. 1992;22(5): 464-9.

41. Wang MQ, Lin HY, Guo LP, Liu FY, Duan F, Wang ZJ. Acute extensive portal and mesenteric venous thrombosis after splenectomy: treated by interventional thrombolysis with transjugular approach. World J Gastroenterol. 2009;15(24): 3038-45.

42. Ferro C, Rossi UG, Bovio G, Dahamane M, Centanaro M. Transjugular intrahepatic portosystemic shunt, mechanical aspiration

thrombectomy, and direct thrombolysis in the treatment of acute portal and superior mesenteric vein thrombosis. Cardiovasc Interv Radiol. 2007;30(5):1070-4.

43. Rosen MP, Sheiman R. Transhepatic mechanical thrombectomy followed by infusion of TPA into the superior mesenteric artery to treat acute mesenteric vein thrombosis. J Vasc Interv Radiol. 2000;11(2 Pt 1):195-8.

44. Ryu R, Lin TC, Kumpe D, Krysl J, Durham JD, Goff JS, et al. Percutaneous mesenteric venous thrombectomy and thrombolysis: successful treatment followed by liver transplantation. Liver Transpl Surg. 1998;4(3): 222-5.

45. Ozdogan M, Gurer A, Gokakin AK, Kulacoglu H, Aydin R. Thrombolysis via an operatively placed mesenteric catheter for portal and superior mesenteric vein thrombosis: report of a case. Surg Today. 2006; 36(9):846-8.

46. Orr DW, Harrison PM, Devlin J, Karani JB, Kane PA, Heaton ND, et al. Chronic mesenteric venous thrombosis: evaluation and determinants of survival during long-term follow-up. Clin Gastroenterol Hepatol. 2007;5(1):80-6.

47. Jona J, Cummins GM Jr, Head HB, Govostis MC. Recurrent primary mesenteric venous thrombosis. JAMA. 1974;227(9):1033-5.

Practice Management

The success of any practice resides in the ability to accurately capture its activity and collect revenue with the minimum cost while still maintaining customer satisfaction. Appropriate coding will allow rapid bill processing, reduce denials, and lower accounts receivable. Improved cash flow cannot help but enhance practice profitability.

Current Venous Coding and Billing

Gary Burns

Three Phases of Peripheral Interventional Billing and Coding

There are 3 phases of reporting venous interventional procedures accurately. They are venous catheter placement (phase 1), diagnostic venogram imaging (phase 2), and venous interventions (phase 3). There are specific reporting requirements for accurate representation of peripheral interventional procedures. Included here is a summary of the key components to each of the phases with regard to representing venous procedures accurately and in compliance with regulators.

Venous Thromboembolic Disease. Contemporary Endovascular Management series. © 2011 Mark G. Davies MD and Alan B. Lumsden MD, eds. Cardiotext Publishing, ISBN 978-1-935395-22-5.

Phase 1: Venous Catheter Placement

There are a few factors to remember when reporting venous catheter placement. First, only the most distal placement in the venous system is reported. For example, if a right common femoral vein is accessed with placement of the catheter to the inferior vena cava (IVC), only the IVC placement is reported. The final destination of the catheter in the IVC includes the initial access and all catheter movement to its end position. Second, only the most distal diagnostic catheter or interventional device will be reported. For example, if a diagnostic catheter is placed for venography but an interventional device is advanced further in the venous vascular system, the interventional device will be reported as the most distal catheter advancement. It then will include all other diagnostic catheter advancements to get it to the vessel of intervention.

It is extremely important to note that a guidance wire placement or end position is never reported as a catheter placement. Also, a sheath is not reported as a catheter position. Again, only report the final end position of a diagnostic catheter or an interventional device. One exception here is when a sheath is used for injection of contrast and venography. It can be classified as a diagnostic catheter position.

Venous Access

There is a code for access to the venous system (36000).* It represents nothing more than a needle puncture to the venous system. This excludes dialysis fistula/graft puncture, which we will discuss later in this document. If more than one access is created in the venous system, each would be reported separately as its own work component.

There is a separate code for access to the venous system with a contrast injection for extremity venography (36005). It represents the venous needle puncture and a contrast injection for extremity venography. From one access with an extremity venography contrast injection, you can only report the 36005. It includes the venous access (36000). However, if you access the right lower extremity for contrast injection venogram (36005) and the left lower extremity for contrast injection venogram (36005), it is appropriate to report each work component.

Venous Catheter Advancement to the Vena Cava (Superior or Inferior)

When a catheter (diagnostic or interventional) is advanced from the access site to the vena cava (inferior or superior), this end position will prevail and include all previous work. There is a code for vena cava catheter placement (36010). This code will include a venous access (36000) and/or venous access with contrast injection for extremity venography (36005). Remember that the end position of the diagnostic catheter or interventional device prevails and includes all other catheter work components to this end path. For example, if a right common femoral vein access was accomplished followed by a contrast injection venography with eventual movement of a inferior vena cava filter, the interventional device would prevail as the most distal end position (36010). This position would include the venous access and the contrast injection venogram.

"Selective" Venous Catheter Advancement to a Superior Vena Cava or Inferior Vena Cava Branch

When venous diagnostic catheters or intervention devices are advanced out of the vena cava to branched vessels arising from the vena cava, there are codes to reflect the complexity of these movements. Any branch vessel that arises off of the vena cava (superior or inferior) is defined as a vascular family. The first branches that arise off of the vena cava are considered first-order selective catheter advancements (36011). If the catheter is manipulated past a first-order bifurcation, the selective movement is considered second order branches (36012).

As with the venous access site (36000)

---

or venous extremity contrast injection (36005) being bundled into the vena cava placement, the SVC or IVC placement will be bundled into the "selective" catheter advancement to a first-order branch (36011). Also, when a selective catheter is advanced to a second-order branch (36012), it is not appropriate to report the first-order selective branch (36011). The first-order branch (36011), the vena cava placement (36010), and the venous access (36000 or 36005) are all bundled into the second-order end position of the diagnostic catheter or interventional device placement.

"Selective" Venous Catheter Advancement to Multiple Superior Vena Cava or Inferior Vena Cava Branches

If the interventional physician manipulates the catheter or interventional device to multiple branches that arise off of the vena cava, each would be reported separately. For example, if a right common femoral access was accomplished with advancement of the diagnostic catheter to the right brachiocephalic vein (first-order branch off of the SVC, 36011) and left brachiocephalic vein (36011), each would be reported separately. Again, remember that the venous access and the vena cava placement would be bundled into the brachiocephalic placements and not reported separately regardless if diagnostic venograms (ie, SVC gram) or interventions (ie, IVC filter) were performed.

"Selective" Venous Catheter Advancement to Multiple Branches Within a Vascular Family

As discussed earlier, a vascular family is a network of venous vessels that arise from the vena cava (superior or inferior). We have also noted that each vascular family with a selective diagnostic catheter or interventional device would be reported separately. Once in a vascular family a physician will encounter the first-order branch (36011) that arises off of the vena cava. This first-order branch vessel will bifurcate into a second-order branch (36012). Again, we already established that only the end position can be reported.

When a physician works to manipulate catheters or interventional devices selectively into multiple families arising off of the vena cava, then each is reported separately.

However, it is important to note that any further advancement of a selective catheter or interventional device past second-order bifurcations does not have a code to reflect this higher level of work component. Remember, one distal end position path represents only one code assignment. The second-order advancement includes all distal placements in a vascular family. For example, if a physician accesses the right common femoral vein with advancement to the inferior vena cava and then superior vena cava to the right brachiocephalic vein vascular family with final selective manipulation to the right basilic vein, only the second-order placement (36012) is reported. This represents one pathway and only one end position of a diagnostic catheter placement or interventional device.

A noted exception to the above is when a physician selectively advances a diagnostic catheter or an interventional device to multiple second-order branches within a vascular family, it is appropriate to each end pathway separately. For example, if a physician accesses the right common femoral vein with advancement to the inferior vena cava and then superior vena cava to the right brachiocephalic vein vascular family with final selective manipulation to the right subclavian vein and right internal jugular vein, each of the 2 separate pathways would be reported. The second-order right subclavian vein (36012) and separate pathway end position to the right internal jgular (36012) are reported. This represents 2 pathways and 2 end positions of a diagnostic catheter placement or interventional device. Again, report both work components.

It is important to note that only intentional catheter positions are reported.

Application of Modifiers for Catheter Placements

To accompany the complex rules listed in phase 1, it is important to note that there are some key factors relating to payor submission requirements of your work components. Any guidance offered here should be validated with each of your payors. All payor rules for modifiers should be adhered to, assuring accurate representation of your work. We can report a few basic guidelines related to phase 1.

Modifiers are code attachments to further recognize your complex work. It will be necessary to report a modifier when procedure codes are duplicated as well as when a higher value code is reported with a lower-valued code.

Duplicate Codes

When reporting the same procedure code twice on a claim, you will invariably need a modifier appended to one of your codes to ensure that a payor recognizes the duplicate

nature of your complex work components. For example, when performing a right leg venogram and a left leg venogram from two separate venous access sites, both are reported (36005 + 36005). However, a payor will rarely recognize both access sites with injection codes without a modifier to show 2 access sites were performed. This is primarily because the codes are relatively generic. Code 36005 is a venous access for extremity contrast injection venogram. The code is not specific to right or left leg access and injection. Thus, a modifier 59 (distinct procedure or separate access site with contrast injection in this case) must be appended. The modifier will only need appended to one of the codes that are duplicated (ie, 36005 + 36005-59).

High-Value Codes with Lower-Value Code

When reporting codes of a high-value nature (second-order selective catheter placement, 36012) with a lower-valued code (first-order selective catheter placement, 36011) a modifier 59 (distinct procedure—separate branch placement) is necessary to report the complexity of a procedure. The modifier will only be needed on the lower-valued code (36012 + 36011-59). For example, if a right common femoral vein access was accomplished and the catheter was advanced to the right brachiocephalic vein (first-order branch, 36011) and the left subclavian vein (second-order branch, 36012—separate vascular family) a modifier is necessary to reflect the 2 separate vascular families selectively catheterized.

Phase 2: Diagnostic Venogram Imaging

There are 3 key components to diagnostic venography imaging. First, contrast must be injected. Second, images must be captured and stored. Third and finally, the physician must document an interpretation of the vascular vessels.

Guiding injections to ensure that an interventional device is in position prior to the interventional technique is not considered diagnostic imaging. Road-mapping imaging techniques are also not considered diagnostic imaging. Postinterventional follow-up imaging is considered part of the interventional technique and again not diagnostic imaging because these imaging techniques tend not to have revealed the initial diagnostic interpretation of the endovascular disease.

A physician must create an initial disease assessment interpretation of a contrast injection whether patent, totally occluded, and anything in between to qualify for reporting a code for diagnostic imaging. And remember, a stored image will validate your work components.

Venography reporting is not impacted by the amount of contrast injected or the number of images stored. It is solely based on the disease assessment of the vessel.

Selective Venography

There are some venography codes that reflect the narrative of selective venography in the narrative of the procedure. For example, selective bilateral renal venography reflects this narrative. When the narrative of the venography code reflects the "selective" terminology, a catheter position within the vessel is necessary to report the imaging procedure. As in the selective bilateral renal venography (75833) procedure, 2 catheter positions are required within the renal veins (ie, right renal vein and left renal vein) to accompany the imaging code. It is noted that the IVC gram (75825) is not included in the code narrative for selective bilateral renal veno-

gram, and thus, can be used as an additional imaging component if the 3 components for diagnostic venography imaging are met (ie, contrast injection, image capture, physician interpretation).

Venous Imaging Performed at the "Same Time/Same Session" as the Venous Intervention

Guidelines have been established in the past few years by payors to limit diagnostic imaging reimbursements at the same time of the interventional procedure. Thus, when a physician performs a diagnostic venography at the same time as the interventional procedure the physician must append a modifier to reveal that venous imaging was not done previously. The modifier established to reveal that the venogram was a diagnostic study that leads to the intervention is 59 (distinct procedure). For example, if a right lower extremity unilateral venogram (75820) was performed and a venous angioplasty followed at the same session, the physician must append the modifier 59 to the venography (75820-59) to show that the interpretation lead to the interventional procedure.

If the procedure is staged where the venography was performed at a separate session than the intervention, the repeated venogram should not be reported a second time. However, if there is a change in the clinical findings, it would be appropriate to report the venography with the modifier 59 to establish it as a distinct imaging component at the time of intervention.

Phase 3: Venous Interventions

The third phase of accurate billing and code capture is the reporting of venous interventions (angioplasty, stent, IVC filter placement, IVC filter removal, thrombectomy, ablation, and dialysis graft/fistula declot). Guidelines have been established for each intervention separately, and then a complex set when multiple interventional techniques are used for clinical treatment of venous disease. When reporting most venous interventions, a companion imaging component will accompany the surgical code assignment. For example, the venous balloon dilation is labeled as a surgical work component (ie, 35476). There is a supervision and interpretation imaging component that accompanies the surgical work (75978). These 2 companion codes will travel together for each vessel treated with balloon dilation.

Venous Angioplasty

Only one procedure code is established for venous angioplasty (35476). However, this code would be reported for each venous vessel treated. The venous vessels zones of treatment are established from venous bifurcation to bifurcation. It is not reported for each size of balloon utilized for dilation. It is also not reported for each dilation at the same disease site or each dilation within the same vessel zone, but at different disease sites within a vessel.

For example, if a physician dilates a right brachiocephalic vein (35476 + 75978) and a right subclavian vein (35476 + 75978), each is reported separately because of the bifurcation from the brachiocephalic to the subclavian with the internal jugular. In fact, if a venous dilation was also performed in the

superior vena cava (35476 + 75978) it would be established as its own zone of treatment and added as a separate work component. Thus, a physician would report the superior vena cava, right brachiocephalic, and right subclavian as separate work zones for venous angioplasty.

It is important to note that each of the other phases of procedure capture are not included in this interventional technique and should be reported separately. Add the catheter placement to the interventional zone as well as any diagnostic imaging performed to assess disease prior to intervention in the venous vessels.

Modifier Adjustments

As discussed earlier, when a code is duplicated but reported correctly it must be appended with the modifier 59 (distinct procedure) to establish the separate work zones. In the above example, the reporting would be as follows: 35476 + 75978 (superior vena cava), 35476-59 + 75978-59 (right brachiocephalic), 35476-59 + 75978-59 (right subclavian). It is important to note that other modifiers may be required by payors to further establish these separate work zones. Our recommendation is offered because we find it most consistent with coding guidelines and payor acceptance across the country. Also, note that the first set of codes is not modified (ie, superior vena cava). Only the following codes that duplicate the initial set are modified.

Venous Stent

The code established for venous stent is the same that is used for arterial-based stent procedures (37205—initial vessel treated by stent deployment, 37206—additional vessel treated by stent deployment). Intravascular stent is reported in the same manner as venous angioplasty. Each vessel zone treated by intravascular stent is reported. It is important to note that a physician can only report the initial vessel treated by stent deployment (37205) once during an interventional procedure. Each vessel after the initial vessel treated by stent deployment is considered an additional vessel treated (37206).

The venous vessels zones of treatment are established from venous bifurcation to bifurcation. It is not reported for each size (ie, diameter or length) of stent placed in the venous vessel. Nor does it reflect any difference in the deployment methods (ie, balloon expandable or self-expanding). It is also not reported for the number of stents placed in the same vessel zone. It is reported once for each vessel treated by stent deployment. One initial (37205) vessel treated and the remaining vessels treated with stent deployment past separate bifurcations are the additional vessels (37206). The additional vessel treated (37206) can be reported multiple times but only once within a vessel.

There is a supervision and interpretation imaging component that accompanies the surgical work (75960). These 2 companion codes will travel together for each vessel treated with stent deployment (37205 + 75960 initial vessel, 37206 + 75960 additional vessel, 37206 + 75960 additional vessel, etc).

For example, if a physician places a stent in the right brachiocephalic vein (37205 + 75960) and a right subclavian vein (37206 + 75960), each is reported separately because of the bifurcation from the brachiocephalic to the subclavian with the internal jugular. In fact, if a venous stent was also performed in the superior vena cava (37206 + 75960), it would be established as its own zone of treatment and added as a separate work component. Thus, a physician would report the superior vena cava, right brachiocephalic, and right subclavian as separate work zones for venous stent deployment.

Modifier Adjustments

As discussed earlier, when a code is duplicated but reported correctly, most payors will require a modifier appended (ie, modifier 59 distinct procedure) to establish the separate work zones. Our recommendation is offered because we find it most consistent with coding guidelines and payor acceptance across the country. It would be appropriate to consult each of your payor guidelines for modifier submission requirements.

It is important to note that each of the other phases of procedure capture are not included in this interventional technique and should be reported separately. Add the catheter placement to the interventional zone as well as any diagnostic imaging performed to assess disease prior to intervention in the venous vessels.

Venous Angioplasty Followed by Stent Deployment

When combining multiple interventional techniques like venous angioplasty followed by stent deployment, documentation is necessary to establish each interventional procedure as its own separate work component. For instance, if the balloon angioplasty yielded a suboptimal recoiled residual stenosis, a predilation and postdilation percentage assessment of the disease would reveal the reason for further intervention with the stent. Also, if a balloon angioplasty resulted in a vessel dissection, then the multiple interventional techniques are established by the result of the initial procedure. In each of the balloon results (ie, residual stenosis, dissection) both interventions are reported. It is not appropriate to modify and angioplasty from a stent deployment. They are independent procedures that are commonly not bundled by payors.

For example, a proximal right subclavian vein 90% stenosis was dilated with an angioplasty balloon (35476 + 75978). On follow-up imaging a 50% residual stenosis was identified. After several attempts with multiple dilations at the same site within this vessel (no additional codes), a 50% residual stenosis remained. This was followed by a stent deployment (37205 + 75960). Both procedures are reported with their companion supervision and interpretation components. No modifiers are necessary to separate these individual work components.

Along with the predilation and postdilation percentages, it is also good documentation principles to establish the location of the disease within a vessel as proximal, midlevel, or distal. These documentation principles assist in revealing the complexity of treatment in the venous system without the visual reference of a set of venography images.

It is important to note that each of the other phases of procedure capture are not included in this interventional technique and should be reported separately. Add the catheter placement to the interventional zone as well as any diagnostic imaging performed to assess disease prior to intervention in the venous vessels.

Predilation and/or Postdilation of Stent Deployment

Any predilation performed to be able to place a stent at a venous stenosis is considered part of the stent deployment and not a separate work component. Remember, a venous angioplasty followed by a documented suboptimal result (ie, residual stenosis or dissection) and stent deployment is considered as their own separate work components (venous angioplasty + stent deployment).

Any postdilation performed within a stent at the same session as the deployment is considered part of the initial stent deployment. Obviously, if balloon dilation is performed within in-stent stenosis then the angioplasty can be reported as its own work component. It is often noted that there is no suboptimal result to a stent deployment when a balloon is needed to further expand a stent.

A physician can only report both work components (angioplasty + stent) when there is a suboptimal result of angioplasty and the desired outcome was not accomplished. The dissection or residual stenosis (best reported in pre- and postpercentage) reveals the distinct work components and meets the separate guidelines for reporting angioplasty and stent.

Inferior Vena Cava Filter Placement

When placing an IVC filter all 3 phases (placement, imaging, and intervention) can be reported. Venous access (ie, either jugular access or common femoral vein access) is accomplished with placement of the diagnostic catheter to the IVC (36010) for venography imaging. Remember, sizing of the vena cava and mapping the location of the renal veins are not considered part of diagnostic imaging. Thus, a physician must establish a diagnostic assessment of thrombus or false passages in the IVC. A normal IVC is acceptable as long as the documentation reflects no thrombus disease present or duplicated IVCs. When a diagnostic IVC study is reported, a modifier 59 (distinct procedure) is necessary to establish it as its own work component (75825-59).

Once the imaging is established and the physician deploys the vena cava filter,

2 work components are established to report the procedure (37620 + 75940). Follow-up venography after the placement of the filter is considered part of the assurance of accurate deployment and not reported as a separate work component. Also, the reporting of a permanent or temporary removable filter does not reflect any different work component.

Inferior Vena Cava Filter (IVC) Removal

When an existing IVC filter is no longer necessary to capture venous thrombosis, some of the 3 phases (placement, imaging, and intervention) may be reported. Venous access (ie, usually jugular access) is accomplished with placement of the filter capture device to the IVC (36010). Remember, if a diagnostic venogram is not accomplished but contrast is injected to locate the position of the filter, no diagnostic imaging is reported.

Once the location is established and the physician retrieves the vena cava filter, 2 work components are established to report the procedure (37203 + 75961, considered foreign body retrieval). Follow-up venography after the removal of the filter is not considered a separate work component.

Venous Thrombectomy

Venous thrombectomy includes any infusion/injection of thrombolytic agents during the mechanical removal of thrombus in the venous system. It also is not delineated by vessel as with angioplasty and stent deployment. Any mechanical thrombectomy during one date of service is all included in one procedure work component (37187). When the calendar date changes to a subsequent day, and a mechanical device is utilized for thrombectomy, a separate work component can be established (37188). All fluoroscopic guidance to assist in the thrombectomy is not reported separately.

It is noted that these are not the procedures utilized for dialysis/fistula thrombectomy interventions. Also, there is no supervision and interpretation component attached as a component to this procedure.

Endovenous Ablation

Endovenous ablation of incompetent veins in the extremity is divided into 2 interventional techniques (ie, radiofrequency and laser). Each are further divided into first vessel treated and second with all other vessels treated in an extremity. All imaging guidance to treat the incompetent veins is not considered a separate work component.

Radiofrequency Ablation

Radiofrequency endovenous ablation first vessel (36475), second, and subsequent veins treated in the same extremity through separate access sites (36476) reflects the further division within this interventional technique.

Laser Ablation

Laser endovenous ablation first vessel (36478), second, and subsequent veins treated in the same extremity through separate access sites (36479) reflects the further division within this interventional technique.

Also, there is no supervision and interpretation component attached as a component to this procedure.

Conclusion

Venous physician work components are complex. Most venous vascular procedure reporting can be divided into the 3-phase approach outlined in this document (catheter placement, diagnostic imaging, and venous intervention). The above is an attempt to guide a physician though the maze of complex procedure reporting requirements, as well as offer suggestions for documentation quality. In no way is it possible to list all scenarios for venous procedures. Each physician must have a high-quality support system (ie, certified medical coders) that understands the guidelines for each payor. Without a high-quality support system, a complex venous procedure involving multiple work components may reflect payments that do not reveal all the procedures performed by the physician.

Index

*Figures are indicated by f
and tables by t following the page number.*